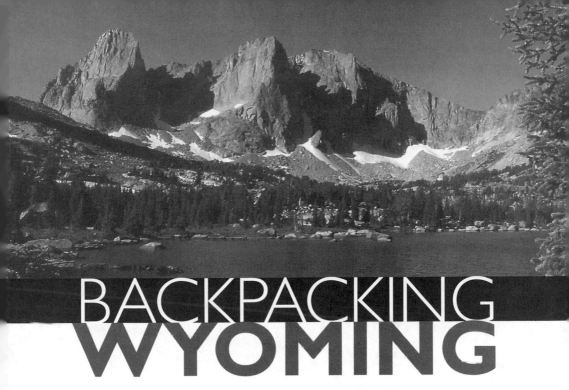

BACKPACKING
WYOMING

*From Towering Granite Peaks
to Steaming Geyser Basins*

DOUGLAS LORAIN

 WILDERNESS PRESS ... *on the trail since 1967*

BERKELEY, CA

Backpacking Wyoming:
From Towering Granite Peaks to Steaming Geyser Basins

1st EDITION 2010

Copyright © 2010 by Douglas Lorain

Front and back cover photos copyright © 2010 by Douglas Lorain, except photo of
    paintbrush, which is copyright © 2010 by Christine Ebrahimi
Interior photos, except where noted, by Douglas Lorain
Maps: Douglas Lorain
Cover and book design/layout: Larry B. Van Dyke
Book editor: Laura Shauger

ISBN 978-0-89997-505-4

Manufactured in the United States of America

Published by: **Wilderness Press**
               1345 8th Street
               Berkeley, CA 94710
               (800) 443-7227; FAX (510) 558-1696
               info@wildernesspress.com
               www.wildernesspress.com

Visit our website for a complete listing of our books and for ordering information.
Distributed by Publishers Group West

Cover photos:
    (front, top) Meadow above North Piney Lake, Wyoming Range (Trip 22)
    (bottom, from left) Upper Paintbrush Canyon, Grand Teton National Park (Trip 12);
                Shoshone Geyser Basin, Yellowstone National Park (Trip 4);
                Rock Lake Peak, Salt River Range (Trip 23)
    (back) Grand and Middle Teton from below Avalanche Divide,
        Grand Teton National Park (Trip 12)

Previous page: Warrior 1 and 2 and Warbonnet Peak over Lonesome Lake,
                Wind River Range (Trip 17)

SAFETY NOTICE: Although Wilderness Press and the author have made every attempt to
ensure that the information in this book is accurate at press time, they are not responsible
for any loss, damage, injury, or inconvenience that may occur to anyone while using this
book. You are responsible for your own safety and health while in the wilderness. The fact
that a trail is described in this book does not mean that it will be safe for you. Be aware that
trail conditions can change from day to day. Always check local conditions, know your own
limitations, and consult a map.

"I have a hunger for nonhuman spaces, not out of any distaste for humanity, but out of a need to experience my humanness the more vividly by confronting stretches of the earth that my kind has had no part in making."

— Scott Russell Sanders,
The Paradise of Bombs

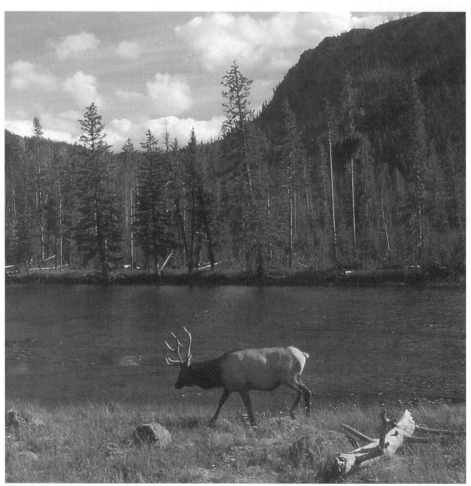

Bull elk, Yellowstone National Park

ACKNOWLEDGMENTS

The help of many people made this book possible. Special thanks go to the following persons:

My occasional hiking partner—Dave Elsbernd.

Forest Service and Park Service personnel, who provided information, read drafts, or otherwise shared their considerable expertise—Craig Cope, Rob St. John, Sid Smith, Matt Walter, Paul Willard, and James Williams.

The people at Wilderness Press who continue to enthusiastically publish my books and do such a stellar job of turning my initial disjointed writing and mapping efforts into something useable and readable for you, the reader. On this book, particular thanks go to Roslyn Bullas, Laura Shauger, and Larry Van Dyke.

I also want to thank the nice people at Hot Springs County Memorial Hospital in Thermopolis, Wyoming, who helped me through a nasty bout of giardia I picked up in the Wyoming backcountry.

Most of all, forever and always, I thank my wife, Becky Lovejoy, who endured months alone having to take care of the dog and house while her husband traipsed off into the wilds in search of new trails. Her love and encouragement are invaluable to this book and to my life.

While the contributions and assistance of the persons listed above were invaluable, all of the text, maps, and photos herein are my own work and sole responsibility. Any and all omissions, errors, and just plain stupid mistakes are strictly mine.

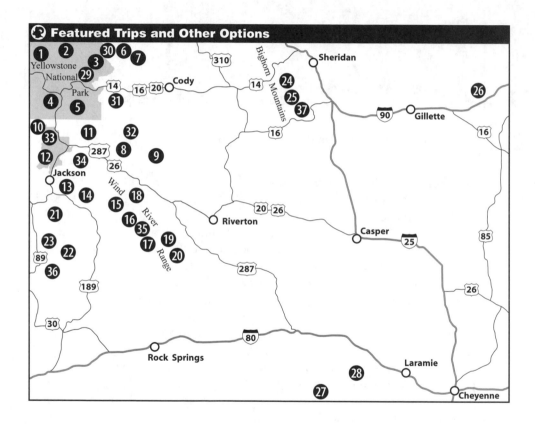

Featured Trips and Other Options

CONTENTS

Summary of Featured Trips xii

Preface xiv

Introduction 1

    How to Use This Guide 2

    General Tips on Backpacking in Wyoming 5

FEATURED TRIPS

YELLOWSTONE NATIONAL PARK • 15

  1   Bighorn Pass & Sportsman Lake Loop **17**

  2   Black Canyon of the Yellowstone River **24**

  3   Lamar River to Hoodoo Basin **31**

  4   Shoshone Lake Loop **39**

  5   Heart Lake & Two Ocean Plateau Loop **45**

BEARTOOTH MOUNTAINS • 55

  6   Beartooth Plateau Loop **57**

  7   Clarks Fork Yellowstone River Canyon **63**

SOUTH ABSAROKA RANGE · 71

8 Emerald Lake 73
9 Greybull River & Burwell Pass Loop 78

GRAND TETON NATIONAL PARK & VICINITY · · · · · · · · · · · · 87

10 Bitch Creek Loop 89
11 Teton Wilderness Loop 95
12 Grand Teton Loop 104
13 Granite Creek & Granite Highline Loop 113
14 Brewster Lake & Gros Ventre River Loop 119

WIND RIVER RANGE · 129

15 Green River Lakes & Titcomb Basin Loop 131
16 Central Wind Rivers Loop 141
17 Lonesome & Baptiste Lakes Loop 152
18 Glacier Trail 163
19 Dickinson Park & Bears Ears Trail Loop 168
20 Stough Lakes & Middle Popo Agie River Loop 174

WYOMING & SALT RIVER RANGES · · · · · · · · · · · · · · · · · 183

21 Little Greys River Loop 185
22 North Piney Creek Loop 192
23 Mount Fitzpatrick Loop 198

BIGHORN MOUNTAINS · 207

24 North Bighorn Mountains Loop 209
25 South Bighorn Mountains Loop 215

BEAR LODGE MOUNTAINS · 223

26 Sundance to Ogden Creek Loop 225

SOUTHERN WYOMING MOUNTAINS · · · · · · · · · · · · · · · · 231

27 Encampment River Trail 233
28 Snowy Range High Lakes Loop 238

OTHER BACKPACKING OPTIONS

29   Pelican Valley & Wapiti Lake Loop   **247**

30   Crandall Creek & Papoose Ridge Loop   **248**

31   Eagle Creek to Eagle Pass   **249**

32   Ishawooa Creek & Deer Creek Pass Loop   **250**

33   Moose Creek & Owl Creek Loop   **251**

34   Mount Leidy Highlands   **252**

35   Wind River Highline Trail   **253**

36   Lake Alice & Fontenelle Mountain Loop   **254**

37   Circle Park Loop   **255**

Appendix: Organizations & Agencies   257

Index   263

About the Author   272

SUMMARY OF FEATURED TRIPS

TRIP NUMBER & NAME	PAGE
BEST IN MAY & JUNE	
2 Black Canyon of the Yellowstone River	24
7 Clarks Fork Yellowstone River Canyon	63
26 Sundance to Ogden Creek Loop	225
27 Encampment River Trail	233
BEST IN JULY	
8 Emerald Lake	73
9 Greybull River & Burwell Pass Loop	78
10 Bitch Creek Loop	89
11 Teton Wilderness Loop	95
13 Granite Creek & Granite Highline Loop	113
20 Stough Lakes & Middle Popo Agie River Loop	174
21 Little Greys River Loop	185
22 North Piney Creek Loop	192
23 Mount Fitzpatrick Loop	198
28 Snowy Range High Lakes Loop	238
BEST IN AUGUST	
1 Bighorn Pass & Sportsman Lake Loop	17
6 Beartooth Plateau Loop	57
12 Grand Teton Loop	104
14 Brewster Lake & Gros Ventre River Loop	119
15 Green River Lakes & Titcomb Basin Loop	131
16 Central Wind Rivers Loop	141
17 Lonesome & Baptiste Lakes Loop	153
18 Glacier Trail	163
19 Dickinson Park & Bears Ears Trail Loop	168
24 North Bighorn Mountains Loop	209
25 South Bighorn Mountains Loop	215
BEST IN SEPTEMBER & OCTOBER	
3 Lamar River to Hoodoo Basin	31
4 Shoshone Lake Loop	39
5 Heart Lake & Two Ocean Plateau Loop	45

| RATINGS (1–10) | | | LENGTH | | ELEVATION GAIN |
SCENERY	SOLITUDE	DIFFICULTY	DAYS	MILES	
7	5	6	3–4	22–32	1450–3200′
8	7	6	3–4	23	3100′
6	9	5	2–5	17	2700′
7	7	6	2–4	15–18	500–1300′
8	8	8	3–5	27	3800′
10	9	8	3–6	46	9300′
8	7	6	3–5	25–31	4750–6900′
7	8	7	5–7	60–64	6000–7900′
8	6	7	3–5	33	6400′
9	6	5	4–6	31–53	5000–8000′
7	9	8	3–5	31–33	7200–8100′
7	9	5	3–5	33	6700′
8	9	9	4–7	39	12,000′
9	4	5	2–4	22	3400′
8	5	6	3–5	46–55	6550–9750′
10	5	6	3–6	21–26	3300–4800′
10	3	8	5–8	49–61	9100–11,800′
10	8	8	4–7	37	9200′
10	5	6	6–14	71	10,100′
10	6	7	6–10	62–80	7700–10,100′
10	3	5	4–7	39–58	7500–10,000′
8	3	6	4–7	44	8000′
10	4	7	3–6	37–38	5500–5800′
8	5	5	4–6	33–40	4000–5100′
8	3	7	3–6	31	5800′
7	8	7	4–6	48–55	4100–6700′
6	5	5	3–5	40	2900′
6	8	7	5–10	62–72	5750–9000′

PREFACE

Authors of guidebooks face a dilemma. Without dedicated supporters the wilderness would never be protected in the first place. The best, most enthusiastic advocates are those who have actually visited the land, often with the help of a guidebook. On the other hand, too many boots can also be destructive. It is the responsibility of every visitor to tread lightly on the land and to speak out strongly for its preservation.

Americans have long recognized the unique nature of Wyoming's wild character and the value of protecting these resources for future generations. Consider the fact that this one state contains our country's (and the world's) first national park (Yellowstone), its first national monument (Devils Tower), and its first national forest (Shoshone). But while Wyoming has millions of acres of land that is now officially set aside in national parks or wilderness areas, the job of protecting Wyoming's precious wildlands is far from complete. You are strongly encouraged to join in the efforts to protect more of the state's ever-dwindling roadless terrain from the headlong push to drill, dig up, pave over, or otherwise destroy every piece of "useless wilderness" that remains. Not only must some areas be set aside for permanent protection, the remaining lands (the vast majority of the state's acreage) needs to be managed in a more sustainable and environmentally friendly manner. One excellent grassroots organization working to achieve these ends is the Wyoming Wilderness Association; you are strongly encouraged to join them in their efforts (see p. 258 for contact information). But even land that is officially protected as wilderness needs continued citizen involvement. Issues like use restrictions, grazing rights, mining claims, and entry fees continue to present challenges. Remember that *you own this land*. Treat it with respect and get involved in its management.

To their credit, many of the agency officials who reviewed this material stressed the need for hikers to leave no trace of their visit. But especially in already crowded backcountry areas, the time has come for us to go beyond the well-known "no trace" principles and leave behind a landscape that not only shows no trace of our presence, but is in *better* shape than before we visited it. Here are some guidelines:

- **Be scrupulous to leave no litter of your own.** Even better, remove any litter left by others (blessedly little these days).

- **Do some minor trail maintenance as you hike.** Kick rocks off the trail, remove limbs and debris, and drain water from the path to reduce mud and erosion. Report major trail-maintenance problems, such as large blowdowns or wash-outs, to the land managers so they can concentrate their limited dollars where those are most needed.

- **Always camp in a place that either is compacted from years of previous use or can easily accommodate a tent without being damaged.** Sand, rocks, or a densely wooded area are best.

- **Never camp on fragile meadow vegetation or immediately beside a lake or stream.** If you see a campsite "growing" in an inappropriate place, be proactive: Place a few limbs or rocks over the area to discourage further use, scatter "horse apples," and remove fire-scarred rocks.

- **Never feed wildlife, and encourage others to refrain.**

- **Do not build campfires.** I have backpacked countless thousands of miles in the last couple decades and built just one fire (and that was only in an emergency). While there are still places in the lower-elevation forests of Wyoming where you could build a small campfire with a clear conscience, you simply don't need a fire to have a good time, and it damages the land. When you discover a fire ring in an otherwise pristine area, scatter the rocks and cover the fire pit to discourage its further use.

- **Leave *all* of the following at home:** soap—even biodegradable soap pollutes; pets—dogs and bears do not get along and even well-mannered pets are instinctively seen as predators by smaller wildlife; anything loud; and any outdated attitudes you may have about going out to "conquer" the wilderness.

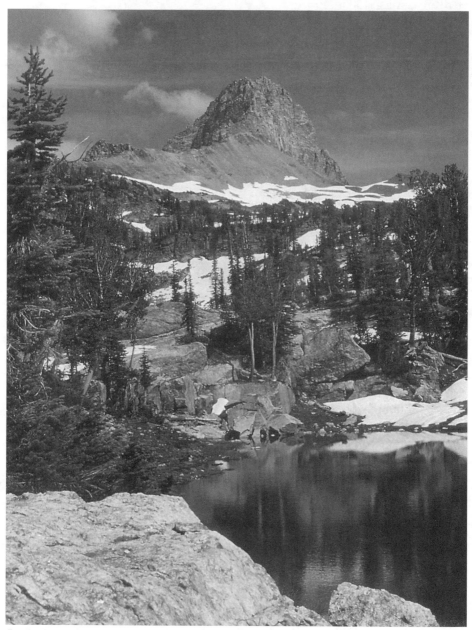

Buck Mountain over Alaska Basin, Jedediah Smith Wilderness (Trip 12)

INTRODUCTION

No offense to those of you from elsewhere in the country (with the possible exception of Alaska), but you ain't seen nothin' until you've hiked in Wyoming. Your home state probably has some terrific backpacking areas, but Wyoming is so full of stunningly beautiful scenery, abundant and interesting wildlife, and outstanding long trails that you could spend several lifetimes backpacking here and only scratch the surface of the Cowboy State's wonders.

Beginning with the day that the first Native American migrated into this area, through the days of the earliest white explorers, and all the way to the present, Wyoming has always been a terrific place to "get away from it all." Consider the fact that when measured by its area, Wyoming is the ninth largest state in the country. In population, however, the state ranks almost dead last. If you do the math, that adds up to one heck of a lot of wide open spaces. In fact, Wyoming proudly boasts that it contains the most isolated place in the entire Lower 48 (based on its distance from the nearest road), in southeast Yellowstone National Park. It is not surprising, then, that some of our country's best long-distance backpacking is found in Wyoming.

There are many ways to see and appreciate the beauty of Wyoming, including dayhikes, rafting trips, bicycle tours, or even from your car. The focus of *this* book, however, is on the best ways for *backpackers* to see the state. Most of Wyoming's best scenery is far from roads and can be seen and truly appreciated only by those willing to hit the trails. After many years and thousands of trail miles, I have selected what I believe to be Wyoming's very best backpacking trips. The focus is on *longer* trips — from 3 days to 2 weeks. These are beyond a simple weekend outing, but they make *terrific* vacations, and give you enough time to fully appreciate the scenery. Best of all, you'll have the chance to really get to know and love the state and the outstanding wildlands that comprise so much of its area.

HOW TO USE THIS GUIDE

Each featured trip begins with an information box that provides a quick over-view of the hike's vital statistics and important features, which lets you rapidly narrow your options based on your preferences, your abilities, how many days you have available, and the time of year.

Scenery: My subjective judgment of the trip's overall scenic quality, on a 1 (an eyesore) to 10 (absolutely gorgeous) scale, this rating reflects my personal bi-ases in favor of wildflowers, photogenic mountain views, and clear streams—all qualities Wyoming has in embarrassing abundance. If your tastes run more to-ward lush forests or rolling grasslands, then your rating may be quite different.

Solitude: Since solitude is one of the things that backpackers seek, it helps to know roughly how much company you can expect. This rating is also on a 1 (bring stilts to see over the crowds) to 10 (just you and the bears) scale.

Difficulty: Yet another subjective judgment, this rating warns you away from the most difficult outings if you're not in shape to try them. The scale is *rela-tive only to other backpacking trips*. Most Americans would find even the easiest backpacking trip to be a very strenuous undertaking. So this scale of 1 (barely leave the La-Z-Boy) to 10 (the Ironman Triathlon) is only for people already ac-customed to backpacking.

Mileage: This is the total mileage of the recommended trip in its *most basic form* (without added side trips). I have never, however, seen the point of a "bare bones," Point-A-to-Point-B kind of trip. After all, if you're going to go, you may as well explore a bit. Thus, for many trips, a *second* mileage number (in paren-theses) includes distances for recommended side trips. These side trips are also shown on the maps and included in the "Possible Itinerary" section at the end of the trip description.

I have made every reasonable effort (and some *unreasonable* ones) to ensure that the mileages shown are accurate. Users should *not*, however, assume that the numbers are exact. Wilderness maps for Wyoming rarely (if ever) include mileages, and the distances given on trail signs, especially outside of the national parks, are often contradictory and usually unreliable. In addition, many trails in Wyoming have a disturbing tendency to disappear, forcing confused hikers to wander around in search of the tread.

When exact mileages were not available, the distances used in this book are based on a combination of map extrapolation and my own pedometer readings. These numbers can be considered accurate to within a margin of error of perhaps +/- 5%.

Elevation Gain: For many hikers, how far UP they go is even more important than the distance. This box shows all of the trip's ups and downs in a *total* eleva-tion gain given in feet, not merely the *net* gain. As with the mileage section, a second number (in parentheses) includes the elevation gain of recommended side trips.

Days: A *rough* figure for how long it will take the average backpacker to do the trip, this estimate is based on hiking an average of about 10 miles per day. Also considered were the spacing of available campsites, not-to-be-missed side trips, and the trail's difficulty. Hard-core hikers may cover as many as 25 miles a day, while others saunter along at 4 or 5 miles per day, a good pace for hikers with children. Most trips, therefore, can be done in more or fewer days, depending on your preferences and abilities.

Map(s): Every trip includes a map that is as up-to-date and accurate as possible. These maps use bold lines to indicate the main route and all recommended side trips, so you can get an instant overview of the hike. As every experienced hiker knows, however, you'll also need a good contour map of the area. This entry identifies the best available map(s) for the described trip.

Season: There are *two* seasonal entries shown for each trip. The first tells you when a trip is usually snow-free enough for hiking (which can vary considerably from year to year). The second lists the *particular* time(s) of year when the trip is at its very best—when the flowers peak, the fall colors are at their best, or the mosquitoes have died down, and so on.

Permits and Rules: In Yellowstone and Grand Teton national parks all overnight hikers are required to obtain and carry permits and land managers enforce strict quotas on backcountry campsites. Outside of these parks, however, hikers will encounter few restrictions and in the rare instances where permits are required they are typically free at the trailhead. Some areas have specific regulations that prohibit the use of fires, restrict the number of people allowed in each party, or have seasonal closures due to bear activity. These and other rules are noted in this section.

Contact: This section lists the local land agency responsible for the area covered by this hike. You can contact it to check on road and trail conditions before your trip. Turn to the appendix (p. 257) for the mailing addresses, telephone numbers, and websites (if applicable) of all relevant Wyoming land agencies.

Unfortunately, you should not always expect to get useful or reliable information from these agencies. For the national parks the information is usually very good and frequently updated. The U.S. Forest Service, however, has fewer resources and far fewer wilderness rangers, so the information you receive is often out of date, not very specific, and usually less reliable. Forest Service websites in Wyoming are typically very general and are practically useless for gathering up-to-date information.

Special Attractions: This section focuses on attributes of a particular trip that are rare or outstanding. For example, almost every trip has views, but some have views that are *especially* noteworthy. The same is true of areas where you have a better-than-average chance of seeing wildlife, excellent fall colors, and so on.

Challenges: The flip side to the "Special Attractions" section lists the trip's special or especially troublesome problems. Examples include areas with

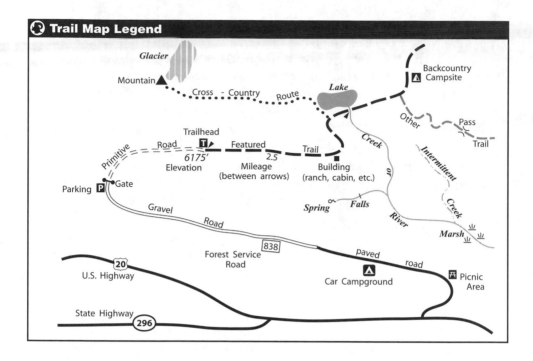

Trail Map Legend

particularly abundant mosquitoes, poor road access, difficult river fords, lots of grizzly bears, or limited water.

Possible Itinerary: Given at the *end* of each trip and intended as a planning tool, the itinerary includes daily mileages and total elevation gains, as well as recommended side trips. Although I have hiked every mile of every trip in this book, many were not done exactly as written here. If I were to *re*-hike a trip, however, I would follow the improved itinerary shown here.

Variations: This self-explanatory section (included only with select trips) suggests the best ways to lengthen, shorten, or otherwise alter the recommended trip.

SAFETY NOTICE

The trips in this book are long, often difficult, and go through some of the most remote wilderness terrain in the U.S. On some trips it is not uncommon to travel for days without seeing another human being. In the event of an emergency, supplies and medical facilities may be several days away. Anyone who attempts these hikes must be experienced in wilderness travel, properly equipped, and in good physical condition. While backpacking is not inherently dangerous, the sport *does* involve risk. Because trail conditions, weather, and hikers' abilities vary considerably, the author and the publisher cannot assume responsibility for the safety of anyone who takes these hikes. Use plenty of common sense and realistically appraise your abilities so you can enjoy these trips safely.

References to "water" in the text attest only to its availability, not its purity. Treat or filter all backcountry water before drinking it.

GENERAL TIPS ON BACKPACKING IN WYOMING

This book is not a "how to" guide for backpackers. Anyone contemplating an extended backpacking vacation will (or at least *should*) already know about equipment, the "no-trace" ethic, conditioning, how to select a campsite, food, first aid, and all the other aspects of this exciting sport. There are many excellent books covering these subjects. It *is* appropriate, however, to discuss some tips and ideas specific to Wyoming.

1) The winter's snowpack has a significant effect, not only on when a trail opens, but also on peak wildflower times, the volume of water in streams you'll have to ford, and how long seasonal water sources are available. The best plan is to check the snowpack on April 1 (the usual seasonal maximum), and note how it compares to normal. This information is available by contacting the Snow Survey Office in Casper at (307) 233-6744, or by checking the snow survey website at *www.wy.nrcs.usda.gov/snow*. If the snowpack is significantly above or below average, adjust a trip's seasonal recommendation accordingly.

2) Trail maintenance in the more isolated parts of Wyoming is often not done as regularly as in many other western states. Some trails are cleared only once every few years and many get no maintenance at all. Expect to encounter downed logs or other obstacles as you hike, and don't expect signs at many trail junctions. Watch the map and the surrounding terrain closely to locate these junctions.

3) A bit of advice for urbanites visiting the Wyoming backcountry: In rural Wyoming (and, for that matter, in much of the rural American West) the *correct* pronunciation of the word *creek* is "crik," with a short "i" rather than a long "e." Keep this in mind so you don't end up sounding like "ignorant city folk."

   Also, when you are passing an oncoming car on rarely used rural roads, acknowledge the other driver with a small wave, whether you know the person or not. Failing to do so identifies you as a rude city visitor.

4) When driving on rural roads, beware of free-ranging livestock, which typically show little fear of cars and have a habit of loitering in the road. It may take considerable patience, honking, and/or swearing to get the animals to move. Calves are particularly notorious for darting in front of cars when you least expect them to. In addition, ranchers regularly use the roadways to push their herds of sheep and cattle between pastures. Be prepared to occasionally get stuck behind (or in the middle of) slow-moving masses of smelly livestock.

   Wildlife may also be present on the road and, especially in Yellowstone National Park, frequently have almost no fear of cars or humans. Drive slowly and be alert for elk, bison, and other critters crossing the highway. Hitting one will, not only kill the innocent animal, it may also total your car and cost you several thousand dollars.

5) Hunting is a long-standing tradition in Wyoming and an important part of the local economy. The overwhelming majority of hunters are responsible citizens who take their sport seriously and respect other users. Still, with all those guns in the woods, it is prudent for hikers to take reasonable precautions. General elk-hunting season, which usually draws the most hunters, begins around October 15 (although in a few parts of the state the season starts as early as September 5) and runs through sometime in November. General deer-hunting season is more variable, but typically occurs in October and November. Smaller but locally significant numbers of hunters also pursue bighorn sheep, mountain goats, pronghorns, moose, and black bears usually in the fall (although there is a spring bear hunt as well), but hunting season varies from place to place and year to year.

Check the latest hunting regulations and seasons for the area you plan to visit by obtaining a synopsis. These hefty handouts are available at most ranger stations and sporting goods stores around the state. For safety, anyone hiking on public lands during hunting season (particularly those doing any cross-country travel) should carry *and wear* a bright red or orange cap, vest, pack, or other conspicuous article of clothing. Hunting is prohibited in national parks, so these precautions are not necessary on those lands.

6) Although Wyoming's black bears (especially those outside of the national parks and parts of the Wind River Range) are generally shy, they are common throughout the state's mountains and forests. To keep them shy, and to protect your precious supplies, hang all food, garbage, and other odorous items at least 10 feet off the ground and 4 feet from the nearest tree trunk, so the bruins cannot reach it. In grizzly country aim for 12 feet up and 5 feet away from the trunk. This procedure will also protect your food supply from an even more common, destructive group of thieves—chipmunks. If you are camping above treeline, especially in grizzly country, use a bear canister.

7) Many of the trails in Wyoming were originally designed for (and are still largely used by) equestrians. Often little regard was given to hikers and the difficulties that pedestrians have in crossing larger streams. As a result, hikers frequently have to ford streams (large and small) on the trips described in this book. In late spring and early summer, rivers and creeks run high with snowmelt, which makes fording them cold, potentially dangerous, and frequently impossible. The typical stream depth for the recommended season of the hike is noted in the trip description, but it can vary considerably from year to year.

If a ford looks too deep, too swift, or too dangerous when you get there, don't risk it! Turn around and head back the way you came. Lightweight wading shoes or sandals give you better traction, protect your feet from cuts and scrapes, and allow you to keep your boots and socks dry. Trekking poles to provide a third and fourth leg of support are also highly recommended. To help you plan, I have noted all significant or potentially difficult fords in the text and labeled them on the maps.

8) Based on its average elevation above sea level, Wyoming is the highest state in the U.S. The air is literally different here—more specifically, it's thinner. Local hikers who already live at fairly high elevations are usually pretty well acclimated to the altitude. But out-of-state visitors may struggle for oxygen when they arrive at a Wyoming trailhead that is 9000 or more feet above sea level, especially when they realize that they must climb to reach their destination. Even residents of the larger, relatively low elevation cities in eastern Wyoming such as Cheyenne or Casper, may take a few days to become accustomed to the much higher mountains of western Wyoming.

Until you get acclimated, plan to experience symptoms such as shortness of breath, lack of appetite, and headaches. Most of the time these symptoms of altitude sickness are merely inconvenient, although they will probably slow your progress and make you uncomfortable. If symptoms become severe, however, you may need to retreat to lower elevations and possibly even cancel your trip. If you have the time, take a few dayhikes in the area to get your lungs accustomed to the thin air before tackling a longer trip in the high mountains.

9) Thunderstorms, especially in the mountains of Wyoming, are so common you should expect them almost every afternoon in mid- to late summer. Lightning safety is a lengthy topic, but avoiding the problem is the best plan. Always schedule your daily travels so you will be below treeline by 2 P.M. and never travel along exposed ridges when a storm is in the area. If a thunderstorm catches you unaware (a frequent occurrence, since the storms often develop very quickly and seemingly out of nowhere), the best rule of thumb is to crouch down in a lower area on the leeward side of a boulder and away from isolated trees. Wear rubber-soled boots or hunch down atop a foam sleeping pad. Finally, have your group spread out so that if one person gets struck others will be unharmed and can help the victim.

10) The weather in Wyoming, especially in the mountains, is often wonderful, with highs in the comfortable 70s and lows in the 40s. But it can also be extremely cold and potentially dangerous. Be prepared for freezing weather and snow at any time of year. Hypothermia is a major concern, so bring several layers of warm clothing, stay out of the cold wind, try to remain reasonably dry, watch members of your party for symptoms (such as shivering, slurred speech, stumbling, and lack of manual dexterity), and always remain well hydrated. Treat mildly hypothermic persons with high energy snacks, warm drinks, and a cheery campfire. In more severe cases, plenty of skin to skin contact in a warm sleeping bag is the best plan.

11) Finally, a melancholy note about a natural phenomenon sweeping the American Rockies, including most of the forested areas of Wyoming: Mountain pine beetles and, to a lesser extent, spruce budworms are chewing their way through the conifer forests of the Cowboy State and are killing tens of millions of trees. In many areas, most of the mature trees have already been killed, leaving the hillsides covered with a rather ugly patchwork of brown,

black, and green. These cyclical bug infestations have occurred for millennia, however, so we have reason to hope that the forests will eventually return to their former health.

BE BEAR AWARE: HIKING IN GRIZZLY COUNTRY

Although Wyoming is justly famous for a great variety of wildlife, the most famous (or infamous) wild animals here are its bears. Depending largely on how many bad horror movies you have seen, you may or may not be happy about the possibility of encountering one of these powerful native residents on the trail. But such encounters occur fairly frequently, so hikers need to be familiar with the proper procedures to ensure the safety and survival of both humans and bruins.

All bears are intelligent, curious, powerful, potentially dangerous, and seem constantly hungry. But you should deal with grizzlies and black bears differently, so the first step in being bear aware is knowing how to identify the two species. Black bears are somewhat smaller than their more famous cousins, with adults usually weighing between 150 and 350 pounds, while adult grizzlies tip the scales at between 350 and 1,000 pounds. When you come around a corner in the trail and unexpectedly find yourself face-to-face with a bear, however, both species look awfully big (and stubbornly refuse to hop up on a scale to be carefully weighed), so size is not a reliable indicator in the field. Similarly, color is a poor way to identify the animals because both species range in color from very light brown to almost jet black.

A better way to tell the bears apart is by field marks. Black bears have a straight, sloping face and snout, relatively tall ears, and a rear end that sticks up slightly higher than their shoulders. Grizzly bears have a dished-in face, relatively short and rounded ears, a rear end that slopes downward and is lower than their front, and a prominent hump at their shoulder. Grizzly tracks are noticeably larger than black bears (frighteningly so, in fact), and often show the marks of the bear's 3- to 4-inch claws.

Although black bears inhabit all the forested mountains of Wyoming, grizzly bears are found only in the northwest part of the state, especially in and around Yellowstone National Park. Grizzly bear numbers have increased noticeably in the last couple of decades, however, and their range has been expanding. Today, you might reasonably expect to encounter grizzly bears on any hike from the northern Wind River Range and Gros Ventre Wilderness through northern Grand Teton National Park, all of Yellowstone Park, and into the Beartooth and Absaroka ranges. Grizzly bears are fairly common on Trips 1 through 11 in this book.

Black bears are generally shy around humans, but they are still potentially dangerous, especially once they obtain human food and associate hikers with yummy snacks. Grizzlies are more unpredictable than black bears and are usually more aggressive. Attacks by either species are rare (statistically, hikers in Wyoming have a much greater chance of being killed in a car accident than of being mauled by a bear), but they get lots of publicity when they occur and are common enough that hikers need to take some reasonable precautions. Unfortunately, coming up with hard-and-fast rules in dealing with bears is difficult because individual bears act differently in different situations. There are, however, some generally agreed-upon recommendations that hikers should follow.

Without question, the best strategy is to avoid bears in the first place, and especially to avoid attracting them to you or your camp, but you should:

- **Never approach any bear** (getting a close-up photograph just isn't worth it), and be especially careful to stay away from any female bear with cubs.

- **Never approach or linger around an animal carcass.** Bears, especially grizzlies, often feed upon and aggressively defend carcasses against intruders.

- **Never camp near a carcass or in an area with obvious signs of recent bear activity,** such as fresh diggings, tracks, torn-up stumps, or scat, even if your permit says you are supposed to camp there.

- **Always check at a ranger station about recent bear sightings and activity** for the area you plan to hike in. In Yellowstone National Park, trails and campsites are sometimes closed due to bear activity, and these closures should always be respected.

- **Especially in grizzly bear country, make noise while you hike.** A large percentage of bear attacks occur when a bear is surprised by a hiker. When a bear hears a hiker coming up the trail, however, they will usually leave the area. When I hike alone in bear country, I carry an aluminum can with pebbles in it that I shake every 50 to 100 yards.

- **In grizzly country, travel in a group and stay on the trail.** Bears almost never attack groups of more than three people, and a surprisingly large number of attacks occur when people are traveling cross-country. In certain bear management zones of Yellowstone National Park, hikers are not allowed to travel off-trail and are strongly encouraged to travel in groups.

- **Never hike at night, when bears are most actively searching for food.** It is also better to avoid late evenings and early mornings.

- **Leave all particularly smelly foods at home.** Remember that bears can smell *many* times better than you can, so if *you* are able to smell something, it's a sure bet that a bear can smell it from a long way away.

- **Since dogs and bears do not get along, it is generally unwise to hike with your dog in bear country.** Dogs are not allowed at all in the backcountry of Grand Teton or Yellowstone National Parks.

- **In camp, store all your food** (and other odorous items, such as hand lotion, toothpaste, and garbage) out of reach from bruins and *a minimum* of 100 yards from your sleeping area. You should also sleep at least 100 yards away from where you cooked your food.

- **Store your food either in a bear-resistant canister** (available for rent at many ranger stations and now required in Grand Teton National Park) **or hang your food** either from a camp's established bear pole or from a narrow tree limb that is at least 10 feet off the ground and 4 feet away from the trunk. In grizzly country, make those numbers 12 feet from the ground and 5 feet from the tree trunk.

If all of these avoidance strategies fail and you encounter a bear, here are some recommendations:

- In grizzly country it is increasingly common for people to carry bear spray (approved by the Environmental Protection Agency) in a hip holster that is immediately ready for use. The idea is that, in the event of an attack, you should spray toward the bear's face starting when the charging bear is about 30 feet away from you. If you have time to pull it out. If you have practiced and know how to use it. If you do not panic and can manage reasonably good aim in a very stressful situation. And if you do not have a cross wind or (much worse) wind blowing toward you, then it may effectively deter a bear. But that's a lot of "ifs," so *never* think of bear spray as an alternative to employing common sense and following the other advice listed here.

- If you encounter a lone black bear and it has not seen you, back away on the trail around a bend and make plenty of noise. Most of the time the bear will leave the area once it knows a human is there and you can cautiously continue hiking.

- If you see a lone grizzly bear and the terrain allows, you might try to make a wide detour around the area on the downwind side of the animal. If that is not possible, you should probably turn around.

- If you encounter a grizzly bear with cubs, abandon the trail entirely and return the way you came.

- If the bear sees you but is a reasonable distance away and makes no aggressive moves (such as huffing or clacking its teeth), stand your ground. If it is a black bear, make some noise and it will almost always run away. If it is a grizzly bear, alter your route to move away from the bear's area. If it is a grizzly bear with cubs, then slowly back away and leave the way you came. Your trip in this area, at least, is over.

- In the rare instance that a bear approaches or charges you, the experts all say to remain calm and **do not run**. You cannot outrun a bear and running encourages them to chase you. This advice may sound impossible to follow, but as someone who has been charged *twice* by grizzly bears, I can attest that on both occasions I was so completely petrified I could not have moved if I had wanted to. Try to talk to the bear in a soothing voice, back away slowly, and never look the bear directly in the eye. Most bear charges are "bluff charges" meant simply to scare you out of their territory; the bear will turn away shortly before it reaches you.

- If a black bear attacks you, use bear spray if it's available and fight back with anything you have (your walking stick, a rock, your fists, etc.). Frequently a black bear will decide it just isn't worth it and go away.

- If a grizzly bear attacks you, use bear spray if it's available and then play dead. Drop to the ground and lay flat on your stomach, with your hands clasped behind your neck. You probably won't have time to take it off in any event, but the experts say to leave your pack on for added protection. Do not provide *any* resistance. You can't win and the movement will only encourage the bear to continue mauling you. Wait for the bear to leave the area before you get up, tend to any injuries, or make any other movement.

- The only instances where experts advise fighting back against a grizzly bear is when a bear attacks after stalking you as prey or drags a person out of a tent at night. In such circumstances the person being attacked or dragged away will almost certainly be killed, so you may as well fight back, since you really have nothing to lose. Fortunately, such events are *extremely* rare, so don't lose any sleep over it.

- When you return from your trip, report any potentially dangerous bear encounters to the local land managers.

All of that said; *do not* be so afraid of bears that it ruins your trip. Remember that bear attacks are very rare and certainly *not* worth missing out on the spectacular backcountry of Wyoming.

Grizzly track, Miller Creek Trail (Trip 3), Yellowstone National Park

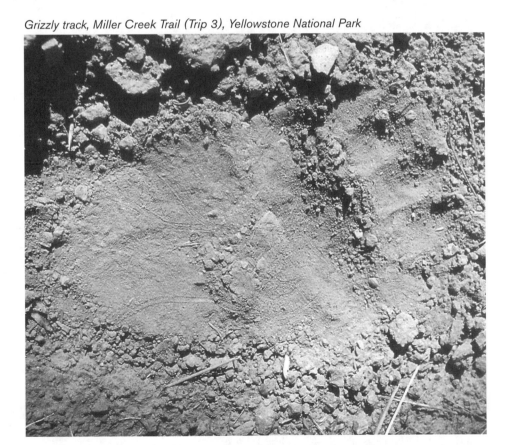

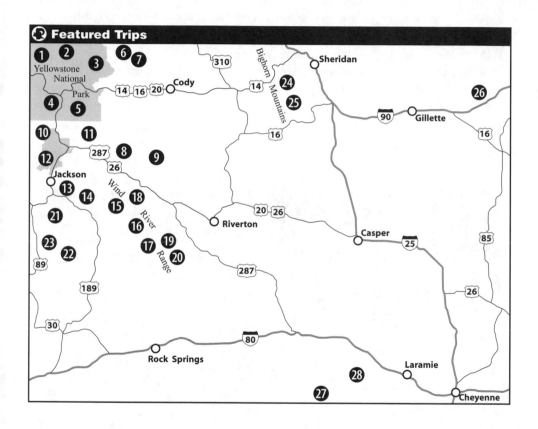

FEATURED TRIPS

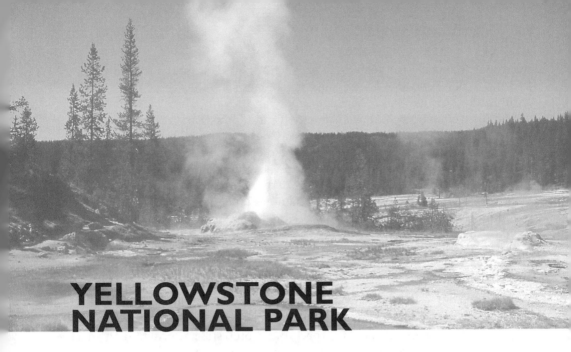

YELLOWSTONE NATIONAL PARK

Although small parts of Yellowstone National Park are in Montana and Idaho, the vast majority of the world's first (and, arguably, still its best) national park is in the Cowboy State. So while Wyoming has numerous outdoor wonders of which it is rightly proud, Yellowstone is unquestionably at the top of the list. And how could it not be? With its thousands of geysers and other thermal features, unusually large and beautiful mountain lakes, countless waterfalls, sublime mountain scenery, colorful canyons, and amazingly abundant wildlife, Yellowstone literally has it all.

Approximately 1,000 miles of trails provide access to the park's countless backcountry attractions, so a person could easily spend years hiking here and never see it all. Surprisingly, while the roads are often bumper-to-bumper with traffic and the roadside nature trails are elbow-to-elbow with tourists, many (even most) of the longer trails in the park are rarely traveled. Solitude, in other words, is surprisingly easy for the backpacker to obtain. The park has a quota on backcountry use and requires that all overnighters stay at designated campsites. Once you obtain a permit you are assured of a good place to camp that your party will have all to themselves. For a fee, you can reserve a permit, and while a reservation is advisable for the more popular trails (see individual hikes for details), for lesser-used trails it is often possible to get a free permit even as late as the day you start to hike. Keep in mind, however, that specific campsites and trails may be closed due to bear activity or wildfires at any time. Even hikers with a reservation may be told that the hike they planned to do is now impossible. If you are flexible, however, you can usually get a permit for another area and still have a great time.

Second only to its geysers, probably the most outstanding feature of Yellowstone National Park is its incredible array of wildlife. Although seeing these

Photo: *Geyser in Shoshone Geyser Basin (Trip 4)*

magnificent animals is a big attraction for hikers, it is important to remember that the park is *not* a zoo! The animals are not tame and they certainly are not in secure cages. Critters have the right-of-way and should always be considered armed (as well as hoofed, clawed, antlered, and toothed) and dangerous. Bison, for example, may look like shaggy, big-headed domesticated cattle, but don't be fooled. These 2,000-pound giants are unpredictable and extremely dangerous. Although many people worry about grizzly bears in Yellowstone, bison are statistically much more dangerous. While grizzly maulings are rare, almost every year people are gored, trampled, and sometimes killed by bison. In some areas it is common for bison to lie right on or beside the trail. *Always* walk well around the creatures. Moose and elk should also be avoided, especially during the fall rut when the bulls become territorial and quite aggressive.

Park rules require visitors to stay at least 25 yards away from any large animal, and at least 100 yards away from any bear. Bears with cubs or near a carcass they may be defending, rutting bull moose, and any animal that appears agitated should be given even more room. Smaller animals, such as squirrels, weasels, and foxes, don't require that kind of space, but should still be left alone and, most important, *never* fed. Not only may they bite you, but in the long run receiving human food will hurt the animal's chances for survival in the wild. For information about safety when hiking in bear country, see the separate section in the Introduction (p. 8).

Although most of the best long trails in Yellowstone National Park are described in this book, one outstanding area has been omitted—the lush and waterfall-rich Bechler River country, also known as Cascade Corner, of southwest Yellowstone. An excellent and popular one-way trip starts at the Lone Star Geyser Trailhead near Old Faithful (see Trip 4) and goes 34 miles down the impressive Bechler River Canyon to an exit point at either Bechler Ranger Station or Cave Falls. Unfortunately, this trip requires a very long, complicated car shuttle. Since this area is easier to reach by both road and trail from Idaho, I describe the route in *Backpacking Idaho*, which is also available from Wilderness Press.

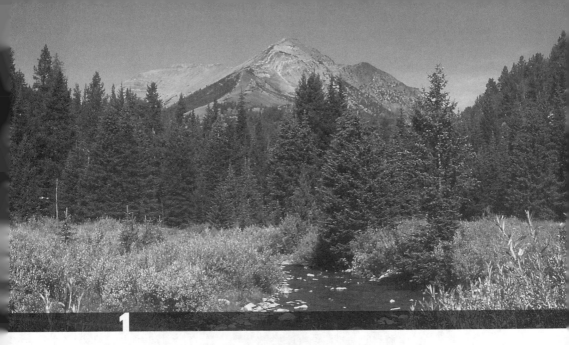

BIGHORN PASS
& SPORTSMAN LAKE LOOP

RATINGS: Scenery 8   Solitude 5   Difficulty 6
MILES: 45.7 (54.7), including a 3.9-mile roadwalk
ELEVATION GAIN: 6550´ (9750´)
DAYS: 3–5
MAP: Trails Illustrated *Mammoth Hot Springs-NW Yellowstone National Park*
USUALLY OPEN: Mid-July to October
BEST: Late July to mid-September
CONTACT: Yellowstone National Park
SPECIAL ATTRACTIONS: Good mountain scenery; plenty of wildlife

PERMIT

A permit is required. Advanced reservations are recommended. The nearest location to pick up a permit is the Mammoth Hot Springs Ranger Station.

RULES

Fires are allowed only at specified camps. All food and other odorous items must be stored away from bears *at all times*. Most of this trip is in the Gallatin Bear Management Area, where off-trail travel is prohibited from May 1 to November 10. Because of the bears, a minimum group size of four is recommended and solo hiking is discouraged.

Photo: Electric Peak over Gardner River

TAKE THIS TRIP

Some of the best mountain scenery in Yellowstone National Park is in the Gallatin Range, a cluster of 10,000-foot peaks filled with snowy summits, colorful wildflowers, sparkling lakes, and all the other attractions typically found in the mountains of the American West. This being Yellowstone, however, these mountains also boast a higher concentration of wildlife than places not protected in a national park. So not only can hikers enjoy the usual wildflower-covered meadows and impressively tall peaks, they will also probably see elk, bison, moose, and possibly bears and wolves, along with many smaller animals.

The loop described here visits many of the Gallatin Range's most outstanding scenic attractions, including lovely Sportsman Lake, miles of beautiful lower-elevation meadows, and wonderful viewpoints at Bighorn Pass and Electric Divide. It also provides access to side trips to such places as Electric Peak and Cache Lake and visits a wide variety of habitats. All in all this is perhaps the most diverse, scenic, and enjoyable longer backpacking trip in the park.

CHALLENGES

Grizzly bears are very common—camp and act accordingly.

HOW TO GET THERE

The trailhead is in the northwest part of Yellowstone National Park along the spur road into Indian Creek Campground. The campground turnoff can be reached either by driving north 12.9 miles from the Norris Geyser Basin junction or south 8.9 miles from Mammoth Hot Springs. In either case, turn west at the sign for Indian Creek Campground, drive over a bridge, and almost immediately thereafter reach the signed Bighorn Trailhead. Parking is on the right.

DESCRIPTION

The slightly uphill trail begins by going west through a forest of young lodgepole pines that are slowly recovering from the massive fires of 1988. Most of the trees are only about 15 feet tall, so shade is something of a rarity. The extra sunshine allowed in by the shorter trees, however, has led to fine wildflower displays from late June to early August and generally better views. After 0.1 mile you come to a junction. Go right on Bighorn Loop and soon walk past several car campsites in Indian Creek Campground. At 0.3 mile follow the campground's loop road for 10 yards before veering left back onto the trail.

The path soon comes to an unsigned junction with an abandoned section of the Howard Eaton Trail near the edge of a huge rolling meadow. Keep left on Bighorn Pass Trail, which stays along the south edge of the lovely meadow not far from meandering Indian Creek. Looking straight ahead across the meadow to the west you can see (from left to right) Antler Peak, the gap of Bighorn Pass, Bannock Peak, and the long sloping ridge of Quadrant Mountain. To the right (north-northwest) is the more pointed summit of Electric Peak. Wildlife is common in this meadow with lots of elk and perhaps even a moose or two if you are lucky.

At 0.9 mile you pass Camp 1B1, then keep going west, mostly in meadows, to an ankle- to calf-deep ford of Indian Creek at 2.3 miles. The trail then crosses about 1.5 miles of rolling country covered with sagebrush, grasses, and wildflowers where you have fine views to the west of the Gallatin Range and a good chance of seeing bison. About halfway into this lovely section you ford Panther Creek, a stream you will follow for the next few miles. Once the rolling meadow ends, you head gradually uphill in a wide canyon that features increasingly forested terrain. Unlike most of Yellowstone, the forest here has very few lodgepole pines, with lots of Engelmann spruces, subalpine firs, and some western white pines instead. Panther Creek is always nearby and the forest is broken by several small meadows. Both moose and elk are common here and, with binoculars, you may spot a few of the bighorn sheep that call nearby Quadrant Mountain home. The vegetation mix is also excellent bear habitat. This fact, along with the frequent piles of bear scat on the trail, is a useful reminder to stay alert and make plenty of noise while you hike. While not looking for wildlife, you will probably notice the fine views of bulky Bannock Peak to the southwest.

As you gradually gain elevation, the meadows become larger so that eventually the forest comes only in scattered clumps. At 7.2 miles you pass a shallow, marshy pond, then the pace of the climb increases until you reach 9110-foot Bighorn Pass at 8.4 miles. This high point has superb views of the distant Absaroka Range to the east and the sweeping valley of the Gallatin River to the northwest, the upper reaches of which are covered with a skeleton forest of burned snags.

Making your way down into the aforementioned Gallatin River Valley, descend fairly steeply past sheer cliffs on your right for about 1 mile before things level out beside the joyful Gallatin River. From here you enjoy a gentle and pleasant walk, never far from the small stream and mostly in attractive meadows or unburned forest. A quick look at that forest demonstrates that here on the west side of the park, the climate is somewhat wetter than elsewhere in Yellowstone, resulting in thicker greenery and more undergrowth. At about 4.5 miles from Bighorn Pass, as you enter a particularly large meadow, is Camp WB6, a very pleasant spot with nice views of Crowfoot Ridge to the south-southwest. In September, campers can expect to be kept awake by bugling elk throughout the night. Wolves often follow the elk down to these meadows and may also be heard or seen by sharp-eyed hikers.

Below Camp WB6, and still mostly in nearly level meadows, the trail passes Camps WB4 and WB3, both designed for stock users. About 60 yards after you pass less attractive Camp WB1 is a junction. Turn right and steadily climb an open slope of grasses and burned snags for 0.8 mile to a junction with the Fawn Pass Trail. Go left (west) and gradually descend through huge meadows where

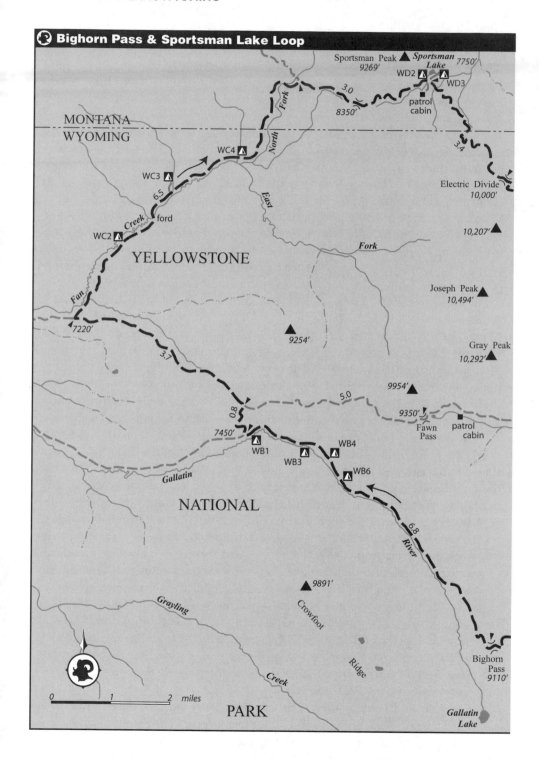

Bighorn Pass & Sportsman Lake Loop

Sportsman Peak ▲ *Sportsman* 7750'
9269'   *Lake*
                    WD2
3.0   WD3
8350'   patrol
                   cabin

3.4

MONTANA
WYOMING   WC4

                North   Electric Divide
WC3   Fork   10,000'

6.5   East
    Creek ford   10,207' ▲
WC2
    YELLOWSTONE   Fork

    Fan   Joseph Peak ▲
                            10,494'

    7220'
                    ▲   Gray Peak
3.7   9254'   10,292' ▲

                        9954' ▲
            5.0
                    9350'
    0.8   Fawn   patrol
7450'   Pass   cabin
        WB1
                WB4
    Gallatin   WB3
                    WB6
    NATIONAL

                        6.8
                    River

                    ▲ 9891'

    Grayling
                Crowfoot

                        Bighorn
            Ridge   Pass
    Creek   9110'

0   1   2 miles
                PARK   *Gallatin*
                            Lake

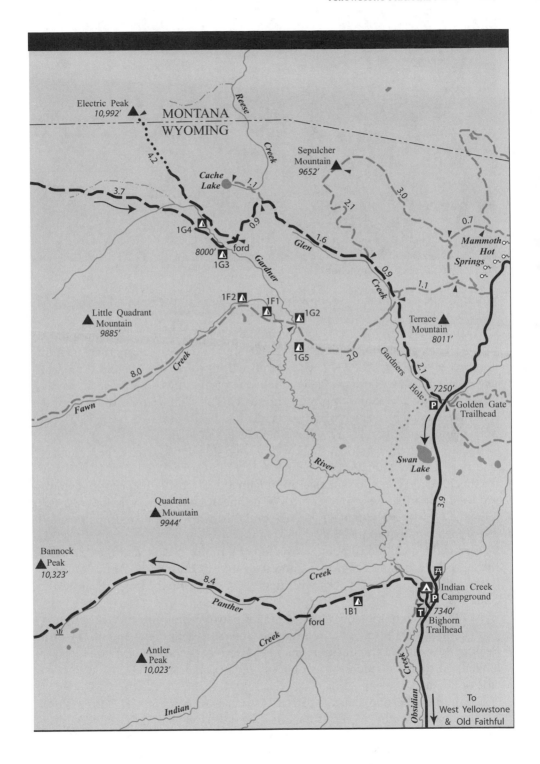

Electric Peak
10,992'

MONTANA
WYOMING

Reese Creek

Sepulcher
Mountain
9652'

Cache
Lake

4.2

3.7

1.1

0.9

3.0

2.1

0.7

Mammoth
Hot
Springs

1G4

Glen

1.6

8000'

ford

1G3

Gardner

Creek

0.9

1.1

Little Quadrant
Mountain
9885'

1F2

1F1

1G2

Terrace
Mountain
8011'

Creek

8.0

1G5

2.0

Gardners

Hole

2.1

Fawn

7250'

P

Golden Gate
Trailhead

River

Swan
Lake

Quadrant
Mountain
9944'

3.9

Bannock
Peak
10,323'

Creek

8.4

Indian Creek
Campground

Panther

ford

1B1

P

7340'
Bighorn
Trailhead

Creek

Antler
Peak
10,023'

Indian

Obsidian Creek

To
West Yellowstone
& Old Faithful

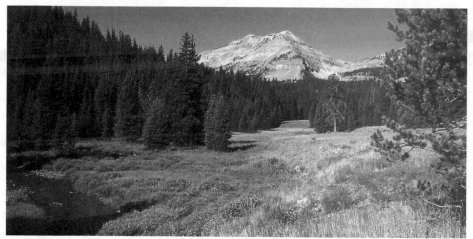

Bannock Peak over Panther Creek

you may see elk and will certainly have good views of the forested ridges in all directions.

At 19.7 miles turn right at a junction onto the Fan Creek Trail. This route heads up the wide, gentle valley of its namesake stream initially in open areas amid sagebrush, scrubby willows, and assorted wildflowers. After 0.4 mile the trail leaves the meadows and gradually climbs the partly forested hillside above the creek. You pass pleasant Camp WC2 and then it's another 0.5 mile, often in muddy areas flooded by beaver activity, to a relatively easy ford of Fan Creek. Moose are a common sight amid the willow flats along the creek.

Sticking with the hillside just above the west side of Fan Creek, the trail takes you northeast to a junction with the side trail to Camp WC3. Immediately after this junction you splash across an unnamed side creek, then continue going gradually uphill to very nice Camp WC4 opposite where East Fork Fan Creek joins the North Fork of that stream. Beyond this camp, you hike uphill through forest for 1.5 miles to a junction.

Turn right, continue climbing to the top of a minor divide, and then descend through the snags and regrowing forest of a 1988 burn zone. About halfway down are a set of switchbacks with fine views of pointed Electric Peak to the east.

At the bottom of the downhill is a ranger patrol cabin, Camp WD2, and gorgeous Sportsman Lake. Set in a large meadow and with views of both Electric Peak to the east and craggy Sportsman Peak above its northwest shore, this lake is well worth an overnight stay or a long lunch stop. Camp WD3 is on the east side of the lake.

To continue the loop, take the path that starts near the Camp WD2 turnoff and go diagonally (southeast) across the meadow until you enter unburned forest on the other side. From here you begin a long, tiring, moderately steep uphill. About halfway up this 2200-foot ascent you go in and out of a burn zone, and then, with more elevation gain, enter a land of sloping grasslands, rocks, snowfields, and scattered whitebark pines and subalpine firs. You top out at 10,000-foot Electric Divide, with its fine views of several mountain ranges in both Wyoming and Montana. Wildlife enthusiasts may see elk, bighorn sheep, or grizzly bears in the Electric Divide area.

From Electric Divide you descend a series of short steep switchbacks and then go more gradually downhill through an enchanting mix of meadows, forest, and several small creeks. At 3.1 miles from Electric Divide is the turnoff to Camp 1G4, then it's only a short distance to Camp 1G3 and a shallow ford of Gardner River. Look upstream here for a fine view of Electric Peak. After the river crossing you climb for 0.2 mile to a junction atop a small ridge.

The trail to the left makes a long, steep climb to the top of Electric Peak. Although this trail eventually deteriorates into a rough scramble route, it is a terrific 8.4-mile side trip if you have the time and energy.

The main trail goes straight at the Electric Peak junction and travels northeast through dense forest for 0.9 mile to another junction, this time with the Cache Lake Trail, another possible side trip. Go straight and gradually descend along small Glen Creek. Most of the way is in attractive but increasingly dry meadows of grasses, wildflowers, and sagebrush on the hillside above the creek. Keep right where the Sepulcher Mountain Trail goes left, and descend along Glen Creek another 0.9 mile to a flat area and a pair of junctions only 100 yards apart. Go straight at both junctions and cross the large, nearly flat, treeless, and often hot expanse of Gardners Hole for a final 2.1 miles to the Golden Gate Trailhead. From here it is a 3.9-mile car shuttle or roadwalk back to the Bighorn Trailhead near Indian Creek Campground.

POSSIBLE ITINERARY

	CAMPS & SIDE TRIPS	MILES	ELEVATION GAIN
DAY 1	Camp WB6	12.9	1900'
DAY 2	Camp WC4	11.8	1000'
DAY 3	Camp 1G3	11.3	3150'
DAY 4	Camp 1G3, with dayhike up Electric Peak	9.0	3200'
DAY 5	Out, including the 3.9-mile roadwalk back to your car	9.7	500'

VARIATIONS ·

A slightly shorter version of this loop, with almost equally good scenery but usually less wildlife, uses the Fawn Pass Trail rather than the Bighorn Pass Trail to cross the Gallatin Range on the westward leg. This route avoids the roadwalk or car shuttle at the end because you start and finish at the Golden Gate Trailhead.

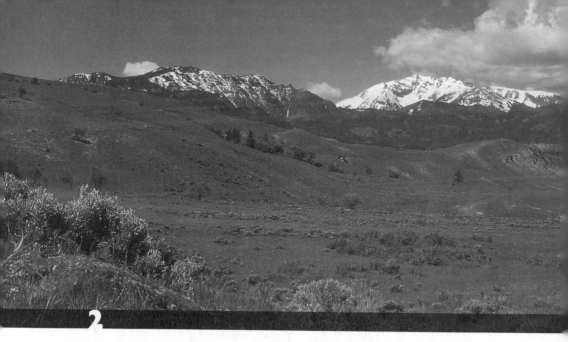

BLACK CANYON OF THE YELLOWSTONE RIVER

RATINGS: Scenery 7   Solitude 5   Difficulty 6

MILES: 32.2 as a loop with the Rescue Creek Trail

22 as a point-to-point hike from Hellroaring Trailhead

ELEVATION GAIN: 3200´ as a loop; 1450´ as a point-to-point hike

DAYS: 3–4

MAPS: Trails Illustrated *Mammoth Hot Springs-NW Yellowstone National Park* and *Tower/Canyon & NE Yellowstone National Park*

USUALLY OPEN: May to November

BEST: May–June and September–October

CONTACT: Yellowstone National Park

SPECIAL ATTRACTIONS: Excellent early and late season hiking; terrific canyon scenery; the thunderous cataract of Knowles Falls

PERMIT

A permit is required. Advanced reservations may help. The nearest location to pick up a permit is the Mammoth Hot Springs Ranger Station.

RULES

Fires are allowed only at specified camps. All food and other odorous items must be stored away from bears *at all times*.

Photo: Electric Peak from lower Rescue Creek Trail

CHALLENGES ·

The canyon can get very hot in midsummer (spring and fall are preferable). A tough ford of Hellroaring Creek (or an extended detour to a bridge) is required if the trip is done as a one-way, point-to-point hike. Grizzly bears are common, especially in the spring.

HOW TO GET THERE ·

To reach the lower trailhead, drive U.S. Highway 89 to Gardiner, Montana, which is immediately beyond the north entrance to Yellowstone National Park. At the first junction after you cross to the east side of a large bridge over the Yellowstone River, turn right (southeast) on Fourth Street (a.k.a. Jardine Road), drive 0.1 mile, and then turn right on gravel White Lane. Proceed one block and reach the signed Yellowstone River Trailhead on the right, just before a church. There is only room here for about four cars to park. Please do not park in the church's parking lot.

If you have a second car and are doing the loop, leave the second car at the Rescue Creek Trailhead, along the north entrance road of Yellowstone Park 0.7 mile south of the north entrance station. Without a second car it is an easy 1.2-mile walk between the two trailheads.

Those doing this as a one-way point-to-point hike can reach the upper trailhead by driving 5 miles south from the north entrance of Yellowstone National Park to Mammoth Hot Springs. Turn east toward Tower Junction, drive 14.8 miles, then turn left (south) at a sign for Hellroaring Trailhead. Go 0.3 mile down this good, dead-end gravel road to the trailhead.

TAKE THIS TRIP

The Black Canyon of the Yellowstone River is a generally overlooked gem in a national park chock full of precious stones. Since they are at the lowest elevations in the park, the trails here open earlier and stay open later than most other park trails, thus providing excellent "shoulder season" hiking. And although there are no geysers or other thermal features to amaze you, the quite dramatic scenery features a powerful river, tall canyon walls, and plenty of wildlife, especially in the spring before the animals move up to the high country.

The most popular itinerary is to do this trip as a one-way mostly downhill hike from the Hellroaring Trailhead with an exit at Gardiner, Montana. This scenario, however, requires two cars and misses the views along the lovely Rescue Creek Trail. A loop trip from the lower trailhead provides a better variety of scenery and still hits all the best parts of the Yellowstone River Trail, especially when you include a dayhike through the upper reaches of the Black Canyon.

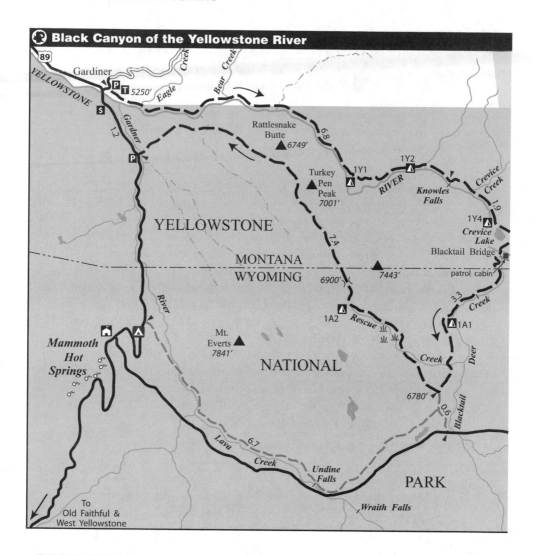

Black Canyon of the Yellowstone River

DESCRIPTION •

From the Gardiner Trailhead, the trail cuts through a narrow 60-yard strip of land between the church property on your left and a private campground on the right to a prominent trail sign. For the next 0.5 mile you cross private land (please stay on the trail), passing the confluence of the small and clear Gardner River with the larger and murkier Yellowstone River to where signs tell you that you are entering Yellowstone National Park. The surroundings are unlike what most people think of when they envision Yellowstone. Here, at the lowest elevations in the park, the only trees are some scattered Rocky Mountain junipers and a few cottonwoods by the river. In fact, the region is a semidesert, complete with sagebrush and prickly pear cactus. In summer it can get very hot in this canyon, but the relatively mild winters make it critical winter range for many of the park's large mammals, including bison, elk, and bighorn sheep.

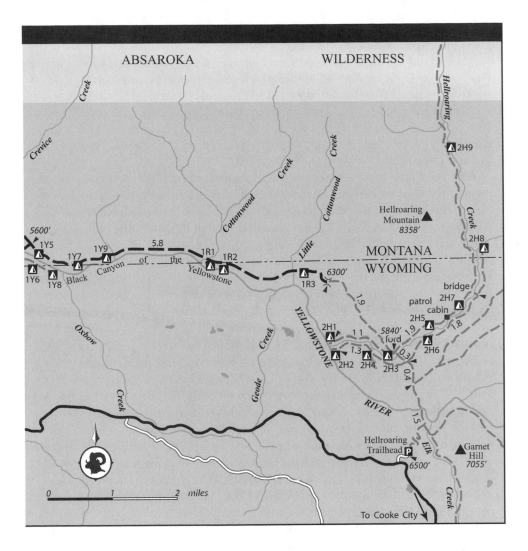

By June most of the large animals have left for higher terrain, so pronghorns and a few mule deer are the only large mammals you are likely to see. Bighorn sheep, however, linger longer than the others, so you may see small herds on the canyon walls through June. One animal you are very likely to see throughout the summer are ospreys, large fish-eating hawks that fly along the river and dive into the water in search of a meal. Other possible wildlife sightings include mergansers, bald eagles, and river otters. If the animals are not around, you can always be content with the nice views of both the river and the snow-capped Gallatin Range to the west.

Throughout its length the gently graded trail follows the slopes on the north side of the Yellowstone River. Although there are many small ups and downs, which add considerably to the trip's total elevation gain, you rarely climb more than 200 feet above the water. At 1.6 miles you reach the first significant landmark at a bridge over large, swift Bear Creek. The rocky canyon walls in this area are a good place to look for bighorn sheep.

Above Bear Creek the environment becomes gradually wetter, so evergreen trees such as Douglas firs and limber pines are increasingly common. The other striking feature is that the canyon walls get noticeably higher and steeper, so the scenery improves. The next landmark arrives at 5.5 miles when you pass Camp 1Y1, a fine riverside site with a lovely little beach. The trail then makes its first significant climb, gaining about 300 feet up an old rockslide well above a twisting and rampaging section of the river.

After returning to river level, the trail traces a gentle course for 0.5 mile beside a stretch of relatively quiet water where you pass Camp 1Y2, which is more exposed and less attractive than Camp 1Y1. At 6.8 miles you reach Knowles Falls. Although the falls is only 15 feet high, when such a large volume of water goes over even a short falls, the scene is very impressive.

The trail now climbs once again, up and over a rocky formation just above Knowles Falls, then crosses cascading Crevice Creek on a bridge. Shortly after the bridge you pass the turnoff to Camp 1Y4, then cross a hillside above tranquil and deep Crevice Lake, which sits in a depression and has no permanent inlet or outlet.

At 8.7 miles is a major junction. The Blacktail Deer Creek Trail, which is the recommended return route for those doing the loop, goes to the right. After a brief 0.2 mile this trail crosses the Blacktail Bridge over the Yellowstone River. This bridge provides access, not only to the return trail, but to a side trail that goes upstream on the south side of the river. This side trail passes a National Park Service patrol cabin before taking you to very attractive Camps 1Y6 and 1Y8. If you are doing the loop hike, the best plan is to set up a base camp at one of these sites, or at one of the other nearby campsites on the north side of the river, and dayhike upstream through the heart of the Black Canyon of the Yellowstone.

Those doing the dayhike should follow the Yellowstone River Trail, which continues straight (upstream) from the Blacktail Deer Creek junction and soon comes to attractive and conveniently located Camp 1Y5. In the next mile you pass two more pleasant campsites (1Y7 and 1Y9) giving you plenty of places to choose from for spending the night in this area. The next few miles are easy and wonderful hiking. Most of the way is on a gentle grassy bench a little above the river. Wildflowers are abundant in the spring, and views of the crags and partly forested ridges on either side of the canyon are inspiring.

At 12.3 miles you take a log over small Cottonwood Creek and immediately thereafter pass the turnoffs to Camps 1R1 and 1R2. After these campsites the trail climbs steadily away from the river, traversing mostly open slopes with good views back down the canyon to the west. Near the top of the climb, hop over Little Cottonwood Creek in a beautiful, gently sloping meadow, and pass Camp 1R3. From here a short section of gentle climbing takes you to a wide, grassy saddle with fine views to the west of the Black Canyon of the Yellowstone and the snowy peaks of the distant Gallatin Range. You can also look east to the even more distant Absaroka Range.

For hikers doing the Rescue Creek Loop, this saddle is the recommended turn-around point for a dayhike from your base camp near Blacktail Bridge. Hikers continuing upstream to the Hellroaring Trailhead should keep hiking east from this pass and descend to a junction just before an often difficult, or sometimes impossible, ford of Hellroaring Creek. By hiking upstream 1.9 miles you can de-tour around this ford to a bridge. Either way, on the other side of the creek you pass several well-signed junctions and side trails leading to fine campsites, then climb for 2.2 miles to the Hellroaring Trailhead.

To return on the recommended loop via the Rescue Creek Trail, cross the Blacktail Bridge and go south on Blacktail Deer Creek Trail tackling an extended, moderately steep climb of a mostly open hillside above boisterous Blacktail Deer Creek. Near the top of the climb you pass a waterfall, although it is easy to miss since the falls cannot be seen from the trail and its sound is lost amid the general roar of cascading water. Above the falls the trail's grade eases considerably and you wander through an enchanting meadow that dries out later in the year but in late spring and early summer is lush and beautiful.

At 2.2 miles from the Yellowstone River you pass the turnoff to Camp 1A1 and then make your way south through open, rolling grassland and sagebrush country. This open area features excellent views, especially to the south of the rounded and often snow-covered Washburn Range. Amid this glorious country, step over tiny Rescue Creek and then walk uphill for 0.4 mile to a junction.

The Blacktail Deer Creek Trail goes straight, but you turn right on the little-used Rescue Creek Trail. This delightful path wanders through open country for 0.6 mile, then crosses trickling Rescue Creek and skirts the right (northeast) side

Canyon rim near Blacktail Bridge

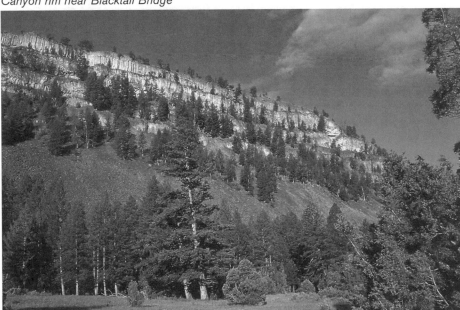

of a large, flat, marshy meadow, a good place to look for breeding sandhill cranes throughout spring and summer. At the head of the meadow is poorly signed Camp 1A2.

From the meadow the trail climbs briefly to a wide, rolling saddle on the southwest side of an unnamed, rounded butte. Look northwest from here for some excellent views of distant Sheep Mountain. You reenter Montana at an unmarked boundary a little below the saddle and then begin a long downhill. The first couple of miles of this descent are in the viewless shade of a forested draw, but then you pass beneath the impressive crags of first Turkey Pen Peak then Rattlesnake Butte and enter drier, more open terrain.

At the bottom of the descent you are back in a semidesert environment, not far above the breaks of the Yellowstone River Canyon. Views to the west of the Gallatin Range and the town of Gardiner are superb. After crossing a relatively dry, nearly flat expanse for about 2 miles, the trail dips down to a bridge over the Gardner River and reaches the Rescue Creek Trailhead. From here it is an easy 1.2-mile roadwalk to the Yellowstone River Trailhead in Gardiner.

POSSIBLE ITINERARY

	CAMPS & SIDE TRIPS	MILES	ELEVATION GAIN
DAY 1	Camp 1Y5	8.9	950′
DAY 2	Camp 1Y5 with dayhike to saddle near Little Cottonwood Creek	11.2	750′
DAY 3	Out, including the 1.2-mile roadwalk back to Gardiner	12.1	1500′

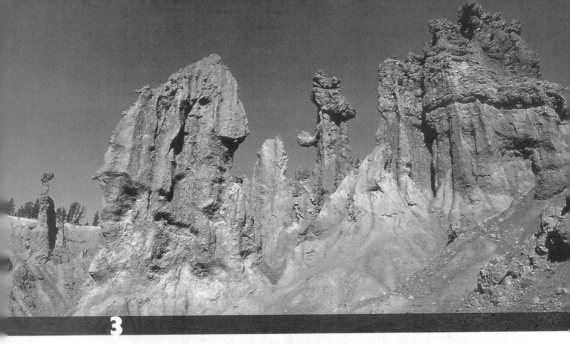

3

LAMAR RIVER TO HOODOO BASIN

RATINGS: Scenery 7   Solitude 8   Difficulty 7
MILES: 47.8 (55)
ELEVATION GAIN: 4100´ (6700´)
DAYS: 4–6
MAP: Trails Illustrated *Tower/Canyon & NE Yellowstone National Park*
USUALLY OPEN: July to October
BEST: Mid-July and September
CONTACT: Yellowstone National Park
SPECIAL ATTRACTIONS: Amazingly abundant wildlife; a remote and uncrowded portion of the park; unique geologic formations

PERMIT

A permit is required. Advanced reservations may help, but aren't usually necessary. The nearest location to pick up a permit is the Tower Ranger Station.

RULES

Fires are allowed only at specified camps. All food and other odorous items must be stored away from bears *at all times*.

CHALLENGES

Grizzly bears are very common—camp and act accordingly. The trail passes through large burn areas.

Photo: Spires in Hoodoo Basin

TAKE THIS TRIP

Although Yellowstone National Park is internationally famous and visited by approximately 3 million people every year, large parts (in fact *most* of the park's vast acreage) see almost no people. The trip up the Lamar River and Miller Creek trails to Hoodoo Basin in the northeast part of Yellowstone is a good example. But while people are scarce, animals definitely are not. In fact, critters, both large and small, are everywhere.

In my tens of thousands of miles of backpacking throughout western North America, I saw more wildlife on this hike than anywhere else. Bison are the most common large mammal (you could easily see hundreds), but you can also expect to encounter elk, pronghorns, deer, black bears, grizzly bears, moose, coyotes, and possibly wolves. In fact, I saw *all* of these animals, and many more, in *one morning!* The scenery is attractive as well, although it is not as consistently great as many other hikes in Wyoming. This trip, therefore, is more for the wildlife lover than the hiker looking to visit only the state's scenic highlights.

HOW TO GET THERE ···

From the junction at Mammoth Hot Springs in the northwest corner of Yellowstone National Park, drive 18.5 miles east to Tower Junction. Turn left and continue 15.1 miles to the Soda Butte Hiker's Trailhead. If you are approaching from the east, the trailhead is 13.8 miles west of the northeast entrance to Yellowstone National Park.

DESCRIPTION ···

The trail descends briefly to a footbridge over Soda Butte Creek and then crosses the huge sagebrush-covered flats of the Lamar Valley. Since this trip starts at a relatively low elevation, this area has a noticeably different feel than most other parts of Yellowstone National Park. Instead of the park's usual lodgepole pines covering a mountain slope or plateau, the vegetation here is dominated by sagebrush and grasses in a broad and incredibly wildlife-rich valley. In fact, except for a smattering of quaking aspens and the few conifers that rim this scenic valley, there are no trees at all. The openness of your surroundings allows for some of the park's best wildlife viewing. Bison are abundant—and their large "paddies" are everywhere, so watch your step. You also stand a good chance of seeing pronghorns, coyotes, mountain bluebirds, and ravens. Lucky hikers might spot a pack of wolves or see a badger (badger holes are everywhere, even though hikers rarely see their residents).

At 1.1 miles go straight at a junction with the alternate horse trail, and then at 1.4 miles keep left at a junction with Specimen Ridge Trail. Immediately after this junction you pass a small bison-trampled spring and then begin a long, gradual uphill still amid grasslands and sagebrush. Eventually the trail tops a rise before descending to a junction with Cache Creek Trail at 3.1 miles. Go straight and descend another 200 feet to a bridgeless crossing of Cache Creek. Several confusing bison trails cross your route in this area, so look for the conveniently placed orange markers to stay on the official trail. Just before Cache Creek, a side trail goes left (upstream) to Camp 3L1. The ford of Cache Creek is wet and can be very difficult in early summer, but by late July it is only about calf-deep and by September you may be able to rock-hop the stream. Immediately after the crossing a spur trail goes right (downstream) to Camp 3L2.

After crossing Cache Creek the trail gradually ascends into increasingly timbered areas and wildlife becomes less visible. You will probably still see some bison and elk and you may spot a bear, but you are unlikely to see herds of animals as large as the ones in the lower valley.

About 1.8 miles of up-and-down hiking beyond Cache Creek takes you to the turnoff to Camp 3L3 and, 0.5 mile later, Camp 3L4. Both of these are very nice sites on benches above the Lamar River. Unfortunately, this region of the park was hit hard by the wildfires of 1988. The areas near the river and on the slopes to the west were completely burned, but on the eastern slopes (where you are hiking) the burn was spotty, allowing for at least some shade. The trail travels through this burn mosaic generally staying on the slopes well above the Lamar River where there are many nice views of the ridges to the west. The trail is often quite dusty from the pounding of bison hooves, but the grade is gentle and not too difficult. Scientifically minded hikers will find the trail here littered with countless piles of evidence that answer the age-old question about what bears do or do *not* do in the woods. Keep an eye out for bruins and make plenty of noise while you hike.

At about 8 miles, not long after entering a severely burned area, you come to Calfee Creek, a clear stream that requires an easy wade if you cannot find a nearby log across the flow. Soon after this crossing you pass the spur trail to the Calfee Creek Patrol Cabin, a picturesque log structure on a meadow-covered bench above the Lamar River. The main trail goes straight and does a little more up and down for 1.1 miles before descending to a junction just before reaching Miller Creek.

The Lamar River Trail goes straight. You, however, turn left, initially staying near Miller Creek, but then going up and down on the hillside above the water. This area is still in the burn zone, so you should expect to encounter lots of snags, some deadfall, and thousands of small regrowing lodgepole pines. About 1.5 miles from the Lamar River is a junction with the steep downhill spur trail to Camp 3M1, a nice creekside site beside a large grassy flat called Appaloosa Meadows. In September, campers here are often serenaded by bugling elk during the night. The sounds of wolves howling might be heard at any time of year.

From the turnoff to Camp 3M1 the Miller Creek Trail continues its now-familiar pattern of ups and downs on the hillside above its namesake stream mostly through recovering burn areas. Along the way you pass turnoffs to Camps 3M2

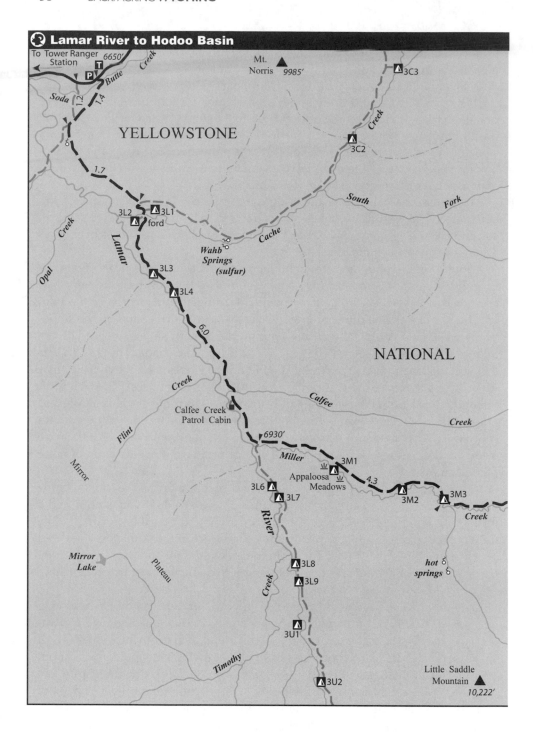

Lamar River to Hodoo Basin

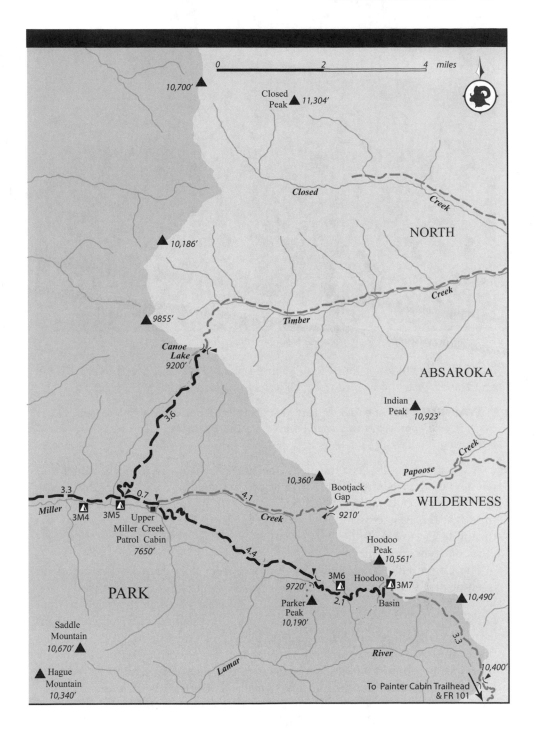

0   2   4   *miles*

10,700'

Closed
Peak 11,304'

Closed   Creek

NORTH

10,186'

Creek

9855'   Timber

Canoe
Lake
9200'

ABSAROKA

Indian
Peak 10,923'

3.6

Creek

10,360'   Papoose

Bootjack
Gap

3.3   0.7   4.1   WILDERNESS
Miller   3M4 3M5 Creek   9210'
                    Upper
                    Miller Creek
                    Patrol Cabin
                    7650'   Hoodoo
                                             Peak
                                             10,561'
                    4.4   3M6 Hoodoo
                                        9720'   3M7
PARK   Parker 2.1 Basin 10,490'
                                        Peak
                                        10,190'
Saddle
Mountain
10,670'
                                        Lamar   River   3.3

Hague
Mountain
10,340'   10,400'

To Painter Cabin Trailhead
& FR 101

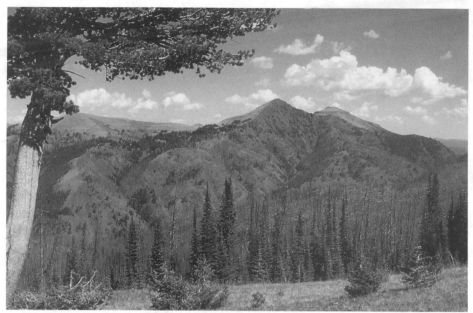

Peak north of Bootjack Gap, from the Hoodoo Basin Trail

and 3M3. Shortly after the second of these camps, the trail drops to creek level and travels near the water through a lovely unburned forest.

WARNING: Be especially alert for bears here, as the sounds from the creek may mask your approach. *I was charged by a startled grizzly here, so please take this warning seriously!*

After about 1 mile near the creek, the trail climbs away from the water and reenters the burned area eventually passing above little-used Camp 3M4 before coming to a creek at 16.5 miles that flows out of a large side canyon. About 0.2 mile past this easy crossing is the turnoff to Camp 3M5. Just 25 yards after the turnoff to Camp 3M5 is the junction with Canoe Lake Trail, a fine side trip that is particularly worth your time.

The Canoe Lake Trail begins by climbing four steep switchbacks across an open or partly burned slope. Watch for grizzly bears on the canyon walls here. Binoculars will help you get a closer look—at least you *hope* the bears are that far away! After about a mile the trail's grade eases considerably when you enter a very attractive forest of lodgepole pines and Engelmann spruces with an understory dominated by grouse whortleberry. The woodsy, gently uphill walk continues for about 1.8 miles before the trail gets steep once again and the tread disappears in a long sloping meadow. To relocate the trail, walk to the top of the meadow where the route is once again obvious. From the end of the meadow it is only about 100 yards to a low ridge just above narrow Canoe Lake, 3.4 miles from the Miller Creek Trail. The meadow-rimmed lake sits in a small basin below a scenic but burned rocky buttress. The trail continues a short distance down to the lake and then 0.2 mile up a grassy swale to a low pass (at the boundary of

Yellowstone National Park) with nice views over the vast expanse of the Absaroka Range.

After returning from the Canoe Lake side trip, turn east up the Miller Creek Trail and continue going upstream for 0.7 mile to an unsigned fork. The right branch goes to Upper Miller Creek Patrol Cabin, a log building that you can see about 150 yards away at the edge of a meadow. Go left at the fork and 100 yards later reach a junction. The Bootjack Gap Trail goes left, climbing in 4.1 miles to the park boundary at the trail's namesake location. Although this is a nice hike, you'll find better scenery if you go right at the junction onto the Hoodoo Basin Trail and soon rock-hop or make a shallow ford of what is left of Miller Creek. The trail is a little washed out at this crossing, but if you angle to the right (downstream) as you cross, you will relocate the tread after about 10 yards.

In the 18 miles since starting in the Lamar Valley your net elevation gain is only 1000 feet. As a result, there is still a lot of climbing to do before you reach the high country. The trail soon succumbs to that necessity by making a long, steady, and rather steep climb in 11 switchbacks sometimes in undamaged forest, but more often over burned and grassy slopes. Views improve rapidly as you climb, especially down the Miller Creek Valley and up to rugged Saddle Mountain to the southwest and Lamar Mountain to the south.

The uphill grade eases after 1.5 miles when you reach the top of a minor ridge and travel through unburned forest and view-packed meadows; the latter make a good place to observe both elk and grizzly bears. After some additional steep climbing, you finally enter the rolling meadows and scattered whitebark pines of the high Absaroka Range. Views seem to extend forever, encompassing countless peaks and valleys in all directions. Don't let the scenery completely distract you; frequent, large piles of scat and some frighteningly huge bear paw prints remind you to stay alert and make plenty of noise while you hike. The trail tops a rounded knob, drops 150 feet to a meadow-covered vale with an intermittent creek, and then slowly ascends through gorgeous high meadows generally heading east-southeast. The trail is faint through these meadows, so look for cairns and orange markers which guide you to a pass on the north side of Parker Peak. There is a small and muddy, but picturesque pond just to the right of the trail here. For adventurous hikers, it is relatively easy and well worthwhile to follow the long, open northwest slope of Parker Peak to its summit, which has amazingly far-ranging views.

From the pass the trail makes a moderately steep switchbacking descent into the beautiful and mostly forested basin holding Camp 3M6 and then switchbacks down a little more (a total of 500 feet down from the pass) to cross a small creek. You then regain virtually all of your recently lost elevation in a series of uphill switchbacks that lead to the top of a ridge. From here you descend 250 feet to the final destination of your hike, Hoodoo Basin. With its hundreds of colorful and wildly eroded pinnacles, spires, and arches, this basin is one of the most fascinating places in Yellowstone National Park. Better yet, the long miles required to get here ensure that you will probably have it all to yourself. Hoodoo Peak provides an impressive backdrop to this unique area. A tiny trickle of water flowing out of the basin is just enough to provide water for Camp 3M7 another 0.2 mile up the trail on the other side of the basin.

> **WARNING:** Be extremely careful if you choose to explore off-trail in Hoodoo Basin because the steep and eroded soils provide for very poor footing. In fact, it is probably better to stay on the trail and avoid damaging this fragile resource.

Although Hoodoo Basin is the logical turnaround point, there is more to explore here. The most worthwhile option is to continue beyond Camp 3M7 climbing for another 3.3 miles through huge sloping meadows with a riot of colorful wildflowers in midsummer and views that seem to extend to eternity. The trail eventually leads up to a view-packed pass at the park boundary.

Once you have had your fill of this lovely area, make the long hike back along the trail you came in on.

POSSIBLE ITINERARY

	CAMPS & SIDE TRIPS	MILES	ELEVATION GAIN
DAY 1	Camp 3M1	10.6	550'
DAY 2	Camp 3M5, including a side trip to Canoe Lake	13.3	1900'
DAY 3	Camp 3M5, with a dayhike to Hoodoo Basin	14.4	3600'
DAY 4	Camp 3L4	11.3	450'
DAY 5	Out	5.4	200'

VARIATIONS ·

With two vehicles and a long car shuttle, you can turn this into a shorter (32 miles) one-way hike. To do so, continue on the trail over the pass southeast of Hoodoo Basin, into Shoshone National Forest and the Painter Cabin Trailhead at the end of Sunlight Creek Road (Forest Service Road 101). Be warned, however, that the last 4.5 miles of FSR 101 get quite rough, so you might prefer to walk it.

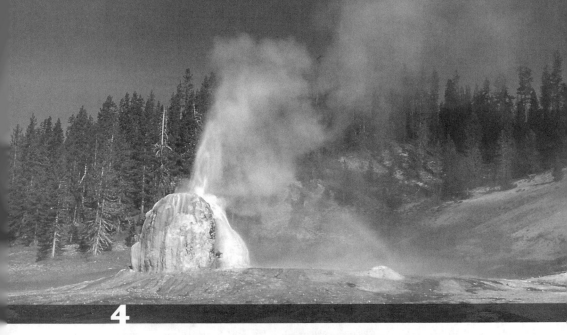

4

SHOSHONE LAKE LOOP

RATINGS: Scenery 6   Solitude 5   Difficulty 5
MILES: 39.5
ELEVATION GAIN: 2900´
DAYS: 3–5
MAP: Trails Illustrated *Old Faithful & SW Yellowstone National Park*
USUALLY OPEN: Mid-June to October
BEST: Mid-July to October
CONTACT: Yellowstone National Park
SPECIAL ATTRACTIONS: A geyser basin without the roadside crowds; a huge and very scenic backcountry lake

PERMIT

A permit is required. Advanced reservations are *strongly* advised. The nearest location to pick up a permit is the Old Faithful Ranger Station. The backcountry office is located near the post office and in the same building as the emergency medical facility in the southwest corner of the large complex of parking lots and buildings around Old Faithful Geyser.

RULES

Fires are allowed only at specified camps. All food and other odorous items must be stored away from bears *at all times*.

Photo: Lone Star Geyser

CHALLENGES

Black bears and a few grizzly bears—camp and act accordingly. Permits are hard to obtain because it's quite popular. Mosquitoes are abundant in early summer. The trail has lots of frustrating and seemingly unnecessary ups and downs and a potentially difficult ford of Lewis River Channel.

HOW TO GET THERE

Drive the Grand Loop Road in Yellowstone National Park to the turnoff to Old Faithful Geyser, the park's most famous and popular attraction. With signs everywhere you simply can't miss it. From the Old Faithful exit go 2.7 miles southeast on the Grand Loop Road to the signed Lone Star Geyser Trailhead on the right. This trailhead is immediately after you drive past the parking lot for Kepler Cascades.

DESCRIPTION

The trip starts by following a wide, partly gravel and partly paved bike path (actually an old road) that travels through a typical Yellowstone forest of lodgepole pines with a few Engelmann spruces. The very gently uphill route parallels the crystal-clear Firehole River, crossing it on a concrete bridge after just 0.4 mile

TAKE THIS TRIP

As the largest backcountry lake in the park (or, for that matter, in all of the Lower 48) and with perhaps Yellowstone's best geyser basin not accessible by roads, it is not surprising that the Shoshone Lake region is one of the most popular backpacking destinations in Yellowstone National Park. The lake is also popular with canoeists and kayakers, who paddle into Shoshone Lake via the Lewis River. Campsites here are often hard to come by, and reservations are strongly advised for anyone contemplating this trip.

Although the lake and geysers make the hike popular and well worth doing, this trip is perhaps not as appealing as some other long hikes in the park. First, the scenery, while very nice, is not as spectacular as that, for example, on Trip 1 through the Gallatin Range or Trip 2 along the Yellowstone River. Secondly, wildlife is relatively uncommon here, at least compared to other trails in Yellowstone. You may see a few moose, elk, or bison, but not in the numbers found on other hikes. Although grizzly bears are present and you should act accordingly, these bruins are somewhat less common here, which may help some hikers sleep a little better at night.

Except for a relatively small area near the southeast corner of Shoshone Lake, this is one of the few longer trails in Yellowstone that largely escaped the massive fires of 1988. As a result, you don't have to worry about hiking through miles of snags with limited shade.

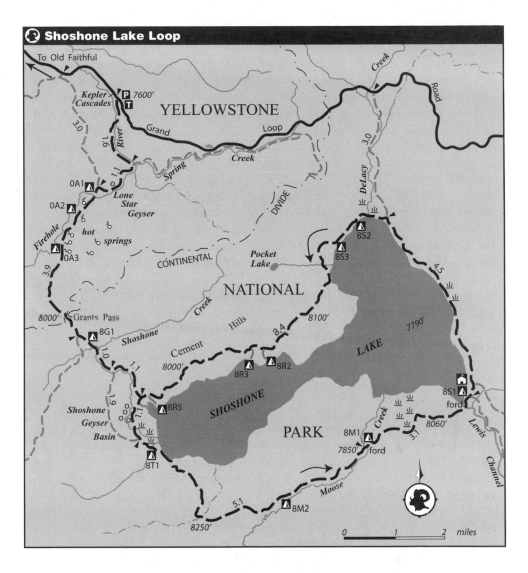

Shoshone Lake Loop

To Old Faithful

Kepler Cascades

P 7600'
T

YELLOWSTONE

Grand

Loop

Creek

River

Spring

Creek

Road

Creek

3.0

1.6

1.1

0A1

0A2

Lone Star Geyser

Firehole

hot springs

0A3

3.9

CONTINENTAL

DIVIDE

DeLacy

3.0

Pocket Lake

8S2

8S3

NATIONAL

8000' Grants Pass

8G1

Shoshone

Hills

8100'

8.4

4.5

7790'

LAKE

1.0

1.1

Cement

8000'

8R3

8R2

1.9

1.7

Shoshone Geyser Basin

8R5

SHOSHONE

PARK

8S1

ford

8060'

Creek

3.1

Lewis

Channel

8M1

7850' ford

8T1

Moose

5.1

8M2

8250'

0   1   2   miles

and never straying far from its banks. At 1.6 miles you stay straight on the bike path where the signed Spring Creek Trail goes left. Your trail now pulls a little away from the river, going through forest and past lovely meadows for 0.8 mile to where the bike path abruptly ends just before Lone Star Geyser. This impressive geyser has a unique 12-foot-tall cone (one of the tallest in the park) and erupts approximately every 3 hours with a 30- to 40-foot plume of hot water. The picturesque scene is well worth seeing, so plan to wait, either now or on the return leg of your journey, to enjoy the show.

After skirting the east side of Lone Star Geyser, the trail goes 0.3 mile through forest to a junction with the Howard Eaton Trail. Turn left and in rapid succession pass Camp 0A1, take a wooden bridge over the now-fairly-small Firehole River, and pass through an area of bubbling hot springs. A short walk beyond these geothermal features takes you to Camp 0A2 and then it is almost a mile of very gentle meadow and forest hiking to Camp 0A3, a lovely and inviting site right next to the Firehole River. After some additional meadow hiking, the trail finally begins to climb, slowly gaining 300 feet to cross the Continental Divide at forested Grants Pass, a wide saddle that is so unassuming it is easy to miss.

From Grants Pass the trail descends a little and then at 6.6 miles comes to a fork. The Bechler River Trail goes right, but you veer left and soon reach Camp 8G1. From here you twice cross meandering Shoshone Creek on rickety logs before following that beautiful grass-lined stream to a junction with a horse bypass trail at 7.6 miles. Go straight on the main trail, which does a few minor ups and downs as it continues following Shoshone Creek for 1.1 miles to a junction with North Shoreline Trail. This trail is the return route of the recommended loop.

In the large meadow to the right of the junction is the Shoshone Geyser Basin, the gases from which you have likely smelled for some time now. Turn right on the hiker-only Geyser Basin Trail and then right again just 0.1 mile later at a junction with a spur trail to the lake. For the next 0.5 mile the trail goes past bubbling springs, around colorful pools, and near geysers of various sizes. It is an impressive display of geothermal activity and a particular treat because, unlike most other geyser basins in the park, this one has no crowds.

WARNING: Hydrothermal features are beautiful but uniquely dangerous with scalding water, deceptively thin soils, and unpredictable eruptions. Stay on the trail in these areas and remain well back from all hot water pools, springs, geysers, and other features.

After passing through the geyser basin, make an easy ankle-deep ford of Shoshone Creek and then cross the large, often boggy (and *buggy*) meadows at the west end of enormous Shoshone Lake. In addition to providing nice views of the lake, these meadows are surrounded by huckleberry bushes, which turn beautifully red and orange in late September.

Kayakers on east shore of Shoshone Lake

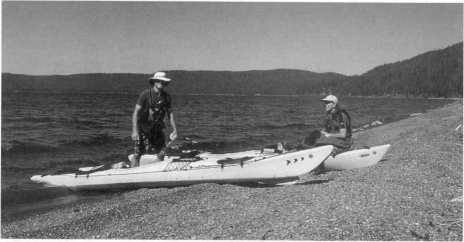

Keep straight at a reunion with the horse bypass trail and then cross more meadows and several little meandering creeks to inviting Camp 8T1. From here the trail closely follows a scenic little beach on the shoreline of Shoshone Lake for 0.2 mile. Although the lake here seems to invite swimming, be prepared for some *very* cold water. The beach ends at the southwest tip of Shoshone Lake, where the trail makes a short but rather steep climb up a mostly forested hillside quickly leaving the lake behind. This ascent is the first of many tiring ups and downs that characterize the entire loop around the lake. The intermittent climb culminates in a moderately steep ascent to the top of a broad forested ridge. From there, the trail gradually descends to the flats above initially unseen Moose Creek.

The trail stays in the forest away from the creek to a junction at 12.9 miles with the side trail to very attractive Camp 8M2. Go straight and continue 1.8 miles amid pines before you finally reach pretty Moose Creek with its meadow-covered shore. In the morning and evening you may see moose feeding among the willows bordering their namesake waterway. On nights in mid- to late September their slightly smaller cousins, elk, will entertain you with high-pitched bugling in the evening and rob you of sleep during the night. Other wildlife commonly seen here include gray jays, belted kingfishers, and red squirrels.

Make a generally easy calf deep ford of Moose Creek and almost immediately pass the short spur trail to spacious Camp 8M1. The trail now quickly climbs about 200 feet and then gradually descends toward a large marshy meadow. Spread out north of this meadow is the broad expanse of Shoshone Lake. The trail stays in the trees around the south and east sides of the meadow and then climbs again (you should be used to the up-and-down pattern by now), slowly gaining another 200 feet over a low ridge. Here is where you first encounter evidence of the 1988 fires, complete with downed trees, a few burned snags, and thousands of young lodgepole pines.

After topping the wide-topped ridge, the trail descends rapidly to the hike's biggest potential obstacle, the ford of Lewis River Channel. In early summer this crossing ranges from difficult to impossible, but by late July the ford is usually less than 2 feet deep and the water is not overly swift.

Once across, you go north along the shore of Shoshone Lake, following signs to Shoshone Lake Ranger Station, and soon veer away from the lake to a junction with Lewis River Channel Trail. You turn left, walk 0.2 mile, and then go straight at the junction with Dogs Head Trail. Now on the Delacy Creek Trail, you soon pass the spur trail to Camp 8S1 and the small A-frame building that serves as the Shoshone Lake Ranger Station.

Keep straight on the main trail and resume your pattern of often frustrating ups and downs as you cross the hillside above the east shore of Shoshone Lake. For the first 1.5 miles you travel in a 1988 burn area, which means that there is little shade. The hiking can be uncomfortably hot on summer afternoons, but the short trees allow for almost continuous views across the great expanse of deep Shoshone Lake. Once it reenters unburned forest, the trail gradually works its way down to lake level where you follow a scenic little rocky beach that separates the lake on your left from a lily-pad-filled swamp on your right. Look for beaver lodges at the north end of this swamp.

After following the beach for about 0.7 mile, the trail climbs onto a forested hillside above the lake and resumes its up-and-down pattern. The ups and downs are usually quite steep, so the hiking is slow and tiresome. Fortunately, the frequent lake views are excellent and keep you going. The last mile of this section is less strenuous and therefore more fun to hike, eventually taking you to the beach at the lake's northeast end where there is a junction.

You turn left onto North Shoreline Trail, which soon leads you to an easy wade across sluggish Delacy Creek. From here the trail follows the beach for 0.5 mile before heading back into the trees near Camp 8S2. Like other lakeshore sites this spot is both scenic and usually quite breezy, the latter helping to blow away the bugs. About 0.5 mile after Camp 8S2, you pass the spur trail to Camp 8S3 and then make a short detour away from the lake. After returning to the lakeshore, you follow the beach for 0.1 mile to the head of a particularly pretty cove. From here you again pull away from the lake, climbing more than 300 feet to a forested ridgetop. After descending the other side of this ridge, you make another frustrating 200-foot climb before immediately losing all that hard-won elevation and coming to the signed side trail to Camp 8R2. Just 0.2 mile later is the side trail to Camp 8R3. Both of these camps are fine lakeshore sites along a very scenic rocky shoreline.

The main trail continues west, gently rolling up and down in viewless forest well away from the lake. Finally, just as you begin to catch glimpses of the lake's meadow-rimmed west shore (and smell whiffs of sulfur from the Shoshone Geyser Basin), you pass the side trail dropping to Camp 8R5 and soon thereafter reach the junction with Shoshone Lake Trail and the close of the loop. Turn right and return the 8.7 miles over Grants Pass and past Lone Star Geyser to the trailhead.

POSSIBLE ITINERARY

	CAMPS & SIDE TRIPS	MILES	ELEVATION GAIN
DAY 1	Camp 8T1	10.1	500'
DAY 2	Camp 8S3	13.4	1500'
DAY 3	Camp 0A3	11.5	850'
DAY 4	Out, with a delay as you wait to watch Lone Star Geyser erupt	4.5	50'

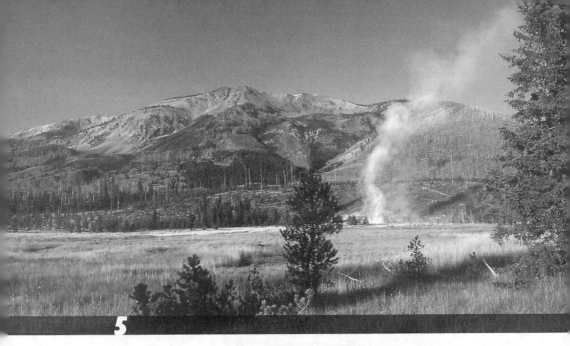

5

HEART LAKE & TWO OCEAN PLATEAU LOOP

RATINGS: Scenery 6   Solitude 8   Difficulty 7
MILES: 61.5 (72)
ELEVATION GAIN: 5750´ (9000´)
DAYS: 5–10
MAP: Trails Illustrated *Yellowstone Lake & SE Yellowstone National Park*
USUALLY OPEN: Mid-July to October
BEST: Mid-August through September
CONTACT: Yellowstone National Park
SPECIAL ATTRACTIONS: Lots of solitude (once you get away from Heart Lake); plenty of wildlife; seemingly endless expanses of wild country

PERMIT

A permit is required. Advanced reservations may help, especially for camps near Heart Lake. The nearest location to pick up a permit is the Old Faithful Ranger Station.

RULES

Fires are allowed only at specified camps. All food and other odorous items must be stored away from bears *at all times*. Due to the bears, access to Heart Lake is prohibited from April 1 to June 30. Off-trail travel in the Two Ocean Plateau

Photo: Mt. Sheridan and steaming Rustic Geyser

45

This trip is for hikers who really want to immerse themselves in the incredible vastness of the Yellowstone backcountry. Although the scenery is pleasant, especially around Heart Lake and in the Snake River Canyon, it doesn't compare to that in many other parts of Wyoming. The main attraction is the opportunity to enjoy solitude amid some of the wildest country left in the Lower 48.

For hikers who want even more, it is possible to extend this hike even deeper into the wilderness on loop trips that go all the way to the Yellowstone River or south into the adjoining Teton Wilderness Area in Bridger-Teton National Forest. Wildlife, as usual in Yellowstone, is common so your chances of seeing moose, elk, grizzly bears, wolves, and other animals are fairly high. The loop trip is equally good in either direction (I describe it clockwise), with the way you go largely dependent upon obtaining a permit.

Bear Management Area requires a permit from July 15 to August 21 and is prohibited the rest of the hiking season. The Trail Creek Trail along the south shore of Yellowstone Lake is closed before July 14, when the bears feed on spawning cutthroat trout.

CHALLENGES

Grizzly bears are common—camp and act accordingly. The trail has several potentially difficult river fords early in the season, lots of mosquitoes in early summer, and many miles of shadeless burned areas. It's difficult to get a permit to camp near popular Heart Lake.

HOW TO GET THERE

The Heart Lake Trailhead is along the south entrance road in Yellowstone National Park. To reach the well-signed trailhead turnoff, drive either 14.2 miles north of the south entrance station or 7.4 miles south of the junction at West Thumb.

DESCRIPTION

The wide, sandy, and sometimes dusty trail departs from the northeast corner of the parking area and travels east through a lodgepole pine forest. Most of the trees here are regrowing from a natural reseeding following the 1988 fires and provide very limited shade. Expect to be uncomfortably warm on hot summer days.

You gain elevation consistently for about 4 miles until you top a barely distinguishable rise. The trail begins a gentle descent to the southeast where you catch your first glimpse down to Heart Lake and your first whiffs of sulfur fumes from the thermal springs along Witch Creek. The hulking peak to your right (southwest) is Factory Hill, at the northeast end of the Red Mountains. In mid- to late September, when the sumac and huckleberry bushes change colors, these mountains live up to their name.

The trail now winds downhill past numerous hot springs and pools in the Heart Lake Geyser Basin. Although there is almost no shade, the way down is attractive and features a couple of quaint log bridges over Witch Creek. Large meadows in the lower valley have fine views of Mt. Sheridan looming to the southwest. At 7.5 miles you pass the two log cabins of the Heart Lake Ranger Station and reach a junction on Heart Lake's sandy shores, the start of the recommended loop.

If you are making a clockwise loop, you will need to turn left (east) at this junction. But first, if you are camping at one of the popular sites along the west side of Heart Lake, turn right. This trail takes you along the beach, crosses Witch Creek on a log bridge, and reaches the first site (Camp 8H6), after about 0.5 mile. The trail also provides access to an unofficial path to Rustic Geyser and the well-maintained Mt. Sheridan Trail. The latter trail is a terrific, view-packed, but difficult and dry side trip. The lookout building atop Mt. Sheridan is staffed during the summer months.

WARNING: Hydrothermal features are beautiful but uniquely dangerous with scalding water, deceptively thin soils, and unpredictable eruptions. Stay on the trail in these areas and remain well back from all hot water pools, springs, geysers, and other features.

Back at the junction beside the Heart Lake Ranger Station, the trail to the east follows the sandy beach along the north shore of large Heart Lake. This is an excellent location for viewing the abundant birdlife that calls this lake home. Common mergansers, white pelicans, and common loons are frequently present, with the last often serenading campers in the evening with the bird's hauntingly wild call. After 0.6 mile on the beach an orange marker indicates where you turn inland away from the water. The trail then wanders through open lodgepole pine forest that is still recovering from the massive 1988 fires, passes the turnoff to Camp 8J1, and comes to the easy ford of Beaver Creek. Almost immediately after this crossing is the turnoff to Camp 8J2, which is reserved for stock parties. Keep left and wander gradually up and down in young forest for about 2 miles until you pass the turnoff to Camp 8J6 and reach a junction.

Veer left at the junction onto Trail Creek Trail, walk 0.1 mile, and then make a log crossing of Surprise Creek just before you reach pleasant Camp 8J3. From here you gradually climb through a sea of snags in a severely burned area where the young trees are too small to provide cooling shade. After about 1.3 miles of this scorched terrain you enter the relatively lush meadowlands beside Outlet Creek and pretty Camp 8O2. The trail follows the meadows beside the meandering willow-lined creek for another 1.6 miles, then just as you are about to reach meadow-rimmed Outlet Lake, it climbs up the ridge to the right (east). At the top of the 450-foot ascent is a meadow at an unnamed pass over Chicken Ridge, which here forms the Continental Divide.

Continuing east, you cross rolling terrain through more of the shadeless, severely burned forests that typify this part of Yellowstone. Eventually the trail meets Grouse Creek and stays on the burned hillside above that slow-moving waterway to the junction with a trail leading to Camps 7G1 and 7G2.

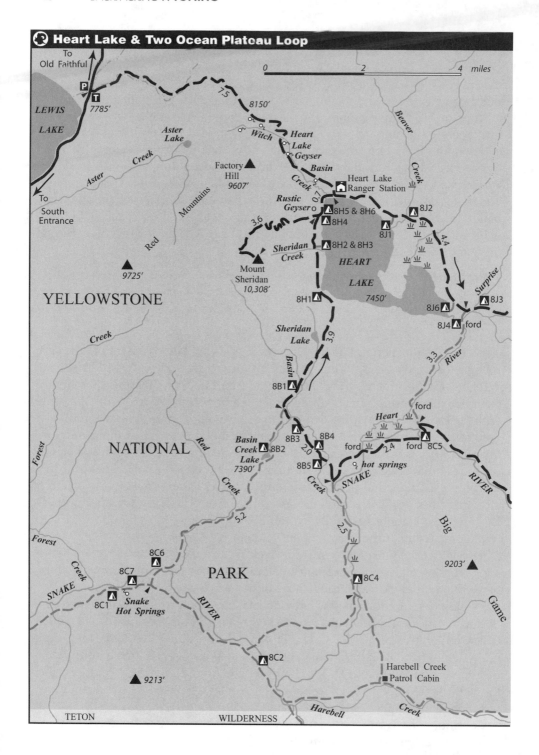

⊙ Heart Lake & Two Ocean Plateau Loop

To Old Faithful

LEWIS LAKE

7785'

To South Entrance

Aster Lake

Aster Creek

Red Mountains

Factory Hill 9607'

9725'

YELLOWSTONE

Creek

NATIONAL

Red Creek

5.2

Forest

Forest

SNAKE Creek

8C7

8C1

8C6

Snake Hot Springs

PARK

9213'

7.5

8150'

Witch

Heart Lake Geyser

Basin

Rustic Geyser

Mount Sheridan 10,308'

Sheridan Creek

8H5 & 8H6

8H4

8H2 & 8H3

Heart Lake Ranger Station

8J1

8J2

HEART

LAKE 7450'

8J6

8J4   ford

8J3

Surprise

4.4

3.6

Creek

0.7

8H1

Sheridan Lake

3.9

Basin

8B1

8B3

8B2

Basin Creek Lake 7390'

8B4

ford

8B5

2.0

Creek

SNAKE

hot springs

Heart

ford

2.4

ford

8C5

River

3.3

RIVER

Big

2.5

8C4

9203'

8C2

Game

Harebell Creek Patrol Cabin

TETON   WILDERNESS   Harebell   Creek

0   2   4   miles

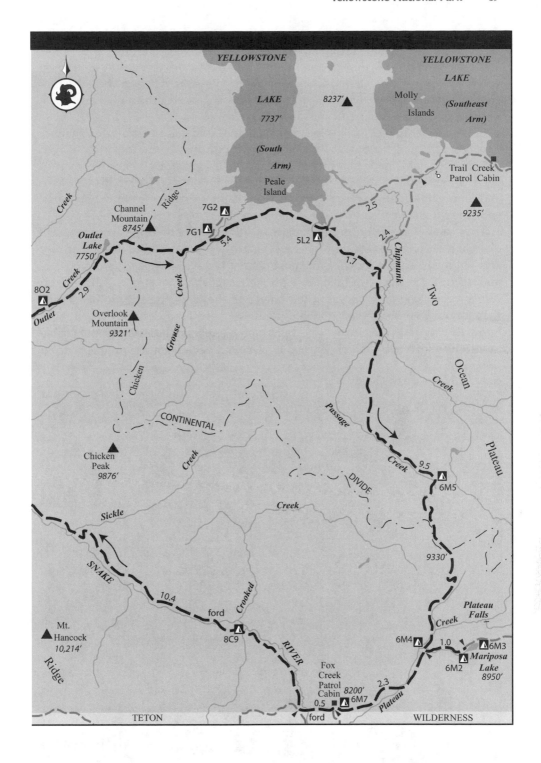

YELLOWSTONE

YELLOWSTONE

LAKE

LAKE

8237'▲

Molly
Islands

(Southeast
Arm)

LAKE

7737'

(South

Arm)

Peale
Island

Trail Creek
Patrol Cabin

Creek

Ridge

Channel
Mountain
8745'▲

7G2

7G1

Outlet
Lake
7750'

5L2

2.5

9235'▲

Chipmunk

5.4

2.4

1.7

Creek

8O2

Outlet

2.9

Overlook
Mountain
9321'▲

Grouse Creek

Two

Ocean

Creek

Chicken

CONTINENTAL

Passage

Plateau

Chicken
Peak
9876'▲

Creek

DIVIDE

Creek

9.5

6M5

Sickle

Creek

9330'

SNAKE

10.4

Crooked

Plateau
Falls

Mt.
Hancock
10,214'▲

ford

Creek

6M4

1.0

6M3

Ridge

8C9

RIVER

Fox
Creek
Patrol
Cabin

2.3

6M2

Mariposa
Lake
8950'

0.5

8200'
6M7

TETON

ford

Plateau

WILDERNESS

You bear right at this junction, take a log over Grouse Creek, and then wander across a charred hillside for about 2 miles with good views of tiny Peale Island and the huge South Arm of Yellowstone Lake. At 20 miles (excluding side trips) you reach Camp 5L2, in a meadow about 200 yards south of the trail beside a tiny creek. Campers at this site may hear wolves howling during the night and/or see sandhill cranes feeding in the meadow.

From the Camp 5L2 turnoff the main trail goes east another 0.2 mile to a junction beside a shallow bay at the southern tip of Yellowstone Lake. Turn right (south) on a faint path that gradually climbs through grassy areas and partly burned forest for 1.7 miles to a junction. Turn right on Two Ocean Plateau Trail and follow this gentle path as it slowly ascends through the meadows and mostly burned forest near sluggish Chipmunk Creek.

The scenery here is subdued—mostly meadows and low ridges with no craggy peaks, cirque lakes, or geysers—but it is truly overwhelming in its enormity and wildness. This is some of the most remote terrain in the U.S., and you certainly *feel* isolated as you hike these trails. In fact the Two Ocean Plateau Trail comes very close to the point in the Lower 48 that is farthest from the nearest road (about 23 miles, as the golden eagle flies). After 1.5 miles you ford or rock-hop babbling Passage Creek and then begin a more consistent and noticeable uphill through open, severely burned terrain. You get a respite from this charred

Beaver dam on Basin Creek

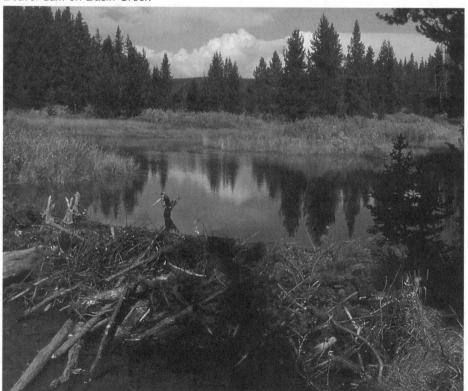

scenery when you follow the upper reaches of Passage Creek for a short time, but mostly the landscape is rather monotonous and not particularly scenic.

Eventually hop over what is left of Passage Creek and immediately keep right at the turnoff to Camp 6M5. A short, steep climb through an attractive, mostly unburned forest leads to a nice viewpoint looking north to Yellowstone Lake and the Absaroka Range; a bit more uphill takes you to a series of large and very beautiful meadows atop the hard-to-discern Continental Divide.

After about a mile the trail leaves the lovely meadows, winds downhill, and follows a small unnamed creek to its confluence with larger Plateau Creek. The trail then leads you to an easy crossing of Plateau Creek shortly before you come to inviting Camp 6M4 and a junction with the South Boundary Trail. A nice side trip from here goes left (east) for 1 mile to Mariposa Lake with its campsites and scenic setting in a large meadow.

The main loop route goes slightly right (southwest) at the South Boundary Trail junction and meanders very gradually downhill through forest and meadows. You make an easy ford of Plateau Creek, and then come to a large meadow with Camp 6M7 and the Fox Creek Patrol Cabin. Directly opposite this cabin is a junction with the Mink Creek Trail, which goes left and after only a few yards leaves Yellowstone National Park.

Go straight at the junction and descend to a ford of the Snake River. In early summer this crossing can be tricky, but by September it is so shallow your ankles may not even get wet. At 0.5 mile from Fox Creek Patrol Cabin, and just 200 yards past the ford, is a junction with the Snake River Trail.

The South Boundary Trail continues straight on a possible longer loop option that takes you over view-packed Big Game Ridge. For the recommended loop, however, turn right and go up and down on the hillside above the lazy Snake River as that stream enters a narrow, quite scenic canyon. After 1.4 miles hop over an unnamed tributary creek just before reaching very nice Camp 8C9. Not long after this camp is the second ford of the Snake River, this one only calf-deep by late summer but often quite difficult early in the season.

The trail spends the next few miles going up and down on the badly burned hillside well above the Snake River. The charred hillside provides no shade, but the lack of trees opens up nice views of the canyon below, towering Mt. Hancock on your left, and distant Mt. Sheridan straight ahead. Eventually the trail switchbacks down to the river and an easy crossing of Sickle Creek. From here you stay near river level as the canyon gradually widens and you leave the worst of the burn zone.

NOTE: Old maps incorrectly show more fords of the Snake River than the rerouted trail now requires.

After walking through a wide meadow-filled lower valley, you come to a junction with the Heart River Trail at 44.6 miles into your trip, excluding side trips. The quickest way to exit is to go right, but this retraces much of your earlier route. For greater variety, and some of the trip's best wildlife habitat, turn left and soon pass Camp 8C5 just before the third ford of the Snake River. In early summer this ford can be very challenging, but by late August people have often placed rocks and logs across the flow to allow for a dry crossing. The trail then goes west-southwest across a nearly flat, open area for 1.3 miles to a final ford of the Snake River, where before about mid-July you will likely get wet up to at least mid-thigh. After this often difficult crossing skirt around the northwest side of a marsh with a cluster of hot springs and then wander through lodgepole pine forest to a junction.

Turn right on Basin Creek Cut-Off Trail and walk 0.4 mile to an easy ford of Basin Creek. In 2008 there was a photogenic beaver dam immediately upstream from this ford. Soon after the crossing is very pleasant Camp 8B5 and a little later Camp 8B4, the latter intended for stock users. The trail then crosses some large meadows with good views north-northwest to Mt. Sheridan and opportunities to see both moose and grizzly bears. You pass Camp 8B3 just before the first of two crossings of Basin Creek and then come to a junction with Heart Lake Trail.

You bear right (north) and walk through a pleasant area of young forest and lovely meadows. The trail crosses several small creeks and takes you past Camp 8B1 before reaching the large meadow holding the glassy waters of Sheridan Lake. The lake's namesake mountain looms impressively over the northwest shore.

From Sheridan Lake cross a minor forested ridge and then descend slightly to Camp 8H1 at the southwest corner of Heart Lake. You then go up and down on the open view-packed hillside above the lake's west shore to a hop-over crossing of Sheridan Creek just before the side trail leading down to Camps 8H2 and 8H3. Go straight and descend nearly to the lakeshore where you pass very inviting Camp 8H4 and come to a junction. The demanding but wonderful side trip up Mt. Sheridan mentioned earlier in the text goes left here.

If you're not going up the peak (or if you already have) continue straight on the main trail, pass Camps 8H5 and 8H6, and follow the lakeshore trail back to the junction near the Heart Lake Ranger Station. Turn left and retrace your steps for 7.5 miles back to the trailhead.

POSSIBLE ITINERARY

	CAMPS & SIDE TRIPS	MILES	ELEVATION GAIN
DAY 1	Camp 8H5	8.2	400'
DAY 2	Camp 8H5, with dayhike up Mt. Sheridan	7.4	2950'
DAY 3	Camp 5L2	13.1	1300'
DAY 4	Camp 6M4	11.4	2200'
DAY 5	Camp 8C9, including a side trip to Mariposa Lake	6.3	400'
DAY 6	Camp 8B5	11.8	500'
DAY 7	Camp 8H5	5.6	500'
DAY 8	Out	8.2	750'

VARIATIONS ·

For an even longer sojourn, skip the Two Ocean Plateau Trail and continue east on the Trail Creek Trail to the Thorofare Trail along the upper reaches of the Yellowstone River. Then hike south to the junction with the South Boundary Trail before going west along that route to its junction with the described loop at Plateau Creek. This option adds about 20 miles and two difficult fords of the Yellowstone River to your trip, but the great expanses of wild scenery make it worth the extra time and effort.

Another option is to forego the Snake River Canyon and continue west on the South Boundary Trail from the junction near the first ford of the Snake River. That route goes over Big Game Ridge in the Teton Wilderness, which offers spectacular views of both Yellowstone Lake to the north and the Teton Range to the south, to the Harebell Creek Patrol Cabin. From there you turn north and follow the Snake River Trail to its junction with the Basin Creek Cut-Off Trail described above.

If you prefer to shorten the trip, follow the described route to the junction of the Heart River and Trail Creek trails at the southeast end of Heart Lake. Go south for 3.3 miles to the junction with the Snake River Trail and continue with the described loop. This 32-mile option skips the Snake River Canyon and the wonderfully wild country around Two Ocean Plateau, but it includes much of the best scenery around Heart Lake and Basin Creek.

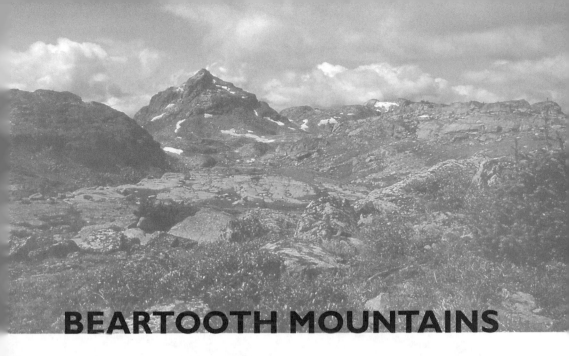

BEARTOOTH MOUNTAINS

Just east of Yellowstone National Park lies a mountain wilderness that is a wonderland for hikers. Although the landscape bears little resemblance to the adjoining park—there are no geysers and only a few bison here—these mountains provide plenty of the kinds of attractions generally missing from Yellowstone. In the Beartooth Mountains backpackers will find dozens of glaciers still sculpting the range's towering granite peaks, huge expanses of alpine rock gardens, and more high mountain lakes than a hiker can shake a stick at. In fact the number of lakes in these mountains is almost unbelievable. From tiny glacial tarns to large sparkling gems, water is practically everywhere. It sometimes seems like more of the surface area in these mountains is covered with water than solid rock. Since most of this magnificent range is in Montana, this book includes only one hike through the Beartooths, but it's a real winner, especially for those who don't mind off-trail travel.

The southern fringe of the Beartooth Mountains includes one of the most dramatic canyons in the state. The powerful but generally little-known Clarks Fork of the Yellowstone River has carved deeply into the dark, mostly granitic rock of this region and created a not-to-be-missed backcountry attraction. Although a long, river-level trail through this canyon is a practical impossibility, the existing high trail offers great views down into the steep defile and generally magnificent scenery.

South of the Clarks Fork stretches the North Absaroka Range, a vast mountain expanse that is protected in a wilderness of the same name. The land here is very different from the Beartooth Mountains with almost no lakes, no granite, and easily eroded volcanic soils. Visitors are few here because of the long road and trail distances, the many difficult stream crossings, and the extremely high concentration of grizzly bears. For years this is where "problem" bears in

Photo: Lonesome Mountain from pass near Arrowhead Lake (Trip 6)

Yellowstone were transported, making the bruins here both more abundant and more aggressive than elsewhere in the state. As a result, most backpackers (including me, your usually intrepid author) don't feel comfortable hiking here and spend far too much time worried about bruins to enjoy the incredible scenery this range has to offer. As a result, this book doesn't recommend any hikes in the North Absaroka Range.

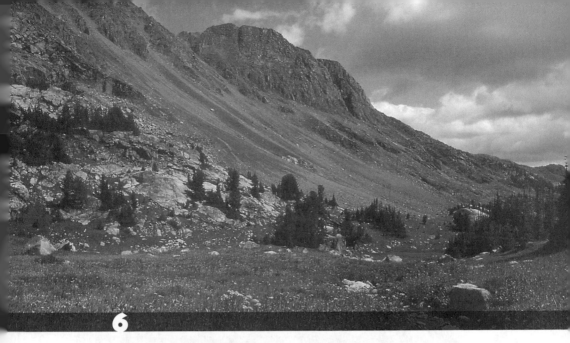

BEARTOOTH PLATEAU LOOP

RATINGS: Scenery 10   Solitude 5   Difficulty 6
MILES: 21.4 (26.4)
ELEVATION GAIN: 3300´ (4800´)
DAYS: 3–6
MAPS: USGS *Beartooth Butte (WY), Muddy Creek (WY), Castle Mountain (MT),* and *Silver Run Peak (MT).* Do not rely solely on the Forest Service's contour map of the Absaroka-Beartooth Wilderness. It is not detailed enough for cross-country travel.
USUALLY OPEN: Mid-July to October
BEST: August through mid-September
CONTACT: Clarks Fork Ranger District, Shoshone National Forest; Beartooth Ranger District, Custer National Forest
SPECIAL ATTRACTIONS: Countless beautiful high-elevation lakes; outstanding mountain scenery; solitude, at least along the off-trail portion.
PERMIT: None required

RULES

All food and other odorous items must be stored away from bears.

Photo: Canyon above Becker Lake

TAKE THIS TRIP

The Beartooth Mountains, which hug the border between Wyoming and Montana northeast of Yellowstone National Park, contain some of the best scenery either state has to offer—quite a statement given the countless natural wonders in this part of the country. During the ice age, large glaciers carved the granite here into steep cliffs, deep canyons, and thousands of cirque basins filled with countless wet meadows and stunningly beautiful alpine lakes.

All those lakes provide plenty of great fishing, swimming (if you don't mind *really* cold water), and places to sit back and revel in the watery scenery. There are also lots of mosquitoes through about early August, plenty of marshy and muddy trails, and hosts of other admiring lake lovers beside any pool or lake that is either near a road or along a popular trail. Hiking here in late summer allows for fewer crowds and *a lot* fewer bugs.

The loop described here includes dozens of beautiful lakes, numerous possible side trips to grand viewpoints and/or sprawling glaciers, plenty of stupendous scenery, and a fair amount of solitude. It also involves a fairly long off-trail section, but the terrain is relatively gentle and most of the way is marked with cairns. With a good map and decent navigation skills, the cross-country section should be fairly easy.

CHALLENGES

Mosquitoes are abundant through July and early August. Extended off-trail travel is required, although most of the route is relatively easy and marked with cairns. Grizzly bears are present—camp and act accordingly.

HOW TO GET THERE

Access to this hike is off the wildly scenic Beartooth Highway (U.S. Highway 212), which is one of the highest elevation paved roads in the U.S. You can reach this road either from Red Lodge, Montana, to the northeast or from Yellowstone National Park and the tiny town of Cooke City, Montana, to the west.

For most Wyoming residents, however, it is easier to reach the trailhead by starting from Cody and taking a side road that intersects the Beartooth Highway near the middle of its route. From Cody, go 16.8 miles northwest on Wyoming Highway 120, then turn left (west) on Wyoming Highway 296, signed as the Chief Joseph Scenic Highway. Drive this very scenic route for 47 miles to its junction with U.S. Highway 212. Turn right (east) and drive 9.3 miles to the turnoff for Beartooth Lake Campground.

Turn left on this good gravel road and proceed 0.4 mile to a fork. Keep right, heading for the campground, drive 0.3 mile, then turn left at a small sign saying

Beartooth Plateau Loop

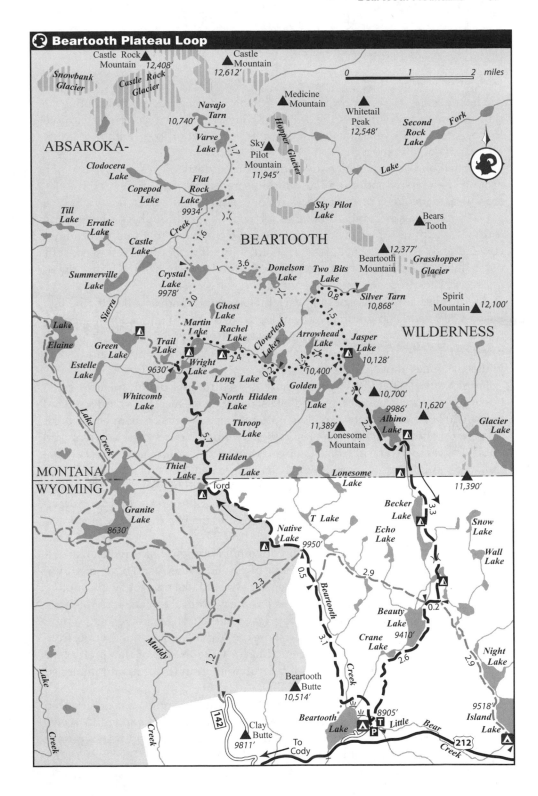

0   1   2   miles

Castle Rock Mountain 12,408'

Snowbank Glacier

Castle Rock Glacier

Castle Mountain 12,612'

Medicine Mountain

Whitetail Peak 12,548'

Second Rock Lake

Fork

Navajo Tarn 10,740'

Varve Lake

Sky Pilot Mountain 11,945'

Hopper Glacier

ABSAROKA-

Clodocera Lake

Copepod Lake

Flat Rock Lake 9934'

Sky Pilot Lake

Bears Tooth

Till Lake

Erratic Lake

Castle Lake

Creek

1.6

1.7

BEARTOOTH

12,377'

Beartooth Mountain

Grasshopper Glacier

Summerville Lake

Crystal Lake 9978'

3.6

Donelson Lake

Two Bits Lake

Silver Tarn 10,868'

Spirit Mountain 12,100'

2.0

Ghost Lake

0.8

1.5

WILDERNESS

Lake Elaine

Green Lake

Martin Lake

Rachel Lake

Cloverleaf Lake

Arrowhead Lake

Jasper Lake 10,128'

Trail Lake

9630'

Wright Lake

2.4

Long Lake

1.4

0.2

10,400'

Golden Lake

10,700'

9986'

Estelle Lake

Whitcomb Lake

North Hidden Lake

Sierra

11,389'

Lonesome Mountain

2.2

Albino Lake

11,620'

Glacier Lake

Throop Lake

5.7

Hidden Lake

11,390'

MONTANA

WYOMING

Thiel Lake

ford

Lake

Lonesome Lake

Becker Lake

3.3

Snow Lake

Granite Lake 8630'

Native Lake 9950'

T Lake

Echo Lake

2.9

Wall Lake

Lake Creek

2.3

0.5

Beartooth

2.9

Muddy

1.2

Beauty Lake 9410'

Crane Lake

Night Lake

3.1

2.6

9518' Island Lake

142

Beartooth Butte 10,514'

Creek

8905'

Beartooth Lake

Little

Bear

212

Clay Butte 9811'

To Cody

Lake

Creek

Creek

TRAILHEAD and go 50 yards to the small trailhead turnaround with its limited parking.

DESCRIPTION •

The trail skirts the meadows on the northeast side of gorgeous Beartooth Lake with stunning views across the water to rugged and very colorful Beartooth Butte. After just 75 yards the trail splits, the start of your loop, with the Beauty Lake Trail going to the right.

Bear left and soon make an ankle-deep ford of Little Bear Creek. Then loop around the marshy and often mosquito-infested north end of Beartooth Lake, cross Beartooth Creek on either rocks or logs, and, 0.1 mile later, turn right on a good trail that heads uphill. Although short sections go through a high-elevation forest of subalpine firs and whitebark pines, you climb mostly through meadows covered with a wide variety of colorful alpine wildflowers. The yellowish cliffs of a ridge that extends north from Beartooth Butte rise west of the trail, providing scenic backdrops to the sloping meadows.

At 3.1 miles a trail branches to the right. Go straight, now on Beartooth High Lakes Trail, and keep gradually ascending for 0.5 mile to a junction just below treeline. The trail to the left goes south to Clay Butte. You go straight and descend briefly to narrow, rock-lined Native Lake. There is a good campsite amid some whitebark pines above the southwest shore.

From Native Lake the trail goes up and down through a delightful just-below-treeline landscape of small tarns and lakes, rocky areas, meadows, and scattered trees. The lakes are mostly nameless but that does not make them any less attractive. At about 6.5 miles you drop rather steeply to an easy creek ford and an outfitter's camp in a meadow just above a deep, rectangular lake. From here the trail goes rapidly uphill, then down, then back up again during a tiring, ruggedly steep 1.2 miles. Just before the top of the second (and longer) uphill, hop over the small outlet to large but unseen North Hidden Lake and resume your previous up-and-down pattern for another mile passing many rocky areas, meadows, and small tarns.

At the bottom of the next significant downhill is Wright Lake, which has several good campsites and sits in the middle of a basin with several other medium-sized lakes. After crossing the outlet creek of Wright Lake on a log, walk another 0.1 mile to where the main trail curves left away from the lake. To see Martin Lake and follow the recommended loop, leave the official trail here and go right on a sketchy use path around the west shore of Wright Lake. About 0.4 mile from the official trail you reach large, scenic Martin Lake. North of this pretty lake with its distinctive island rise several tall, rounded granite buttes and unnamed mountains.

From Martin Lake there are several excellent off-trail options. For experienced scramblers, one highly recommended alternative is the rugged and wildly scenic route that goes north to Crystal and Flat Rock lakes. From there you can scramble over boulder fields and rough alpine terrain up to Varve Lake and Navajo Tarn, then on to the base of Castle Rock Glacier.

For the much easier off-trail loop trip recommended for most backpackers, however, make your way to the northeast corner of Martin Lake and climb along the inlet creek going east. The left (north) side of the creek has fewer boulders and is much easier to navigate. Observant hikers may notice faint traces of a use path where others have made this trek. After 0.5 mile you come to deep and very scenic Rachel Lake, which has some decent campsites and sits directly beneath a dark, cliff-edged butte.

Cross the outlet of Rachel Lake, then walk around the lake's south shore to a braided waterfall feeding into the lake's east end. Still following an obscure use path, sometimes marked with small cairns, make an easy climb to the top of the falls and then travel over tundra and rocks beside the creek to the first of the three large Cloverleaf Lakes. The views across this lake's water to nearby buttes and distant towering peaks are grand. Unfortunately, since you are now above treeline, camping here can be very windy and uncomfortable.

To continue the recommended loop, follow the lake's south shore to an inlet creek at the lake's southeast end and walk 0.1 mile up this creek to the next, equally scenic Cloverleaf Lake. If you have time, the nearby area cries out to be explored. Of particular interest is a small but very beautiful lake that sits in a rocky cirque about 0.2 mile to the south-southwest. A good topographic map is helpful in finding this watery gem.

The main route, still marked with tiny cairns, goes around the south shore of the second Cloverleaf Lake, then up a wide grassy gully. As the gully narrows, the tread becomes more obvious leading you on a gentle uphill grade to the east. At the top is an undulating rocky pass with excellent views to the east and northeast of a pair of tall, flat-topped peaks. You can also look south-southeast to towering and, from this angle, pyramid-shaped Lonesome Mountain.

The cairns lead you north from the rocky pass, going about 0.25 mile across open terrain to narrow Arrowhead Lake, surrounded by rocky cliffs. Briefly skirt the south end of this lake and then go east, climbing to a minor pass from which you can see south to irregularly shaped Golden Lake and east to Jasper Lake and massive, flat-topped Beartooth Mountain. The route now follows cairns going steeply down a gully to very deep, extremely scenic Jasper Lake. If the weather

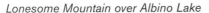

Lonesome Mountain over Albino Lake

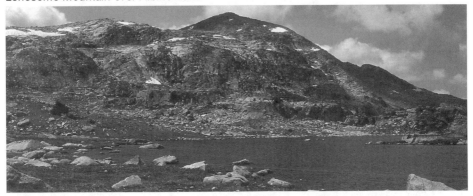

is good, camping at this above-treeline gem allows you to take an extended time to enjoy its many charms. Several excellent cross-country side trips beckon; one superb option goes north-northwest to Two Bits Lake and then up that lake's inlet creek to starkly beautiful Silver Tarn, directly beneath the cliffs of Beartooth Mountain.

To continue the loop, hike along the west side of Jasper Lake, then pick up a use path and climb through a rocky pass to the south. From the top you can see your next destination, huge Albino Lake. From the pass a strenuous, but not technically difficult, scramble route goes southwest up a ridge to the top of Lonesome Mountain.

From the pass an unofficial but easy-to-follow boot trail takes you down to Albino Lake and around its west side. Looking across the water you are treated to stunning views of jagged orange and gray pinnacles and cliffs that rise dramatically to the top of an unnamed peak. The trail loops around the south side of Albino Lake and then crosses the outlet creek to a decent campsite in a grove of small, stunted pines. The path then goes downstream in meadows beside the cascading stream for 1 mile to long, narrow Becker Lake.

The trail takes an up-and-down course above the lake's east side, passes one good campsite along the way, and then climbs to a minor saddle above the lake's southeast end. From here descend to a cluster of lovely, meadow-rimmed lakes, rock-hop the stream between the first two of these lakes, and walk south another 0.4 mile to a junction with the Beartooth High Lakes Trail. Although unsigned, this junction is marked with a large cairn.

Turn right at the junction and quickly drop almost 200 feet to another junction shortly before a creek crossing. Turn left on the Beauty Lake Trail and almost immediately start walking along the east shore of the trail's namesake body of water. As advertised, Beauty Lake is indeed beautiful with its mostly forested shoreline and distant views of Beartooth Butte. The trail now stays in forest as it follows the outlet creek from Beauty Lake to much smaller Crane Lake and then steadily descends back to the wet meadows beside Beartooth Lake. After an easy ford of Little Bear Creek, reach the junction 75 yards from the trailhead. A final left turn here and your trip is complete.

POSSIBLE ITINERARY

NOTE: As with any trip that includes significant off-trail travel, some of the mileages shown here are approximations.

	CAMPS & SIDE TRIPS	MILES	ELEVATION GAIN
DAY 1	Martin Lake	9.7	2000'
DAY 2	Jasper Lake, including cross-country side trips to lake near upper Cloverleaf Lake and to Silver Tarn	8.4	2300'
DAY 3	Out	8.3	500'

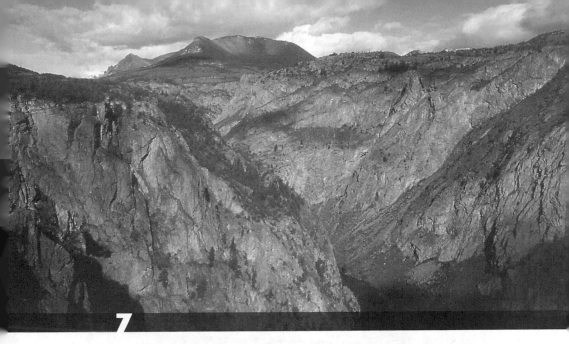

7

CLARKS FORK YELLOWSTONE RIVER CANYON

RATINGS: Scenery 8   Solitude 7   Difficulty 6
MILES: 23.3
ELEVATION GAIN: 3100´
DAYS: 3–4
MAPS: USGS *Bald Peak*, *Beartooth Butte NE*, *Dillworth Bench*, *Muddy Creek*, and *Windy Mountain*. The more general *Shoshone National Forest: North Half* map includes contour lines and is sufficient for most hikers.
USUALLY OPEN: May to late October
BEST: Mid-May to mid-June, September, and October
CONTACT: Clarks Fork Ranger District, Shoshone National Forest
SPECIAL ATTRACTIONS: Dramatic canyon scenery; good early or late season hiking
PERMIT: None required.

RULES ·

All food and other odorous items must be stored away from bears.

Photo: Table Mountain and Clarks Fork Canyon from Dead Indian Trail

TAKE THIS TRIP

The Clarks Fork Yellowstone River winds through some of the wildest, most scenic country in Wyoming, carving a deep, very impressive canyon into the dark rock of the southern Beartooth Mountains. A trail at river level through this canyon is impossible due to the sheer cliffs and raging whitewater, but an alternate path exists, mostly following a high bench almost 1000 feet above the rampaging river.

The trail is a real gem, providing views of both the canyon and the surrounding mountains, and follows the water at river level for 2.2 very scenic miles. As an out-and-back hike from the upper trailhead, this trip hits most of the best scenery and, more important, avoids either a long car shuttle or usually impossible river ford at the lower end.

Although the river's official name is "Clarks Fork of the Yellowstone River," most maps (and all local residents) shorten the name to simply "Clarks Fork," which I use throughout this description.

CHALLENGES

Done as a one-way hike, the trip has logistical difficulties—either a relatively long, rather complicated car shuttle or a difficult, often impossible river ford. Grizzly bears inhabit this area—camp and act accordingly.

HOW TO GET THERE

From Cody, go 16.8 miles northwest on Wyoming Highway 120, then turn left (west) on Wyoming Highway 296, signed as the Chief Joseph Scenic Highway. Drive this wildly scenic route (certainly one of the most spectacular roads in the country) for 23.4 miles to an unsigned turnoff for a dirt road going to the right. (If you reach the Dead Indian Campground, you have driven 0.3 mile too far.) This 0.3-mile road ends at the Dead Indian Trailhead, one of the alternate exit points.

To reach the starting point at the Clarks Fork Trailhead, continue on Wyoming Highway 296 another 21.8 miles to the signed turnoff for the Clarks Fork Trail, just before you reach the sign for Hunter Peak Campground on the left side of the highway. Turn right and drive a steep, narrow gravel road for 0.3 mile to the trailhead.

If you plan to exit at the lower trailhead at the end of Wyoming Highway 292, proceed north from the junction of Highways 120 and 296 north of Cody, following Highway 120 for 12 miles to a junction. Turn left on poorly signed Highway 292 and proceed on this winding road for about 12 miles to where the pavement abruptly ends and the route turns into a rough jeep road. If you have a sturdy four-wheel-drive vehicle you can continue driving, but most cars should be parked near the end of the pavement.

DESCRIPTION ·

The Clarks Fork Trail starts near a horse corral on the northeast side of the small parking lot and travels gradually up and down through sagebrush, grassy areas, and open forests of Douglas firs, Engelmann spruces, lodgepole pines, Rocky Mountain junipers, and quaking aspens. Fantastic views extend in all directions with perhaps the most notable ones to the southwest of Hunter Peak and southeast to the impressive Cathedral Cliffs. Wildflowers abound in late May and June, with larkspur, arrowleaf balsamroot, and, in wetter areas, shooting star being particularly abundant.

At 0.3 mile you pass the first in a series of small marshy lakes, most of which dry up to become wet meadows by late summer. Feeding these lakes are several small creeks that you must hop over. The largest is called Ghost Creek but the others are seasonal and have no name. Early in the season expect the trail in this area to be wet and muddy with the tread badly trampled by horses. At 1.3 miles a faint trail marked with a low pile of rocks splits to the left and goes 0.2 mile to a waterfall. This falls is worth a visit, especially in early summer when heavy snowmelt makes the scene that much more impressive.

At 2.4 miles is a fair campsite immediately before a bridge over rushing Beartooth Creek. Just shy of 4 miles you pass a seasonal pond and then tackle a short, steep uphill. The next couple miles are delightful as you go gradually up and down over a partly forested slope with plenty of wildflowers, a few seasonal creeks, and good views. Especially noticeable is the increasingly steep-walled canyon of Clarks Fork River on your right, although you cannot see all the way

Clarks Fork Canyon near Table Creek

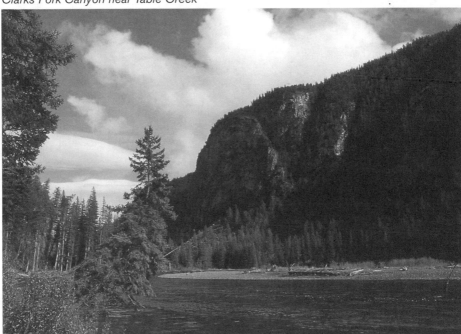

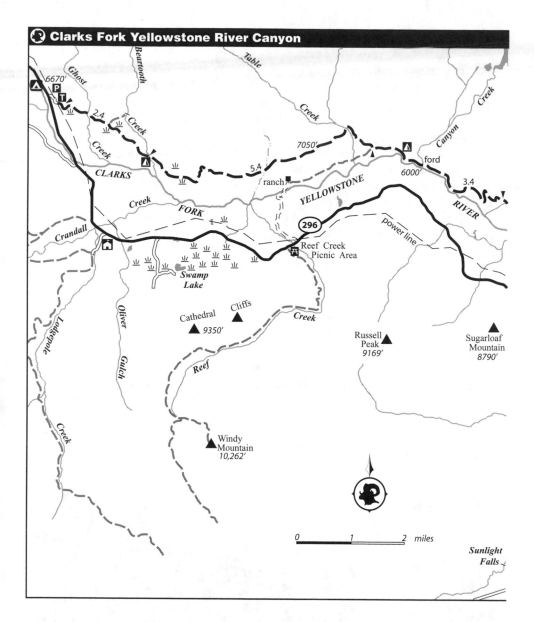

Clarks Fork Yellowstone River Canyon

to the bottom. Pass through a fence at 5.6 miles, and then it's more fun and easy hiking to the log crossing of Table Creek at 6.7 miles.

From Table Creek the trail plummets for a little more than 1 mile to the bottom of Clarks Fork Canyon and a signed junction. The path to the right leads to private land, so turn left on a nearly level path and wander through forest and meadows, soon reaching Clarks Fork. The several possible campsites in this area feature fine views across the river to the cliffs rising above the south bank.

At 8.7 miles you reach Canyon Creek, which may have a log across it, but more likely presents a calf-deep ford in May and June. Past this creek the trail

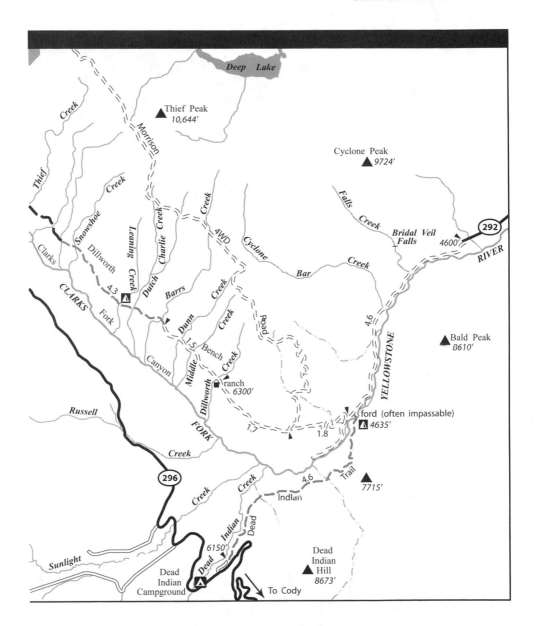

stays near the bottom of the canyon for another 0.9 mile, passing under the towering cliffs of a large rock formation. After only 2.2 miles at river level, the trail leaves the water and for the next 1.3 miles climbs in two long, then two short switchbacks gaining 800 feet to the top of Dillworth Bench.

From this grandstand for the next several miles, you enjoy fine views up and down the canyon and south to the colorful cliffs of Sugarloaf Mountain. The first few miles are easy, lovely hiking as the trail goes gradually up and down in meadows and aspen forests; you hop over several small creeks and pass a few decent campsites. If you are doing this trip as an out-and-back adventure, turn around anywhere along this stretch to return to your base camp near Canyon Creek.

For those continuing on the Clarks Fork Trail, at about 15.5 miles you meet the end of the Morrison 4WD Road, a rough jeep track that hosts the trail for the next few miles as it crosses various small creeks and takes you past a ranch on private land. Views to distant peaks and ridges are nearly constant and there are nice views of Sunlight Basin to the southwest. Unfortunately, you can rarely see down into the deep Clarks Fork Canyon from this road.

At 18.7 miles the road splits. The left fork makes a long, difficult climb to U.S. Highway 212 on the Beartooth Plateau. That road is usually not free of snow and open to traffic until sometime in June. You take the right fork, which goes down a wide gully to the edge of the canyon and switchbacks down a mostly open slope to the river.

Near the river a dead-end jeep road goes upstream about 1 mile before cliffs stop farther progress. On the other side of the river the Dead Indian Trail (a portion of the historic Nez Perce Trail) switchbacks steeply up to a wildly scenic bench with great views down into the Clarks Fork Canyon. That trail then exits the area along an extremely scenic route back to the Dead Indian Trailhead just off Wyoming Highway 296 described in "How to Get There" (see p. 64). *The problem with this option is getting to the other side of the river.* If it is late summer or fall and the river is really low (don't count on it), strong hikers may be able to ford the stream. More likely, this option is simply infeasible. *Always call about this ford's current conditions before your trip.*

Clarks Fork Canyon below Canyon Creek

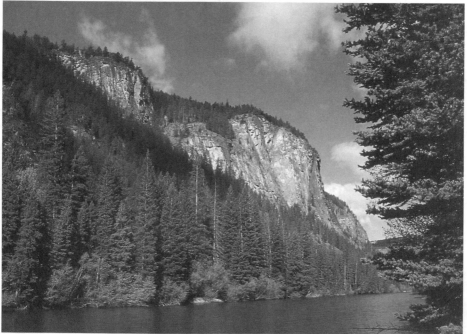

A surer, safer option than fording the river is to continue downstream on the rough jeep road another 4.6 miles to where the road reaches the end of Wyoming Highway 292. This hike can be very hot in midsummer, but the going is relatively easy and quite scenic. Unfortunately, the car shuttle involved is quite long, so the best plan is to make this an out-and-back adventure from the Clarks Fork Trailhead. To see the canyon from another viewpoint, add a dayhike to your trip on the dramatic Dead Indian Trail.

POSSIBLE ITINERARY

	CAMPS & SIDE TRIPS	MILES	ELEVATION GAIN
DAY 1	Near Canyon Creek	8.4	550'
DAY 2	Near Canyon Creek, with dayhike to Dillworth Bench	6.5	1000'
DAY 3	Out	8.4	1550'

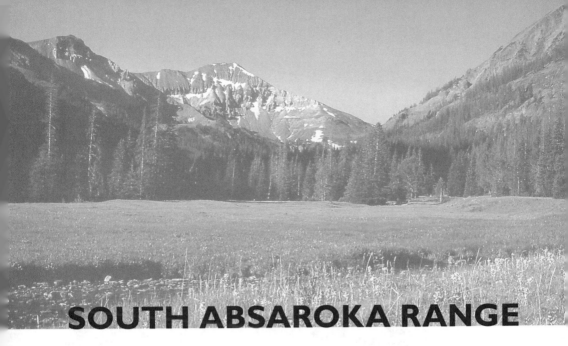

SOUTH ABSAROKA RANGE

ike the northern part of the same mountain complex, the southern Absaroka Range is a contorted landscape of high ridges, impressively deep valleys, open forests, large meadows, and great fishing streams in the rain shadow to the east and southeast of Yellowstone National Park. Unlike the Beartooth Mountains and Wind River Range, these mountains are composed not of granite rock but volcanic strata that have been exposed by erosion. The rock and soil erodes easily, so the trails are subject to frequent washouts. On the other hand, erosion often exposes petrified forests on the hillsides, adding to the area's geologic appeal. Unfortunately, lakes are rare here, because the rock does not hold surface water well.

Also relatively rare are other hikers. Sometimes difficult river crossings, very long trails, and relative isolation restrict most visitors to this land to horse packers and hunting parties, with few pedestrians making the journey to see these mountains. But that is unfortunate, because if you are up for the challenge, hiking here can be a real joy. The scenery is outstanding, the wildlife is abundant (including a healthy population of grizzly bears, so act accordingly), and you can enjoy it all while rarely, if ever, encountering another soul.

Trails in the southern Absaroka Range, most of which is protected in the huge Washakie Wilderness, are often long, poorly signed, and sketchy. Visitors should expect that lesser-used paths will sometimes disappear entirely and be difficult to relocate when they do. In late spring and early summer stream crossings will be challenging at best—think waist- or even chest-deep water that is both cold and fast moving—and often impossible for those not on a horse. By later in the summer, however, trail maintenance (what little is done at all) is complete and the crossings are much more manageable, making hiking here a joy.

Photo: *Along lower Cow Creek Trail (Trip 9)*

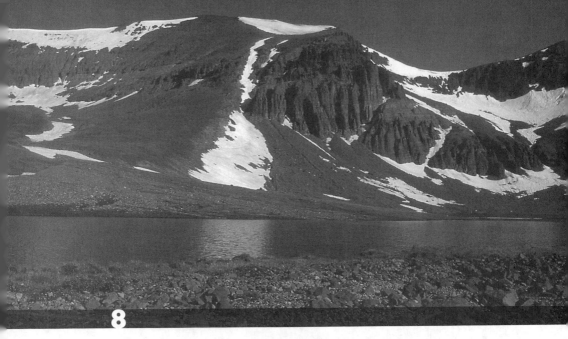

8

EMERALD LAKE

RATINGS: Scenery 8   Solitude 8   Difficulty 8

MILES: 27.4

ELEVATION GAIN: 3800´

DAYS: 3–5

MAPS: USGS *Emerald Lake* and *Snow Lake*

USUALLY OPEN: July to October

BEST: Mid-July to September

CONTACT: Wind River Ranger District, Shoshone National Forest

SPECIAL ATTRACTIONS: Dramatic canyon and mountain scenery; solitude; beautiful, wildflower-filled meadows

PERMIT: None required

RULES

All food and other odorous items must be stored away from bears.

CHALLENGES

Grizzly bears are fairly common—camp and act accordingly. There are some sketchy sections of trail and a total of 20 creek and river crossings, many of which are difficult in early summer.

Photo: Emerald Lake

TAKE THIS TRIP

Emerald Lake is a beautiful little gem in the southern Absaroka Range set in a dramatic meadow-filled cirque beneath peaks topping 12,000 feet in elevation. Since lakes are a rarity in this mountain range, you'd think this beauty would be over-crowded, but in fact it sees so few visitors that the trail often disappears amid the alpine grasses, a testament to the countless other options available to Wyoming residents and to the long, fairly difficult approach trail.

The main problem comes from the numerous stream crossings, which can be a real challenge in the high water of early summer. Still, for the best wildflowers and scenery, July is the ideal time to visit. So come in early to midsummer, but bring a good pair of wading shoes, a sturdy walking stick, strong legs, and the right attitude to enjoy this hike at its finest.

HOW TO GET THERE

From downtown Dubois, three blocks west of where the main road (U.S. Highway 26/287) makes a 90-degree turn, go north on Horse Creek Road, which soon becomes County Road 285. Stay on the main road for 4 miles to the end of pavement, and then follow a good gravel road as it enters the Shoshone National Forest and becomes Forest Road 285.

Pass the turnoff to Horse Creek Campground at 10.8 miles from Dubois, and reach the dispersed trailhead parking area in another 14.8 miles. There is no single parking lot for the trailhead, and corrals and campsites scattered about make it difficult to find the official start of the trail. Look for a trailhead signboard about 50 yards to the left (north) of the road about 0.1 mile before a prominent restroom building.

DESCRIPTION

From the trailhead signboard go north, following signs to Wiggins Fork via Double Cabin, and in about 200 yards come to a calf-to knee-deep ford of Frontier Creek. Although that simple description makes it sound easy, finding the proper trail to the creek, locating the correct crossing point, and picking up the trail on the other side of the ford are all rather tricky. Compounding the problem are numerous livestock trails that crisscross the area. Your best bet is to go upstream about 200 yards from the signboard, cross at a gravelly area, and search for the trail on the other side.

With a little effort you should find a reasonably distinct trail that goes upstream in the forest on the north side of Frontier Creek. Follow this trail for about 250 yards as it pulls away from the creek and takes you to an unsigned junction beside the fence-enclosed log structures of the Double Cabin U.S. Forest Service facility. Go right here on a trail along the edge of a meadow and to a ford of the Wiggins Fork. The water here is swift and usually

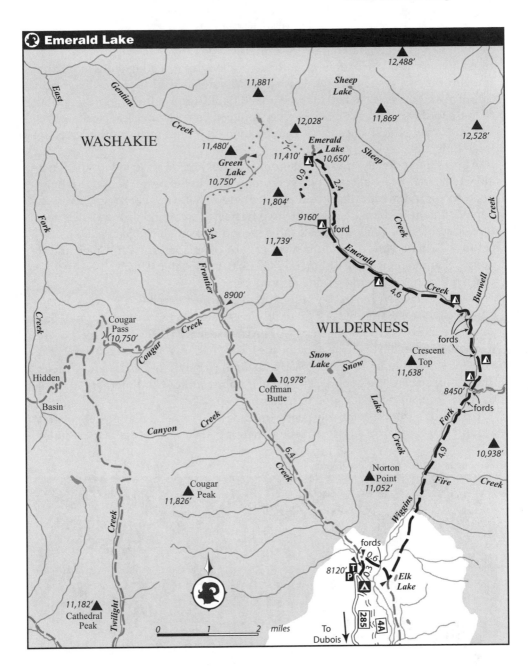

Emerald Lake

higher than knee deep, so be careful. A small sign on the other side of the ford marks the continuation of the trail.

Despite all these early navigation and stream crossing issues, the surrounding scenery is terrific compensation for your efforts. Impressive jagged cliffs and peaks of the southern Absaroka Range rise in three directions and provide outstanding backdrops to the large meadows in the foreground.

Just 0.25 mile after the Wiggins Fork ford, turn left at a junction with Indian Paint Trail and begin walking up the initially wide canyon of Wiggins Fork. The trail soon leaves the meadow for a forest of Douglas firs, lodgepole pines, and Engelmann spruces, enters the Washakie Wilderness, and begins a long, slow uphill. At 5.2 miles is the first of three unavoidable fords of the Wiggins Fork. All of these fords are higher than knee deep and can be tricky in early summer. The last one is the easiest since the stream by then no longer includes the waters of large Emerald Creek.

Almost immediately after the last ford is a trail junction. Go left on the Emerald Creek Trail and walk past two good campsites in the next 0.8 mile that enjoy good access to Emerald Creek and excellent views of extremely rugged Crescent Top Mountain to the west. The next two obstacles are a higher-than-knee-deep ford of swift, clear Emerald Creek and a second crossing just 0.5 mile later. After another 0.2 mile you make a much easier ford of smaller Burwell Creek and finally yet another crossing of Emerald Creek 0.2 mile later. This trail is great for practicing proper stream crossing techniques!

The trail now returns to its gradual uphill in forest, passing a possible campsite about 0.2 mile after the last Emerald Creek ford, then goes another mile to a small meadow with a good campsite. The trail seems to disappear here, but the tread picks up again at the head of the meadow, then travels another 0.8 mile to a very nice campsite immediately before the final (whew!) ford of Emerald Creek. The campsite here is a good place to stay if you want to visit Emerald Lake as a dayhike from a lower-elevation base camp.

Up to this point the relatively gentle trail has made a net elevation gain of only around 1000 feet. You must gain the remaining 1500 feet in the last 2.4 miles,

View near Double Cabin Trailhead

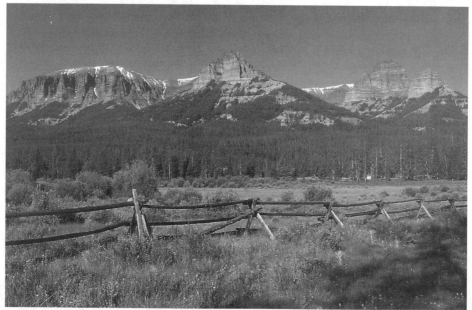

meaning that the trail gets considerably steeper after the last stream ford with several frustrating ups and downs along the way. The difficulty is further enhanced by the fact that the trail frequently fades away in meadows or amid the rocks of stream outwash areas. With persistence, both the steep uphill and navigation concerns are reasonably surmountable.

Over the last mile your efforts are spectacularly rewarded, as you leave the forest and climb steeply over rolling alpine terrain with outstanding views of the surrounding peaks. Elk frequent these meadows during the summer, so watch and listen for these large animals. Your trip ends at starkly beautiful Emerald Lake, an alpine jewel set beneath craggy 12,000-foot peaks. Camping is possible but there are no trees for either shelter or hanging your food. So plan to spend the night here only if the weather is good and you have brought a bear canister to protect your food.

Once at Emerald Lake, don't miss the chance to wander around, especially into the rolling meadowlands to the south-southwest. Here you can admire stupendous views beneath the towering cliffs of the various unnamed peaks and ridges that enclose this high basin.

If you have basic mountain climbing skills and you brought an ice axe, you could turn this trip into a tough loop by climbing through a rugged little pass west of Emerald Lake into the Frontier Creek drainage (see "Variations"). This potentially dangerous route, however, is beyond the skills of the average backpacker and is not recommended for most travelers.

POSSIBLE ITINERARY

	CAMPS & SIDE TRIPS	MILES	ELEVATION GAIN
DAY 1	Emerald Creek at last ford	10.4	1200'
DAY 2	Emerald Creek at last ford, with dayhike to Emerald Lake and explore upper basin	6.6	2400'
DAY 3	Out	10.4	200'

VARIATIONS ·

For another option from the same trailhead that features similarly grand scenery and fewer stream crossings, consider the trail up Frontier Creek to tiny Green Lake. This path has the added bonus of some interesting petrified forests along the way, although many of the best displays have been looted by treasure hunters. Like Emerald Lake, the upper reaches of this hike are incredibly scenic, but the last 3 miles to Green Lake are off-trail and quite rugged. Even so, for determined backpackers the hike is well worth doing.

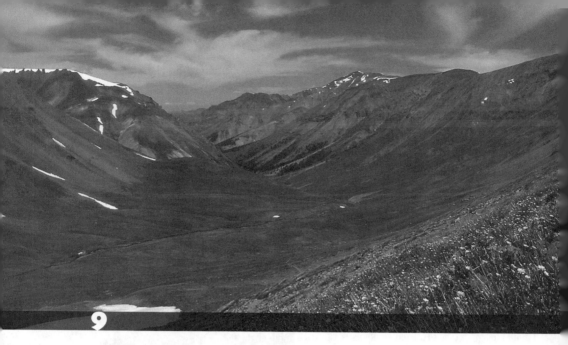

9

GREYBULL RIVER
& BURWELL PASS LOOP

RATINGS: Scenery 10   Solitude 9   Difficulty 8
MILES: 45.8
ELEVATION GAIN: 9300´
DAYS: 3–6
MAPS: USGS *Dunrud Peak, Francs Peak, Mount Burwell,* and *Wiggins Peak*
USUALLY OPEN: July to October
BEST: Mid- to late July
CONTACT: Greybull and Wind River Ranger Districts, Shoshone National Forest
SPECIAL ATTRACTIONS: Dramatic mountain scenery; plenty of solitude
PERMIT: None required

RULES

All food and other odorous items must be stored away from bears.

CHALLENGES

Grizzly bears are in the area—camp and act accordingly. Several trails are sketchy and sometimes hard to follow. The route includes a potentially long (but fun) roadwalk, unless you have an SUV or four-wheel-drive car with superior

Photo: Greybull River Valley and Francs Peak from Greybull Pass

ground clearance that will allow you to drive to the upper trailhead.

HOW TO GET THERE ··············

From the small town of Meeteetse, go east on Wyoming Highway 290, drive 6.8 miles, then turn left on Wood River Road. The pavement ends after 5.3 miles leaving you to drive a good gravel road 10.6 miles to a junction at the border of the Shoshone National Forest. Go straight on Forest Service Road 200.3, which is rather rough but is fine for passenger cars.

Drive 5.2 miles to a parking area on the right just before the road goes downhill to a ford of Jojo Creek. Cars without four-wheel-drive should park here because the remaining road is rough and rocky and requires two potentially engine-swamping fords of the Wood River. By late July the fords become more reasonable, but beware of the possibility of thunderstorms coming through and raising the river level behind you. If your vehicle can handle the road, you can slowly drive another 6.9 miles to the well-developed Kirwin Trailhead.

DESCRIPTION ··················

If you start hiking from the parking area at the end of the reasonably good road, you immediately ford or jump over small Jojo Creek, then walk the road over a huge sagebrush-covered flat with the rather unimaginative (okay, make that *really* unimaginative) name of "The Meadows." Name issues aside, The Meadows does provide terrific views of the peaks ahead and the possibility of seeing both deer and moose. Scattered about The Meadows, and especially along its edge, are trees such as quaking aspens, limber pines, and Engelmann spruces. After 0.4 mile you make a calf-deep ford of Wood River. Another 1.8 miles of mostly flat walking leads you to the second ford of Wood River, after which the road leaves The Meadows and enters increasingly forested terrain.

TAKE THIS TRIP

This hike explores the eastern edge of the vast Absaroka Range, a land of *really* big shoulders. Here huge, mostly treeless mountains rise to impressive heights, canyons thousands of feet deep dissect the range, and enormous meadows fill the valley floors. Compared to almost anywhere you have probably hiked before, everything here is bigger and wilder. Poor road access ensures that few visitors come here, so solitude is another bonus.

Magnificent and long as it is, this loop samples only a tiny portion of this vast, enchanting landscape, leaving plenty to explore on future trips if you like what you see (and it would be hard not to). So if you are prepared to feel (really) small amid mountain giants, this is a land you won't want to miss.

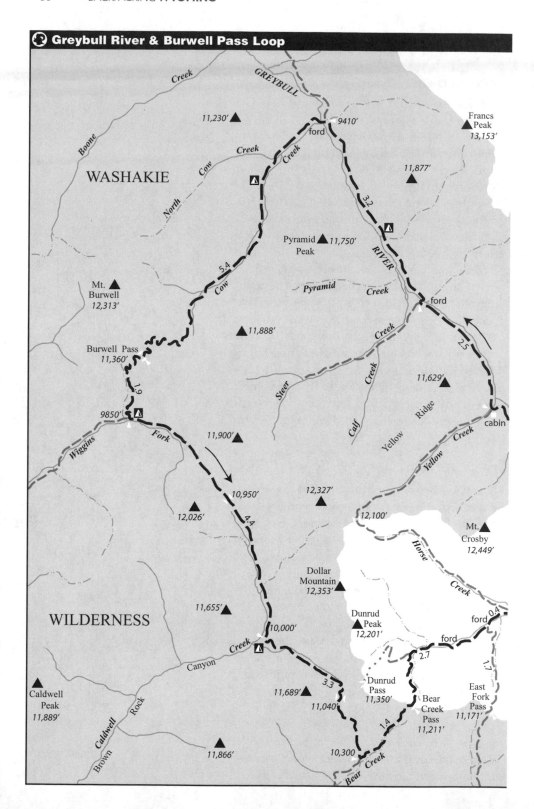

Greybull River & Burwell Pass Loop

Creek

GREYBULL

Creek

Boone

9410'

ford

Francs
Peak
13,153'

11,230'

WASHAKIE

Creek

Cow

North

Creek

11,877'

3.2

Pyramid
Peak

11,750'

RIVER

5.4

Cow

Pyramid   Creek

Mt.
Burwell
12,313'

11,888'

Creek

ford

Burwell Pass
11,360'

Steer

Creek

2.5

Calf

11,629'

1.9

9850'

Ridge

Yellow

cabin

Wiggins

Fork

11,900'

Yellow   Creek

10,950'

12,327'

12,026'

4.4

12,100'

Mt.
Crosby
12,449'

Horse

Dollar
Mountain
12,353'

11,655'

Creek

WILDERNESS

Dunrud
Peak
12,201'

ford   0.4

Creek

Canyon

10,000'

ford

2.7

1.7

Caldwell
Peak
11,889'

Rock

3.3

Dunrud
Pass
11,350'

Bear
Creek
Pass
11,211'

East
Fork
Pass
11,171'

11,689'

11,040'

Caldwell

Brown

11,866'

1.4

10,300'

Bear   Creek

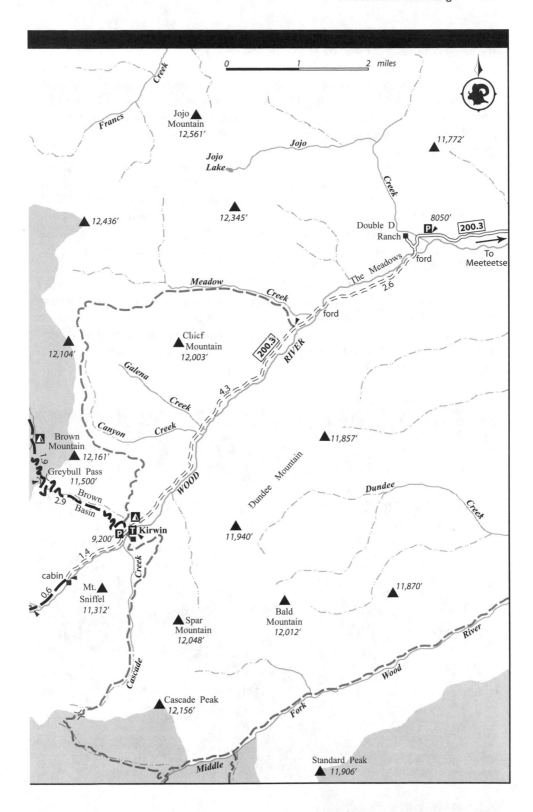

0   1   2 *miles*

Francs Creek

Jojo ▲
Mountain
12,561'

Jojo

Jojo
Lake

▲ *11,772'*

▲ *12,436'*

▲
12,345'

Creek

Double D
Ranch   P ▶   *8050'*   200.3

The Meadows   ford   To
Meeteetse
2.6

Meadow   Creek   ford

▲ *12,104'*

Chief ▲
Mountain
12,003'   200.3   RIVER

Galena   4.3

Creek

Canyon   Creek   WOOD

▲ *11,857'*

Brown
Mountain
▲ *12,161'*

Greybull Pass   Dundee Mountain   Dundee   Creek
11,500'   1.9

Brown   2.9
Basin

▲
Kirwin   ▲
11,940'   *11,870'*
9,200'   P T

1.4

cabin   0.6   Creek

Mt. ▲
Sniffel
11,312'

Spar ▲   Bald ▲
Mountain   Mountain
12,048'   *12,012'*

Cascade   River

Wood

Cascade Peak ▲   Fork
12,156'

Middle

Standard Peak
▲ *11,906'*

Just 0.4 mile after the second ford of Wood River you pass a metal sign on the right announcing the start of Meadow Creek Trail. Continue straight on the increasingly rocky, now up-and-down road all the way to Kirwin at 6.9 miles. In addition to being the location of the official trailhead, this historic townsite features several old but recently restored miner's cabins, a couple of larger mine buildings, a lovely meadow, and absolutely stunning views of massive Mt. Sniffel and other surrounding peaks. There are a couple of decent places to camp not far from the trailhead.

From the west end of the small but well-signed trailhead parking lot you turn onto the Brown Basin Trail and, 15 yards later, come to a junction with the Canyon Creek Trail, which goes to the right and eventually connects with the Meadow Creek Trail. Keep straight and begin a long, steady climb that switchbacks up a mostly open, view-packed slope. The dramatic, craggy pyramid of Mt. Sniffel rising to the southwest above Kirwin townsite is probably the most impressive of the countless memorable vistas.

After the first 15 relatively gentle switchbacks the trail gets noticeably steeper as it climbs through Brown Basin, a steeply sloping grassland tucked beneath the hulks of Brown Mountain to the northeast and Mt. Crosby to the southwest. Among the abundant July-blooming wildflowers in the grasslands here are bistort, lupine, bluebell, phlox, forget-me-not, larkspur, daisy, phacelia, and buttercup—a very partial list.

Yellow Ridge from Greybull Pass

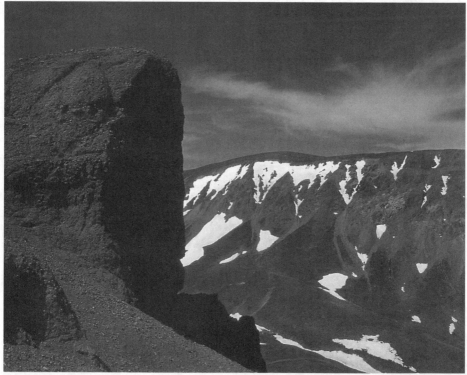

At the head of Brown Basin, and now well above treeline, the switchbacks resume, with 11 well-graded zigzags up to 11,500-foot Greybull Pass. Both the altitude and the views will take your breath away, with stunning vistas down both the Wood and Greybull River canyons. Numerous (mostly unnamed) peaks and ridges rise in every direction, the most colorful of which is aptly named Yellow Ridge to the northwest. While you might expect a pass this high to be snowbound until at least late July, it melts out well before that date. This area is in the rain shadow of such moisture-stealing mountains as the Teton and Wind River ranges to the west, so the clouds have somewhat less precipitation by the time they reach the eastern Absarokas.

Dropping down the north side of Greybull Pass involves 19 short, quite steep switchbacks over rocks and scree to the gentler slopes of the grassy basin below, which has plenty of room for very exposed but also very scenic camping. Still rapidly descending, the often faint trail takes you over the Greybull River (here just a small creek) and then comes to an old miner's cabin very near the mouth of Yellow Creek. An obscure trail that goes up this creek serves as an extremely scenic diversion if you have some extra time. The main trail crosses Yellow Creek and goes through a few patches of trees on its way down the Greybull River for another 2.5 miles to an unsigned junction with the faint dead-end trail up Steer Creek.

Go sharply right at this junction, immediately make an easy ford of the Greybull River, and begin passing to the east of a steep, reddish mountain called Pyramid Peak. Although this section of trail has no established campsites, there are several reasonably good potential sites on flat land not far from the river. Much of the hiking in this section is in burn-scarred areas, but the views are excellent. About 3.2 miles from Steer Creek look for a major side canyon on the left where Cow Creek joins the Greybull River. You want to take the trail up this canyon, but the junction with that path is easy to miss since the signs are placed so that hikers coming *up* rather than going *down* the Greybull River Trail can see them. Once found, the trail takes you down to the confluence of Greybull River and Cow Creek where you make a knee-deep ford of the river and pick up the tread immediately on the downstream side of where Cow Creek joins the flow.

Since the last few hundred yards of Cow Creek cut through a narrow, cliff-lined chasm, the trail is forced to make a steep up-and-down detour to reach the large meadows just above this obstacle. The hiking is now easy as you walk through meadows, hop over North Cow Creek, and generally wander gradually uphill. Several very photogenic, mostly unnamed peaks rise on either side of the canyon. An excellent campsite is on your right about 0.4 mile past the crossing of North Cow Creek.

Hop over Cow Creek at 2.2 and 2.6 miles, respectively, from the Greybull River and then keep slowly gaining elevation until you come to the upper reaches of Cow Creek. Here the pace of your ascent picks up considerably. Soon you are above treeline and climbing over tundralike grasslands, then switchbacking up rocky areas and snowfields to 11,360-foot Burwell Pass. The views, as you might

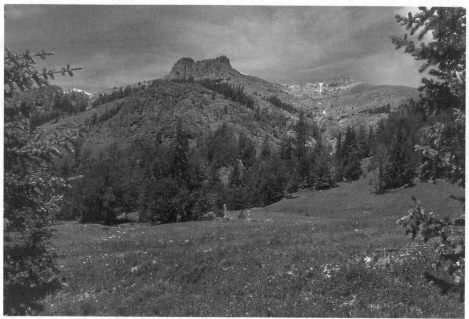

Looking up toward Burwell Pass from Wiggins Fork Trail

expect, are superb down Cow Creek, up to Mt. Burwell, down the Wiggins Fork Canyon, and all around to countless snow-streaked peaks and ridges.

Dozens of mostly gentle switchbacks now lead you down into subalpine meadows and forest and finally to a junction near a stream called Wiggins Fork. Some mediocre campsites are found near this junction. Turn left on the Absaroka Trail and gradually climb once again for about 2.3 miles to a long unnamed pass at the headwaters of Wiggins Fork.

On the south side of the unnamed pass, the trail steadily, but never steeply, descends in rolling grasslands with nice views of the surrounding peaks. The growing stream on your right is Caldwell Creek. About 2.1 miles down from the pass, just as Caldwell Creek turns to the west and enters the impressive defile known as Brown Rock Canyon, the Absaroka Trail leaves the creek and climbs up a hillside to the east. There is a decent campsite in the meadows just before this climb starts.

The trail now rounds a little promontory, enters the canyon of a nameless tributary creek, and steadily climbs to another unnamed pass. From here you are treated to wonderful views of colorful mountains in all directions. From the pass the trail descends a grassy slope where the tread frequently disappears amid the grasses and wildflowers. Look for prominent cairns to help you stay on course. A particularly confusing section is a little more than halfway down where the trail unexpectedly goes uphill to the left. Watch carefully for the cairns here; if you miss one, you will find yourself scrambling blindly in a narrow canyon of loose rock. (Yes, that's the voice of experience—don't ask.) At the bottom of the descent is a junction.

Turn left on the trail to Bear Creek Pass and begin climbing once again over treeless terrain. It's another 900 feet of uphill to the pass, where you are rewarded with terrific views north to the bulky mass of colorful Dunrud Peak and northeast to the depths of the Wood River drainage.

The route into those depths is very steep and often has small, loose gravel, so watch your step. The trail's grade eases near where you pass an obscure but signed trail that goes up a canyon to the left to Dunrud Pass. This trail is not shown on either the USGS or U.S. Forest Service maps.

Cross the growing Wood River three times as you continue to descend, the second two crossings requiring wet feet. Just 0.1 mile before the third crossing you pass a signed junction with the trail to East Fork Pass.

About 0.3 mile after the last Wood River ford, go straight at the junction with the little-used trail up Horse Creek and, 10 yards later, pass through a gate in a wooden fence. Then hop over Horse Creek and walk 0.6 mile to a cabin enclosed by a wooden fence. From here the trail follows a rocky old jeep track so little used that it effectively serves as a wide trail. After 1.4 miles the combination road and trail returns you to the mining cabins and trailhead at Kirwin. If you drove this far, your trip is over. Otherwise you must walk 6.9 miles back along the road to reach your vehicle.

POSSIBLE ITINERARY

NOTE: This plan assumes you start from the lower trailhead at the end of the reasonably good road.

	CAMPS & SIDE TRIPS	MILES	ELEVATION GAIN
DAY 1	Upper Greybull River	10.9	3600'
DAY 2	Cow Creek	8.3	400'
DAY 3	Caldwell Creek	9.9	3000'
DAY 4	Kirwin	9.8	2100'
DAY 5	Out	6.9	200'

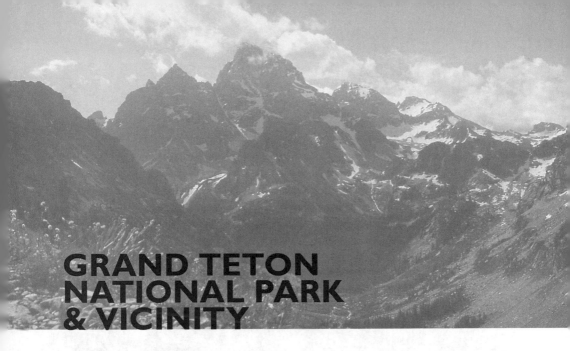

GRAND TETON NATIONAL PARK & VICINITY

Because of thousands of movies, television commercials, calendar covers, postcards, and the like, the Teton Range, especially as viewed from the lowlands around Jackson Hole, is probably the most recognizable cluster of peaks in North America. But despite their familiarity, these mountains remain beyond description, because even if you use every superlative synonym in Mr. Roget's book, you still can never adequately convey their incredible beauty. Far be it from this author to even attempt it. Gather together a large selection of words like *jaw-dropping*, *sky-scraping*, *overwhelming*, and *stupendous*, mix them randomly, and you will do just as well. But for a demonstrably better plan, you simply *must* see these mountains, and better yet hike here, yourself.

What very few hikers realize, however, is that the Teton Range itself is only the spectacular beginning of the backpacking possibilities in this area. Nearby ranges, while perhaps not as chock full of knock-your-socks-off scenery, offer much more solitude, lots of wildflowers, some darn good scenery in their own right, and plenty of wildlife. The Teton Wilderness, for example, northeast of Grand Teton National Park, is a huge land with sprawling meadows, thousands of acres of wildflowers, several waterfalls, and plenty of fine views of rolling forested mountains.

The Gros Ventre Range southeast of the Tetons offers better high-mountain scenery than the Teton Wilderness with lots of lakes, sky-scraping peaks, and some of the most beautiful but little-used hiking trails in the American West. One reason that the trails are so little used is a conspiracy by local hikers to keep this range a secret from out-of-staters (which several locals readily admitted to me.) But if you want to see some of the best that the Wyoming mountains have to offer, you simply *must* ignore the "friendly" advice of the locals to go elsewhere and take at least one extended hike in this outstanding wilderness yourself.

Photo: *Grand Teton from near Lake Solitude (Trip 12)*

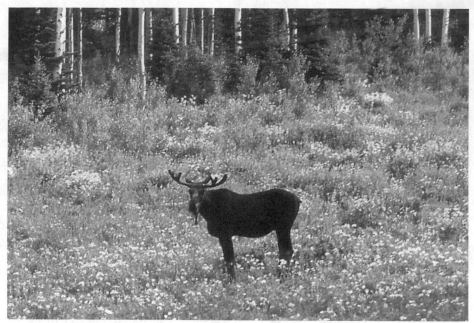

Moose on Deer Ridge, Gros Ventre Range

Even in the Teton Range itself, it is still possible to find solitude, especially in the northern part of the range, which is most easily reached from the west out of Idaho. The peaks here are a little less awe-inspiring than in the more famous southern Tetons and the grizzly bear population is definitely thicker, but the wildflowers are more abundant and crowds are . . . well, there aren't any crowds.

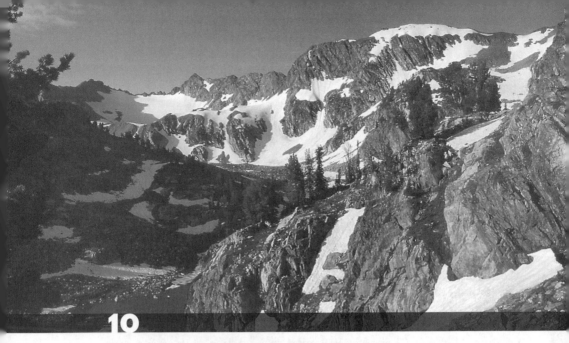

10

BITCH CREEK LOOP

RATINGS: Scenery 8   Solitude 7   Difficulty 6
MILES: 25.4 (31)
ELEVATION GAIN: 4750′ (6900′)
DAYS: 3–5
MAPS: USGS *Hominy Peak, Rammel Mountain*, and *Ranger Peak*
USUALLY OPEN: July to October
BEST: Mid- to late July
CONTACT: Ashton/Island Park Ranger District, Targhee National Forest; Grand Teton National Park
SPECIAL ATTRACTIONS: Rare solitude in the Teton Range; acres of wildflowers in mid-July; excellent views of the Teton Range and beyond

PERMIT

A permit is not necessary for the Jedediah Smith Wilderness, but an entry permit is required for the recommended side trip into Grand Teton National Park. As this is effectively impossible to obtain when you approach by trail from the west, it is easier to simply purchase and carry an annual national parks pass. Spending the night in the park requires an overnight backcountry permit, which can only be obtained in person from ranger stations in the park and is logistically onerous. It is much simpler to make this side trip as a dayhike.

Photo: Glacier Peak

RULES

All food and other odorous items must be stored away from bears. Groups are limited to 20 people. Camps must be located at least 200 feet from any lake and 100 feet from any stream. Camping with livestock is prohibited at or near Camp or Hidden lakes.

CHALLENGES

Grizzly bears are common—camp and act accordingly. Some trails and campsites are regularly traveled by horses. Several miles of the trails are indistinct. Telling people the politically incorrect name of where you went on vacation may make you uncomfortable.

HOW TO GET THERE

Although this entire hike is in Wyoming, the only way to reach the trailhead by road is from Idaho. So, from Jackson, Wyoming, go 32 miles west and north on Wyoming Highway 22, then Idaho Highway 33 to Driggs, Idaho. Continue north on Highway 33 another 10.2 miles to a junction, then turn right on Idaho Highway 32. Proceed 12 miles to a junction with Road 4700E, turn right, and drive 1 mile to a second junction.

Turn right on Road 700N and follow this good gravel road for 3.1 miles to where it enters the Targhee National Forest and becomes Forest Service Road 265. Drive another 0.1 mile to a fork, where you go right, still on Road 265. Remain

TAKE THIS TRIP

The name may be off-putting, but the scenery and solitude in the Bitch Creek drainage in the northwest part of the Teton Range more than makes up for the unsavory nomenclature. Those world-famous jagged peaks of the southern Tetons cannot be seen here, but this loop still includes lots of other high-quality attractions, including, and most especially, many miles of wonderful alpine meadows covered with wildflowers and offering fine views. It also takes you to a scenic little lake perfect for wilderness camping and, from there, gives you the option of a superb off-trail exploration into a wildly scenic but almost never visited corner of Grand Teton National Park. In addition, since the trail leads the hiker through the wettest part of Wyoming, it offers a botanical change of pace with remarkably lush forests and undergrowth more reminiscent of the rainforests of Oregon or Washington than the relatively dry forests of the Intermountain West.

All these highlights can reasonably be explored in a long weekend or extended to a leisurely ramble of as much as a week. All that said, perhaps the most amazing fact is that the trails here, despite their location in the world-famous Teton Range, are so rarely traveled that the tread regularly (and sometimes frustratingly) disappears amid the grasses and wildflowers.

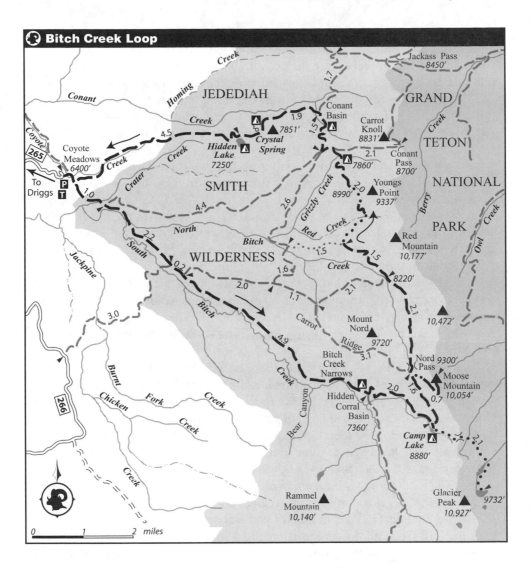

Bitch Creek Loop

on this good but very dusty road for another 9.5 miles to the Coyote Meadows Trailhead. Parking is on the left and the trailhead signboard is on the right.

DESCRIPTION

The trail departs from right next to the signboard and descends for less than 0.1 mile through lodgepole pine woodlands to pretty Coyote Meadows. Wildflowers are abundant right from the start of this hike in both the forest and the meadow. Look for Queen Anne's lace, monkshood, fireweed, false hellebore, lupine, harebell, geranium, yarrow, coneflower, spiraea, goldenrod, sunflower, clover, and a host of others. On the down side, cattle are allowed to graze in Coyote Meadows, so expect lots of cow pies, livestock trails, and noisy mooing.

Cross small Coyote Creek atop a culvert and almost immediately come to a signed but easily missed trail that goes to the left (downstream). Go straight on the main trail and travel through what is, by Wyoming standards, an exceptionally wet, lush forest for 0.25 mile to a junction, the start of your loop.

Go right and gradually ascend a well-worn if somewhat dusty trail through a forest of lodgepole pines, Engelmann spruces, subalpine firs, quaking aspens, mountain ashes, and Douglas firs. At 1 mile, shortly after you cross tiny Crater Creek, is a junction with Conant Pass Trail.

Go straight, descend into the heavily forested canyon of clear, rollicking Bitch Creek, and come to a bridge over that stream's north fork. The gentle trail then goes upstream along mostly unseen South Bitch Creek, generally staying in meadows choked with grasses, wildflowers, and willows. Wildlife lovers should look for beaver activity on the creek, as well as sandhill cranes and moose in the meadows. At 3.2 miles is a junction with the little-used Poacher's Trail.

Continue straight and just 0.2 mile later come to the next junction, this time with a faint trail that goes left toward Carrot Ridge. Go straight once again and travel through a delightful mix of forest and meadows where you gain elevation so slowly you may not even notice. What you will notice is that the surrounding ridges and peaks get more rugged and the scenery commensurately more dramatic as you hike.

At about 7.5 miles you climb around accurately named Bitch Creek Narrows, where the waters of South Bitch Creek rampage through a twisting and, yes, "narrow" cleft of rock. Just above the narrows is the pretty meadow at Hidden Corral Basin, where you will find several scenic campsites.

At the east end of Hidden Corral Basin is a junction. Go left (uphill) on the Camp Lake Trail and begin to climb in earnest. As you gain elevation, your efforts are rewarded with nice views back down to Hidden Corral Basin and southwest to very rugged Rammel Mountain. In addition, during the first half of the climb you cross sloping grasslands that are a riot of colorful wildflowers in mid- to late July. After gaining 1500 feet in 2 miles you reach a junction. The trail to the left goes to Nord Pass and the continuation of the recommended loop.

Before turning that way, however, take the 150-yard trail to the right to visit, or camp at, Camp Lake. This tiny lake sits in a pretty little basin, is surrounded by tree-studded meadows, and lies beneath jagged ridges to the west and reddish Moose Mountain to the east. Despite the lake's small size, it is quite deep, so it has a good population of decent-sized trout, especially near the inlet creek, and is perfect for swimming. True to its name, the lake also has several excellent campsites, although you must set up camp at least 200 feet from the water and livestock are not permitted to camp here at all. In the wet meadows near the lake many varieties of high-elevation wildflowers color the ground. Look especially for aster, shooting star, pink heather, alpine buttercup, elephant head, arnica, marsh marigold, bistort, and Cusick's speedwell.

A rugged but very worthwhile cross-country side trip begins at Camp Lake and takes adventurous types into some outstandingly beautiful alpine scenery. To make the trip, go southeast from the lake, generally staying close to the inlet

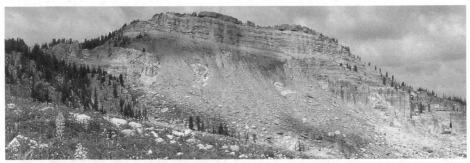

Mt. Nord from trail north of Nord Pass

creek, and climb quite steeply up a mostly forested hillside. If you're observant, you may come across faint traces of a use path from time to time, but don't count on it. After gaining 800 feet you top out at a ridgeline near a small reddish butte. A metal sign announces the boundary of Grand Teton National Park (pets, fire-arms, or campfires are prohibited in the park and you must have a permit to camp). From here make your way south-southeast over a rolling alpine land-scape of ponds, rocky cliffs, snowfields, wildflowers, and excellent views both to the east of the forested hills of the distant Teton Wilderness and south to near-by bulky Glacier Peak. You can easily spend several happy hours wandering around. A good destination is a large glacial lake beneath the steep east face of Glacier Peak, although it requires a tough downhill scramble.

Back at Camp Lake, return to the junction 150 yards northwest of the lake and take the trail toward Nord Pass, which curves to the north-northwest as it as-cends open slopes covered with wildflowers and featuring superb views. To the north you can see orange-tinged, craggy Mt. Nord, to the southwest is Rammel Mountain, and to the west are the vast Snake River Plains of Idaho. In late July and early August wildflowers are abundant here and include white columbine, vetch, bluebell, larkspur, fernleaf, paintbrush, lupine, geranium, flax, and (espe-cially abundant) wild carrot.

Just before the uphill ends at Nord Pass is a junction with the Mount Nord Trail, which goes to the left. Also near here is an unsigned junction with a faint use path that ascends for 0.7 mile to the top of Moose Mountain. The views from the top of this peak make this side trip well worthwhile and even include a part of Jackson Lake to the east.

The main trail goes straight at the junction and soon tops out at grassy Nord Pass. The fine scenery continues as you descend from the pass and travel through alpine meadows at the headwaters of North Bitch Creek that offer excellent views north to Red Mountain, southeast to Moose Mountain, and, most strikingly, west to the orange cliffs of Mt. Nord. The trail is overgrown and obscure in places but a few strategically placed cairns should keep you on course.

After dropping 1050 feet in 2 miles you find yourself right beside small North Bitch Creek at a junction with Carrot Ridge Trail. You could turn left here and exit on this little-used path, but there is plenty of fine scenery still to come on the longer recommended loop, so go straight and begin an intermittent but often very steep climb on a partly forested slope. After 0.6 mile the pace slackens considerably as you make a gentle traverse of a steep slope to the end of a rounded ridge. The trail is very easy to lose here amid a dense growth of tall grasses and wildflowers. The correct course stays level or even climbs a bit as it curves around the ridge and heads generally northeast. The trail remains very faint for the next couple of miles, so you should expect to lose it from time to time and to expend extra energy searching. Good map-reading skills will help a lot.

The proper route takes you up into a very impressive basin beneath aptly named Red Mountain to a crossing of usually dry Red Creek. From there head up the right (east) side of a prominent grassy gully, then climb steeply to a point high on a ridge just west of Youngs Point. About 0.2 mile down the north side of this ridge the tread becomes more distinct again allowing you to follow it steeply down to an easy crossing of Grizzly Creek. There is a mediocre camp at this crossing.

On the other side of Grizzly Creek the trail climbs for 0.15 mile to a junction. Turn left and walk gently uphill for 0.2 mile to a four-way junction in a pretty meadow. You could go straight and be back to the trailhead in just 5.4 miles. If you want to see Conant Basin and Hidden Lake, however, turn right, go over a low rise, and begin going downhill on a recently reconstructed trail with numerous lazy switchbacks and turns. Near the bottom you pass a couple of marshy ponds with a very good campsite then walk another 0.1 mile to a junction in Conant Basin.

Turn left and follow a gentle trail that spends most of its miles in forest but also passes above a couple lovely meadows along Conant Creek. At 1.7 miles from Conant Basin you reach the tiny meadow and excellent campsite at Crystal Spring. The trail then climbs briefly before reaching Hidden Lake. Unfortunately this pleasant forest-rimmed pool has no permanent inlet, so the water level tends to drop dramatically by late summer. Nonetheless, there are two or three nice campsites here and some pretty good fishing.

From Hidden Lake the trail gradually gains about 250 feet to a broad, mostly forested ridgetop with a few openings choked with pungent manzanita. The trail then slowly but steadily descends for 4 miles to a junction with the Bitch Creek Trail and the close of the loop. Turn right and in 0.2 mile return to the trailhead.

POSSIBLE ITINERARY

	CAMPS & SIDE TRIPS	MILES	ELEVATION GAIN
DAY 1	Camp Lake	10.3	2700'
DAY 2	Camp Lake, with cross-country dayhike to lake below Glacier Peak	4.2	1400'
DAY 3	Grizzly Creek, including a side trip up Moose Mountain	8.2	2200'
DAY 4	Out	8.3	600'

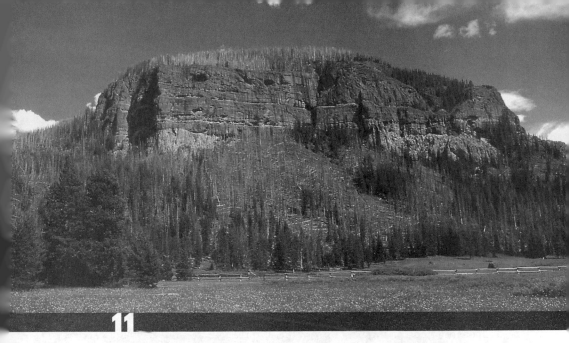

11

TETON WILDERNESS LOOP

RATINGS: Scenery 7   Solitude 8   Difficulty 7
MILES: 60.2 (63.8)
ELEVATION GAIN: 6000´ (7900´)
DAYS: 5–7
MAPS: USGS *Angle Mountain, Crater Lake, Ferry Lake, Joy Peak,* and *Two Ocean Pass*
USUALLY OPEN: Mid-July to October
BEST: Late July to September
CONTACT: Buffalo Ranger District, Bridger-Teton National Forest
SPECIAL ATTRACTIONS: Unusually large meadows with lots of wildflowers in early to midsummer; plenty of wildlife
PERMIT: None required

RULES ···

All food and other odorous items must be stored away from bears. Livestock grazing is prohibited within 0.5 mile of Crater or Ferry lakes.

CHALLENGES ···

The fords of the Yellowstone River and North Buffalo Fork on this route can be very difficult or impossible, especially early in the summer. Grizzly bears are very common—camp and act accordingly. There are miles of horse-pounded

Photo: Hawks Rest

TAKE THIS TRIP

The Teton Wilderness, which stretches along the southeastern border of Yellowstone National Park, is a sprawling land of mostly forested mountains, enormous meadows and marshes, scattered lakes, occasional waterfalls, and high ridges. Unlike its world-famous neighbor to the north, this wilderness has no thermal features, but it shares with the park the same abundance of wildlife, including moose, elk, and both black and grizzly bears. Most of the topography is not wildly scenic in the classic calendar-cover style (although there are a few impressive areas that meet this description), but it is still very beautiful, especially the huge meadows that are filled with colorful wildflowers in early to midsummer.

Many of the numerous loop options in the wilderness are very long and provide days of happy ambling through seemingly endless wildlands far from the rat race of everyday life. Completing the loop recommended here will give you a taste of what this wilderness has to offer and probably whet your appetite for much more. The loop is particularly attractive since it follows generally well-maintained trails, includes two large lakes, and visits some of the wilderness area's best meadows.

The hike also provides access to a geographic oddity: A marsh on top of the Continental Divide feeds creeks that eventually drain to both the Atlantic and the Pacific oceans. Although not very scenic, it's interesting because this is the only place in North America that drains directly into both oceans.

trails. In July there are lots of mosquitoes, especially around the huge marsh at Hawks Rest.

HOW TO GET THERE •

Coming from the east, drive U.S. Highway 26 to a well-signed junction about 3.5 miles west of Togwotee Lodge or 12.5 miles west of Togwotee Pass. Turn right (north) onto Forest Service Road 30050, following signs to Turpin Meadows, and drive this good gravel road for 4.3 miles to a junction immediately after you cross a bridge over Buffalo Fork. Turn right (east), proceed 0.3 mile to a junction with the campground turnoff, then go straight and reach the trailhead in another 0.3 mile. There is plenty of parking here for both horse trailers and hiker's cars.

If you are coming from the west, it is easier to reach the trailhead by turning off U.S. Highway 26 at a junction 3.5 miles east of Moran Junction (near the north end of Grand Teton National Park) and driving paved Forest Service Road 30050 for 10 miles to the junction mentioned above on the north side of the bridge over Buffalo Fork. Turn left (east) and follow the directions given above.

WARNING: This loop includes several stream crossings. Two of these, the North Buffalo Fork and, especially, the ford of the Yellowstone River, are extremely difficult and downright dangerous until at least the middle of July. Even in mid-July the Yellowstone River crossing may be almost waist deep, very swift, and extremely cold. Most hikers should not attempt that ford before late July and even then must be prepared for a potentially tough crossing. At a minimum, wading shoes with good traction and a sturdy walking stick are necessary to complete this loop.

DESCRIPTION

The trail starts at the southeast end of the parking lot beside a large signboard. Initially the terrain supports a lower-elevation vegetation zone dominated by sagebrush, grasses, wildflowers, and scattered lodgepole pines, quaking aspens, and a few firs. Common early summer wildflowers here include lupine, buckwheat, geranium, gilia, and balsamroot. Although often dusty or muddy from heavy horse use, the trail through this landscape is otherwise in good shape and easy to follow.

At 0.3 mile you top a small rise where you can look back west for one of this trip's few views of the rugged Teton Range. At 0.8 mile splash across small Clear Creek and come to a junction. Keep left on the North Buffalo Trail and wander up and down in open forest and meadows. At 2.8 miles you pass a large marshy beaver pond with the rather generous name of Mud "Lake" and then climb to a small ridgetop before descending about 150 feet to large and scenic Soda Fork Meadows.

Walk through Soda Fork Meadows then, at 4.5 miles and shortly after you reenter forest, reach the signed Soda Fork Cutoff Trail that veers right. Keep left and walk a mostly level 0.8 mile to a junction with the main Soda Fork Trail and the start of the recommended loop.

Go straight at the junction and for the next 2.3 miles travel generally uphill to the south edge of huge North Fork Meadows and a junction with the little-used Divide Lake Trail. Keep straight and begin the long, nearly level traverse of North Fork Meadows, which features grasses, wildflowers, willows, ponds, and nice (if not spectacular) views of the neighboring ridges. Detracting somewhat from the otherwise pleasant scenery is the fact that many of the trees in the meadow and on the surrounding ridges have been burned by old forest fires.

You pass a fine campsite on the left about 1 mile into North Fork Meadows and a second not-quite-as-nice camp on the right just 0.5 mile later. After about 2.5 miles you reach the head of the meadows where the trail climbs slightly away from the North Buffalo Fork, then traverses to a good campsite at a junction.

Veer left (uphill) at the junction onto Trail Creek Trail and steadily gain about 800 feet in forest and across open slopes to an undulating pass. The meadows here support a wide array of July-blooming wildflowers including bistort, flax, paintbrush, white columbine, lupine, wild carrot, buckwheat, and numerous others. There are nice views from the pass looking southeast to the rugged ramparts of Joy Peak and Soda Mountain. On the north side of the pass you descend along Trail Creek past beaver ponds and a small waterfall to a junction with

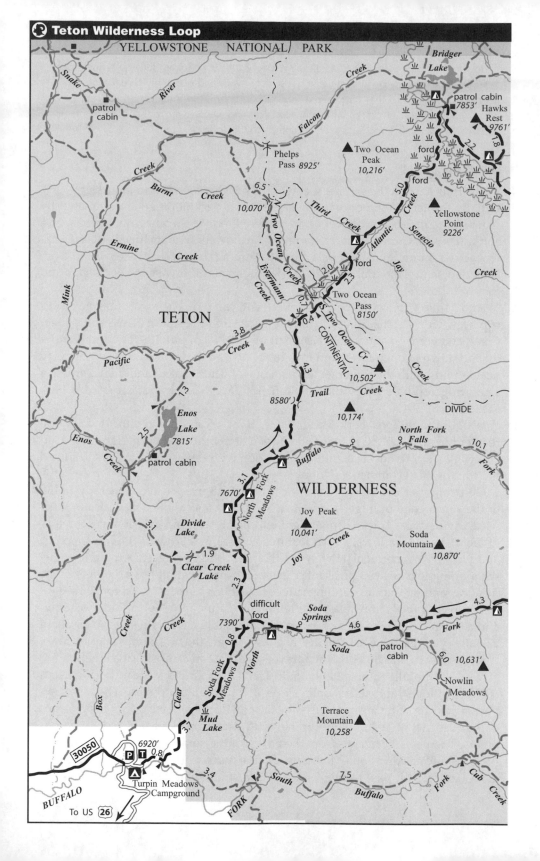

YELLOWSTONE NATIONAL PARK

Bridger Lake

patrol cabin
7853'

Hawks Rest 9761'

Snake

River

patrol cabin

Creek

Falcon

Creek

2.2

1.8

ford

Burnt

Creek

Phelps Pass 8925'

Two Ocean Peak 10,216'

5.0

ford

ford

Ermine

Creek

6.5

10,070'

Third

Creek

Atlantic

Creek

Yellowstone Point 9226'

Semecio

Joy

Creek

Mink

TETON

Evermann

Creek

Two Ocean

Creek

2.0

2.3

ford

Two Ocean Pass 8150'

0.7

0.4

Two Ocean Cr

CONTINENTAL

10,502'

Creek

DIVIDE

Pacific

Creek

3.8

1.3

8580'

4.3

Trail

Creek

10,174'

Enos Lake 7815'

2.5

patrol cabin

Enos

Creek

North Fork Falls

10.1

Buffalo

Fork

WILDERNESS

3.1

3.1

7670'

North Fork Meadows

Joy Peak 10,041'

Soda Mountain 10,870'

Divide Lake

1.9

Clear Creek Lake

2.3

Joy

Creek

4.3

Clear

Creek

difficult ford

7390'

Soda Springs

4.6

patrol cabin

Soda

Fork

6.0

10,631'

0.8

Soda

Nowlin Meadows

Box

Creek

Soda Fork Meadows

North

Mud Lake

Terrace Mountain 10,258'

3.7

30050

6920'

P T 0.8

Turpin Meadows Campground

3.4

South

7.5

Buffalo

Fork

Cub

Creek

BUFFALO

To US 26

FORK

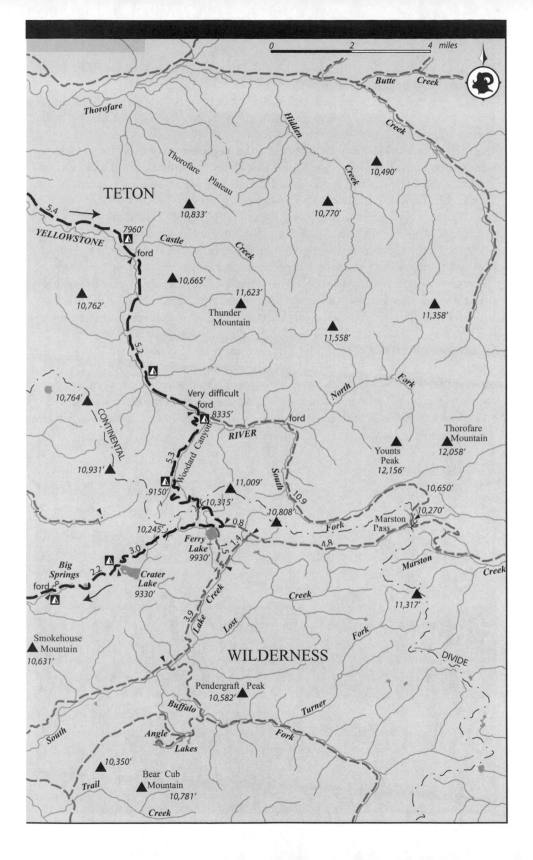

Pacific Creek Trail. Bear right and 0.4 mile later reach a second junction at the southwest end of Two Ocean Pass.

Two Ocean Pass is a unique destination, not because the scenery is all that grand, but because it is a geographic oddity. The "pass" is basically a large, nearly flat, willow-choked marsh, which is fed by both North Two Ocean and South Two Ocean creeks. The marsh, in turn, is the headwaters of both Pacific Creek, which flows into the Snake and Columbia River systems to the Pacific Ocean, and Atlantic Creek, which feeds into the Yellowstone River and eventually the Gulf of Mexico via the Missouri and Mississippi rivers. This is the only place in North America where the two great watersheds merge. That distinction earns Two Ocean Pass official status as a National Natural Landmark.

At the junction you can either go left on the official trail or straight on a slightly shorter and a little more scenic outfitter's trail that skirts the southeast side of the marsh. Both trails cross several small creeks along the way, while the shorter route necessitates an easy calf-deep ford of Atlantic Creek just before the two trails reunite. The shorter, southeast side trail is in better shape and is easier to follow.

Just 0.4 mile past where the two trails reunite, you cross small Third Creek where there is a good campsite. The trail now descends along Atlantic Creek, often on the hillside a little above the stream. This area, and for several miles to come, was burned in the massive fires that hit the Yellowstone ecosystem in 1988, so expect lots of snags and limited shade. A little more than 3 miles down from Two Ocean Pass is a knee-deep ford of Atlantic Creek.

North Fork Meadows

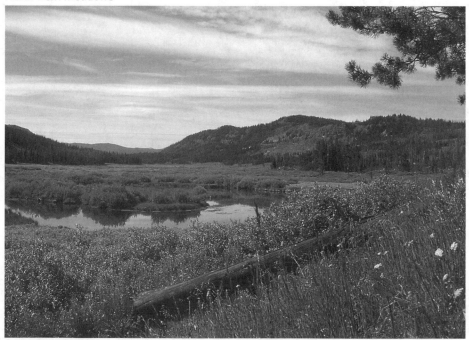

Shortly after the ford of Atlantic Creek you come to the edge of a huge willow-filled marsh where the trail forks. The trail to the right is a dead-end outfitter's path, so bear left and travel across the often muddy marsh to another, this time slightly deeper, ford of Atlantic Creek. The large cliff-edged and fire-scarred butte not far to the northeast is Hawks Rest.

Crossing the remainder of the large marshy meadow between the last Atlantic Creek ford and the Yellowstone River is often difficult before about late July. In early summer expect to struggle through standing water and sucking mud up to a foot deep. In the few drier spots you must contend with a muddy tread that is badly chewed up by horses. The clouds of mosquitoes don't help either. After almost a mile of this miserable hiking/wading you finally cross a large wooden bridge spanning the Yellowstone River. On the other side of the bridge are a junction, a fenced pasture around the Hawks Rest Patrol Cabin, and, blessedly, drier ground. There are numerous good (if badly mosquito infested) campsites in the forest northeast of the bridge. There is even a convenient bear-resistant food storage box here to protect your food.

To continue the loop, from the junction beside the bridge head upstream on the Yellowstone River Trail. The route is frustratingly wet and muddy, especially for the first mile or two in the willow flats near the meandering Yellowstone River and beneath the steep ramparts of Hawks Rest. Bear tracks and scat are numerous here and the thick willows often restrict your visibility to less than 10 feet, so be sure to make lots of noise while you hike. On the plus side, the marshes are filled with wildlife. Moose are often seen and birds are especially common. Look for bald eagles, sandhill cranes, and perhaps a few white pelicans flying along the river. At 2.2 miles from the Yellowstone River bridge there is a very scenic campsite shortly before you cross a small creek. Here a trail goes left on its way up to the expansive views atop fire-scarred Hawks Rest, a worthwhile side trip if you have the time.

Soon after the Hawks Rest junction, the trail leaves the marshy willow flats and spends the next several miles traveling the burned hillside a little above the bottomlands. Since there is almost no shade in this area, the hiking can be hot on a sunny summer day, but it's much drier and more comfortable than the flats below. Views of the river and the encroaching crags and ridges are often excellent. The canyon's first decent campsite comes about 0.3 mile before you reach Castle Creek. This stream is usually spanned by a convenient log, although that's not guaranteed.

From the crossing of Castle Creek the trail goes gradually uphill for about 3.5 miles to an excellent campsite on the Yellowstone River just before a bridgeless crossing of a good-sized but unnamed side creek.

Not quite 2 miles from this creek crossing you come to a pretty meadow where a possibly unsigned but obvious trail goes to the right. Turn onto this trail and very soon come to an intimidating ford of the Yellowstone River. Before mid-July this crossing is close to impossible for hikers, and it remains wet, thigh-deep, and very swift for much of the summer. It is *slightly* easier to cross about 150 yards downstream from the official crossing. Try to time your crossing for the morning when the river is lower because of reduced snowmelt during the night. There are decent campsites on both sides of the crossing.

NOTE: If the ford looks too dangerous, your best bet is to extend the hike an extra day by taking the trail to Marston Pass (see map on p. 99).

Once across the river (whew!) the trail switchbacks up a slope, then takes you into impressive Woodard Canyon, which you gradually ascend to a high basin with camping beneath several streaking waterfalls. You make an easy ford of the canyon's main creek here and begin a long switchbacking ascent into high, rolling alpine terrain. Just after the snowmelt in about the second week of July, this entire area, all the way up to an unnamed pass, boasts great displays of alpine buttercups and marsh marigolds.

From the pass you can look down upon starkly beautiful Ferry Lake, often icebound until late July. A shortcut that angles to the right from the pass is very steep and buried by dangerous snowfields until late July. Especially in early summer it is safer to go left at the pass and ramble down a fairly gentle trail to a junction near the northeast end of Ferry Lake. This is where you meet the trail coming in from Marston Pass, if you skipped the Yellowstone River ford and chose the longer route to Ferry Lake. Camping is not recommended at Ferry Lake since the area is very exposed, has no trees for cover or shade, and is surrounded by sloping ground.

Take the trail that goes west from Ferry Lake, keep straight at a junction with the steeper shortcut trail from the pass, and then ascend over alpine terrain and snowfields past a pretty tarn to a rolling pass. Go up and down across this rolling pass for about 1 mile to a secondary pass and then begin a steep descent. From this secondary pass you have the trip's second glimpse of the distant Teton Range, but the views of the closer ridges and canyons are more likely to draw your attention.

At the bottom of a short but steep switchbacking descent is the meadow above deep Crater Lake. It is easy to walk over to this scenic lake, which has an island and is surrounded on three sides by imposing rocky buttresses and ridges. Unfortunately, camping is only mediocre at this lake, with the best sites a long way from the water to the west.

West of Crater Lake the trail descends into rocky and increasingly forested terrain to a lovely but unnamed jade-green lake with views across the water to the dark cliffs of Soda Mountain. From there it is another 0.9 mile of downhill to the numerous good campsites beside a pretty meadow above aptly named Big Springs.

Ford the newly emerged Soda Fork just below Big Springs and then work your way downhill for about 1 mile to some very scenic meadows with good campsites and fine views of the nearby mountains. The trail stays in these meadows for about 1.4 miles and then goes into forest on the hillside farther away from the Soda Fork, crossing several small streams, all easily splashed across, hopped over, or crossed on logs.

About 0.5 mile after passing a small shallow pond, you go straight at the junction with Nowlin Meadows Trail and then continue traveling west through forest. The trail eventually makes its way down to the willowy bottomlands along the Soda Fork where you may be fortunate enough to see a moose. Along the edge of this meadow you walk past small, mineral-rich Soda Springs and then pass the unsigned and easy-to-miss junction with Soda Fork Cutoff Trail where there is a good campsite. About 0.3 mile after this campsite is a ford of North Buffalo Fork. Although not as difficult as the Yellowstone River crossing, in mid-July this is a challenging, thigh-deep ford. In addition, the rocks here are covered with slippery algae, so watch your footing. About 0.2 mile after the ford is the junction with North Buffalo Trail and the close of the loop. Turn left and retrace your steps 5.3 miles to the trailhead.

POSSIBLE ITINERARY

	CAMPS & SIDE TRIPS	MILES	ELEVATION GAIN
DAY 1	Above North Fork Meadows	10.7	1100'
DAY 2	Hawks Rest	12.0	900'
DAY 3	Castle Creek, including a side trip up Hawks Rest	11.2	2200'
DAY 4	Upper Woodard Canyon	7.7	1500'
DAY 5	Meadow below Big Springs	9.3	1800'
DAY 6	Out	12.9	400'

VARIATIONS •

Either because the Yellowstone River ford is too dangerous or you want a longer trip, skip Woodard Canyon and take the longer route around Marston Pass. This change adds 11.2 miles and a full day of hiking, but requires only a much easier ford of the North Fork Yellowstone River and visits the wildly scenic basin at the headwaters of South Fork Yellowstone River. This basin, however, is thick with grizzly bears, so be sure to travel in a group and make plenty of noise.

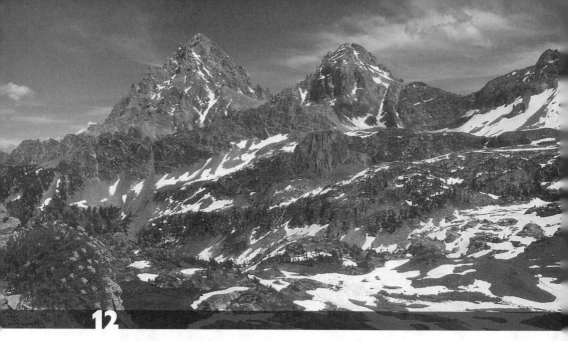

12

GRAND TETON LOOP

RATINGS: Scenery 10   Solitude 3   Difficulty 8
MILES: 48.5 (61)
ELEVATION GAIN: 9100´ (11,800´)
DAYS: 5–8
MAP: Trails Illustrated *Grand Teton National Park*
USUALLY OPEN: Mid-July to mid-October
BEST: Late July and August
CONTACT: Grand Teton National Park
SPECIAL ATTRACTIONS: Some of North America's best mountain
     scenery; wildlife; wildflowers
PERMIT: Required. Reservations are *strongly* advised.

RULES

Camping is allowed only in designated camping zones or sites. Fires are allowed only at specified camps. All food must be stored away from bears at all times. Starting in 2008, all backpackers are required to use bear canisters for storing food and other odorous items. The canisters are available on loan from the ranger stations at Moose Junction and Colter Bay.

CHALLENGES

Black bears are common—camp and act accordingly. The trails and camps are very popular, so obtaining a permit is difficult.

Photo: Tetons from near Hurricane Pass

HOW TO GET THERE •••

From the bustling resort town of Jackson, go north on U.S. Highway 89 (John D. Rockefeller Jr. Memorial Parkway) for 12.5 miles to Moose Junction. Turn left on Teton Park Road and soon come to a visitor center the entrance station into Grand Teton National Park. Turn into the visitor center and go to the wilderness desk to pick up your backcountry permit (preferably reserved well in advance). Permit in hand, drive through the entrance station and go north another 6.3 miles, then turn left at a sign for Lupine Meadows Trailhead. Proceed 1.5 miles on this washboarded gravel road and park in the huge lot for the road-end trailhead.

> **NOTE:** Along most of its trails, Grand Teton National Park employs camping "zones," in which backpackers are allowed to select their own site somewhere within that zone. Some of these zones extend for miles, so precisely where you end up spending the night in your "zone" depends on your preferences in a site, what places are already occupied by other hikers, and your ambition level. Because exact campsite locations are flexible, the daily distances and elevation gains shown in the itinerary (on p. 112) are only approximations.

DESCRIPTION ••

Although equally dramatic in either direction, the spacing of campsites makes a counterclockwise circuit preferable, so begin by walking 0.4 mile back north along the gravel entrance road, and then turning left onto the unsigned Moose Ponds Trail just before the road crosses a trickling creek. Follow this little-used

TAKE THIS TRIP

For nearly any backpacker who has been there, the Teton Range is on their short list of the most spectacular mountains they have ever visited. In fact, in many cases that is a short list of *one*. With their jaw-dropping views, sky-scraping peaks, acres of wildflowers, plenty of wildlife, and amazing sunsets and sunrises . . . well, if it wasn't cheating to rate them higher than 10 on this book's scenery scale, then the Tetons would come in somewhere around 18. This wonderful loop visits all the major highlights of this range and provides access to several side trips that lead to some outstanding lesser-known wonders.

Given the amazing scenery, it is not surprising that the trails here are very popular. If you haven't reserved a permit (a big mistake, especially in July and August) you will have to show up *very* early and wait in line to get one of the permits set aside for hikers on a first-come, first-served basis. Be flexible about which campsites you want to use, and be prepared to wait an extra day or two to get a permit for the area you want to visit. The backcountry office at the Moose Junction Visitors Center opens at 8 A.M., although hikers without a reservation should arrive well before that time to get in line.

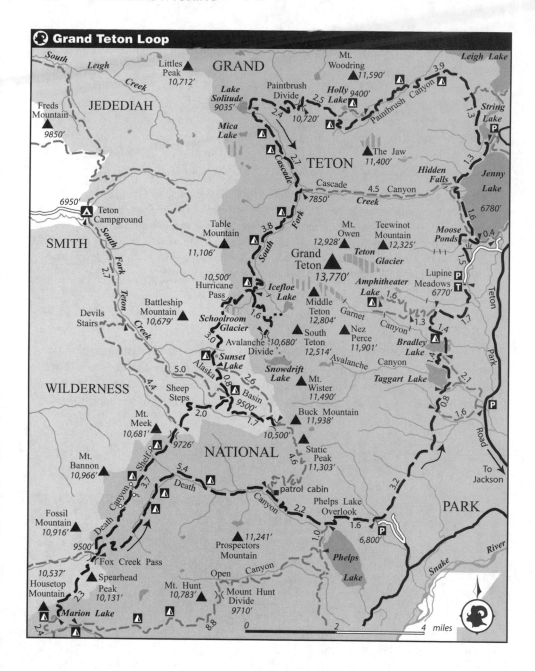

Grand Teton Loop

path as it goes gradually through a lovely lower-elevation valley environment of quaking aspens, lodgepole pines, Engelmann spruces, a few Douglas firs, grasses, and wildflowers. After making a bridged crossing of a small creek, the trail loops around the marshy Moose Ponds. Don't be surprised if you see the pond's namesake animal feeding here, especially in the morning. Even if there are no moose around, you can always enjoy an excellent view across the marsh to craggy Teewinot Mountain. The grassy areas near the marsh host many wild-flowers, including coneflower, goldenrod, harebell, cow parsnip, birchleaf spiraea, and aster. Atop a small ridge just east of Moose Ponds is a junction.

Turn left on a wide, heavily used trail and go 0.15 mile to a second junction where you bear right on the extremely popular lower loop trail around Jenny Lake. Expect to encounter large numbers of dayhikers over the next few miles. After about 1.3 miles you pass a series of junctions with short spur trails to the lake, boat ramps, and other destinations. Stay on the main lake trail on the forested hillside above Jenny Lake, generally following signs to String Lake. The trail goes up and down a bit but is easy throughout. In late July and August look for blooming monkshood (a tall blue wildflower) and ripe thimbleberries (which look and taste like tart raspberries). The trail passes along the fire-damaged northwest shore of Jenny Lake and then follows the lake's cascading inlet creek up to a junction shortly before you reach still-unseen String Lake.

Turn left and cross a mostly open hillside above narrow, marshy String Lake, whose shore is choked with lily pads. At 5.7 miles is a junction. Veer left (uphill), following signs to Paintbrush Canyon, and soon climb out of the lower-elevation vegetation zone with its characteristic sagebrush and aspens and enter a mountain zone with firs and manzanita.

The trail now makes a long and very gradual uphill into Paintbrush Canyon, an extremely impressive defile with towering peaks on both sides. At about 7 miles the trail enters the Lower Paintbrush Camping Zone (the first legal place for you to camp), passing several signed spur trails to possible campsites. Although all of these sites are comfortable, convenient locations for the first night, the views here are not as spectacular as those in the Upper Paintbrush Camping Zone about 3 miles ahead. In the middle of the lower camping zone, a trail bridge takes you over Paintbrush Canyon's rampaging creek, after which it's more uphill, now mostly over open rocky slopes where you can look across the canyon to numerous waterfalls streaking down the steep, north-facing slopes.

The trail now makes a series of short switchbacks climbing into ever-more-spectacular mountain terrain, featuring meadows, rocky cliffs, wildflowers, snowfields, and generally terrific alpine scenery. At 9.6 miles you reach a junction with the trail to Holly Lake, a pleasant pool, with a possible campsite and nice swimming. The main trail goes left at the junction and ascends through gorgeous alpine country into the Upper Paintbrush Camping Zone. There are great campsites here with terrific views of the surrounding peaks and ridges. Camping is allowed only on the left (south) side of the trail until the upper junction with the Holly Lake Loop. Wildlife sightings are common on this trail, with black bears often seen in the lower canyon, marmots and pikas at higher elevations, and Clark's nutcrackers, western tanagers, and various other birds found throughout. Common wildflowers in the alpine meadows of Upper Paintbrush Canyon include gentian, grass of Parnassus, Lewis monkeyflower, aster, spiraea, arnica, and, of course, paintbrush.

The trail ascends through rocky terrain and past a small lake to the upper junction with Holly Lake Trail, where you go left and continue uphill. Only a few hardy conifers, especially whitebark pines, survive here and you eventually leave even those trees behind as you climb into the world of rocks, snow, and tufts of grass to 10,720-foot Paintbrush Divide, the highest point on this circuit with the views to match that distinction. For birders this is a good place to look for black rosy finches, a bird that thrives at these high altitudes. On the down side, the pass often remains blocked by snow until late July or even August. Hikers traveling before that time should ask about current conditions when they pick up their permit. An ice axe may come in handy.

From the divide you descend long switchbacks on an open hillside with great views of hulking Grand Teton to the southeast, the deep U-shaped canyon of Cascade Creek to the south, and shimmering Lake Solitude in a basin to the west. Despite the seemingly harsh environment, countless wildflowers, including a lovely white columbine, grow here. The long switchbacks eventually take you to stunningly beautiful but misnamed Lake Solitude, which sits in a classic mountain setting with lots of wildflowers, cliffs around the shore, and tiny rocky islands. Camping is strictly prohibited and horses are not allowed near this heavily used lake.

The trail descends from the lake, crossing the flower-banked outlet creek and several more small streams that converge to form North Fork Cascade Creek. About 0.7 mile below Lake Solitude, you enter the North Fork Cascade Camping Zone, which has numerous signed spur trails to extremely scenic campsites. Views of the tall canyon walls here are almost as good as those in Paintbrush Canyon, and the view to the southeast of huge Grand Teton is a real jaw-dropper. The camping zone ends just before a bridged crossing of the creek, after which you descend into increasingly forested terrain for almost 1 mile to a second bridged crossing of the creek. Just 0.1 mile later is a major junction.

The more heavily used trail goes left on its way down Cascade Canyon to Jenny Lake. For this loop, however, you turn right on South Fork Cascade Trail, following signs to Hurricane Pass. This trail steadily ascends the west side of fast-moving South Fork Cascade Creek, which more closely resembles a series of small interconnected waterfalls than a "cascade." After 0.6 mile you enter a small, lower basin and the start of the South Cascade Camping Zone, through which you will hike for the next few miles. The trail then climbs a series of short switchbacks taking you into a lovely middle basin, which provides outstanding views of the tall double summit of towering Table Mountain.

From the bottom of the middle basin the trail goes very gradually uphill for 0.5 mile and then ascends a series of switchbacks to an impressive upper basin with numerous terrific campsites, nearby waterfalls, and fine views of Table Mountain, South Cascade Canyon, and a portion of Middle Teton.

About halfway through this gorgeous upper basin is a signed junction and the start of the not-to-be-missed side trip to Avalanche Divide. To make the side trip, turn left on a narrow path that gradually ascends a series of irregularly spaced switchbacks as it climbs for 1.6 miles from meadows to well above treeline at the 10,680-foot divide. Along this scenic trail you pass several shallow ponds and enjoy terrific views of South Teton, but the view from trail's end at Avalanche

Divide is the real attraction. Grand, Middle, and South Teton (all of which look sandy colored from this angle), as well as Table Mountain and Jackson Hole, are all prominently on display, while below you to the east is the scenic basin holding Snowdrift Lake. That lake is well worth a downhill cross-country scramble to visit. If all this isn't enough, there is yet another great destination in this area, Icefloe Lake. To reach it, return on the trail from Avalanche Divide about 0.5 mile, then leave the trail and scramble uphill to the north-northeast over meadows and rocks for about 0.6 mile to this stark, often icebound gem. The view over the lake of Middle and Grand Teton is truly outstanding.

After returning from the side trip to Avalanche Divide and Icefloe Lake, continue up the South Fork Cascade Trail through lovely meadows to a sign announcing the end of the South Cascade Camping Zone. From there you climb a series of switchbacks past the small and rapidly melting Schoolroom Glacier to Hurricane Pass, set in a rolling tundralike environment well above treeline. The view here can hold its own against that from any other place in North America. To the west are the wheat fields and potato farms of Idaho and the numerous cliffs and alpine valleys of the western Tetons. To the north is nearby Table Mountain and more distant Mt. Moran. But the real jaw-dropper is to the east, where you have an eye-level look at Grand, Middle, and South Teton scraping the clear blue sky. Although the view is best in the afternoon, when the sun is behind you and on the peaks, this is also when thunderstorms often build in these mountains, which is no time to be above treeline.

The trail goes left at the pass, climbing a bit more to a 10,500-foot high point where signs indicate that you leave Grand Teton National Park and enter Targhee National Forest and Jedediah Smith Wilderness. Wildlife you might see in this harsh alpine environment includes marmots, ravens, and water pipits. The wildly scenic route descends gradually past the impressive crags of Battleship Mountain and then descends several short switchbacks to a huge sloping meadow alive with colorful wildflowers in late July. At the bottom of this meadow you pass shallow but very scenic Sunset Lake and its several good but often crowded campsites.

From Sunset Lake the trail climbs about 200 feet to a junction atop a minor ridge, where you go straight on the main trail and contour for about 0.4 mile before descending a series of switchbacks into Alaska Basin. This lovely basin is a delightful mix of meadows, small lakes, scattered trees, and rocky outcroppings with numerous possible campsites scattered around the basin. Wilderness rules prohibit horse camping, any camping within 100 feet of water, and all fires.

Near the north end of the basin you pass a junction with a trail going sharply right to South Fork Teton Creek. You go straight and then, 150 yards later, reach a second junction at the start of a fun possible side trip to Buck Mountain Pass. To make the side trip, turn left and go gradually uphill through the upper part of Alaska Basin past shallow ponds and small lakes. Once above this inviting area, the trail slowly winds up into ever-more-stark, rocky terrain. After 1.7 miles go right at a junction and make a final short uphill push to reach the park boundary at Buck Mountain Pass, which has fine views down to Jackson Hole and of the nearby summits of Buck Mountain and Static Peak. If you still have energy, continue on the trail another 0.9 mile to the even higher views from Static Peak Divide, the highest point in Grand Teton National Park reachable by a maintained trail.

Back in Alaska Basin, the trail goes south, traveling up and down over meadows and amazingly flat rocky areas polished by ancient glaciers. Since the tread often disappears on these rocky surfaces, watch for cairns and rocks lining the path to stay on course. The trail crosses South Fork Teton Creek just below a nice campsite at the south end of Alaska Basin and then gradually loses elevation before making seven uphill switchbacks on a section of trail locally known as the Sheep Steps. From here a bit of gradual climbing through open alpine terrain leads to a junction.

Go straight and walk 0.3 mile up to 9726-foot Mount Meek Pass. Signs announce your reentry into Grand Teton National Park, but you may not notice them since your attention is more likely to turn to the view. Most appealing are the views north of the cluster of jagged summits making up the Tetons and to the southwest along the sheer cliffs that rise both above and below a strip of surprisingly gentle terrain called Death Canyon Shelf. This shelf between the towering cliffs on your right and the steep drop-off on your left hosts the trail for the next few miles. Most of the shelf is a designated camping zone and the sites are wildly scenic. Water is spotty at best, however, with only a few tiny springs and creeks along the way. Many of these creeks disappear into rocky sinkholes on the shelf only to reemerge as springs on the cliffs below. Death Canyon Shelf appears to be the center of Grand Teton National Park's marmot population, as these chubby, whistling fur balls seem to be everywhere. You may also be fortunate enough to spot a friendly long-tailed weasel. Some of the most common varieties of the abundant wildflowers on the shelf include pink geranium, blue lupine, yellow marigold, and sky-blue flax. The shelf's most outstanding feature, however, is the view, especially down into steep-sided Death Canyon to the east. At the south end of Death Canyon Shelf you reach Fox Creek Pass, where there is a junction. The main loop trail goes left (northeast and downhill), but for a fine side trip, consider continuing south for 2.3 miles on the very scenic Teton Crest Trail, which wanders over rolling meadowlands before dropping to Marion Lake. This shallow gem has good campsites and a fine setting beneath the tall, striated cliffs of Housetop Mountain.

After returning to the junction at Fox Creek Pass, you turn northeast and immediately descend a series of fairly steep switchbacks down for 1 mile into the huge meadow-covered bowl at the head of Death Canyon. At the bottom of the switchbacks, cross a creek and turn to follow it downstream. About 1 mile later you enter the Death Canyon Camping Zone, which you will travel through for the next several miles. Although the campsites in the upper part of the zone are more scenic, the ones at the lower end of the zone are more convenient for hikers looking to make the final day's hike back to the car a more reasonable length.

Despite its ominous name, Death Canyon is a joy, with a mix of huge meadows, strips of forest, plenty of wildlife, and dramatic views up from the willow flats near the creek to the precipitous canyon walls. The trail remains quite gentle, so the walking is not only scenic but relatively easy. The trail crosses the creek twice on log bridges and passes numerous signed spur trails leading to designated campsites along the way. As the canyon curves to the right (east) it becomes increasingly wooded and the stream drops more steeply in boisterous cascades. The lower canyon is particularly steep and dramatic with contorted walls that tower thousands of feet on either side. Views are frequent and remarkable. You leave the camping zone at yet another log bridge over the creek and continue in forest and meadows to the log patrol cabin at the junction with the Alaska Basin Trail. Go straight and begin descending numerous rocky switchbacks with open views of the stupendous walls to the south and east down toward large and tranquil Phelps Lake.

Near the bottom of the switchbacks you reenter the park's lower vegetation zone, with its characteristic thimbleberries, cottonwoods, Douglas firs, lodgepole pines, and quaking aspens. Wildflowers here differ from the alpine types and include horsemint, coneflower, and balsamroot, all growing on slopes covered with sagebrush. While still on the hillside well above Phelps Lake, you reach a junction with the Valley Trail. Go straight (slightly uphill) and ascend two long switchbacks to Phelps Lake Overlook at the top of a spur ridge. From here the wide, heavily used trail goes gradually downhill in open forest to a junction about 100 yards from Death Canyon Trailhead.

With two cars (or one person to guard the packs while another hikes on) you can end your hike here. Otherwise, hike north on the Valley Trail as it goes very gradually up and down through an open forest of Douglas fir, quaking aspen, and lodgepole pine at the base of the Teton Range. You cross a few intermittent streams along the way, but this is generally dry country, especially by late July

Clouds above the mouth of Death Canyon

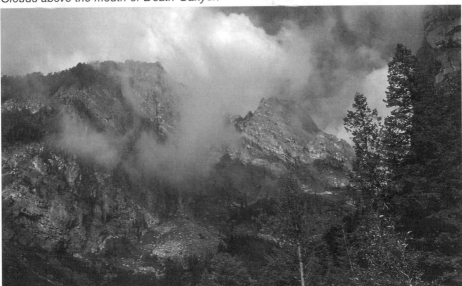

and August when the high country is free enough of snow to make this loop possible. After 3.2 miles go straight at a junction with the Beaver Creek Trail then climb some lazy switchbacks over a mostly shadeless ridge recovering from an old burn and drop to a junction near a bridge over the outlet of Taggart Lake. This lovely, medium-sized lake is a popular destination for dayhikers, so don't expect to be alone. What you can expect is the feature that draws all those day-hikers, fine reflections in the lake's forest-rimmed waters of the rugged spires of the Teton Range.

The trail goes north along the east shore of Taggart Lake then climbs two long switchbacks over an ancient moraine to a junction near the southeast shore of Bradley Lake. Slightly smaller than similar Taggart Lake, Bradley reflects the top of Grand Teton and has a comfortable campsite on its north shore that is open only to hikers doing the loop around the Tetons.

To finish the hike, continue on the Valley Trail as it crosses a bridge over a part of Bradley Lake, climbs northwest to the top of a ridge, then levels out in a mead-ow and comes to a major junction. A very busy but extremely scenic trail goes left on its way up to popular Amphitheater Lake and Garnet Canyon (a worthwhile side trip), but you turn right and descend the top of a small ridge before looping north and ending your journey back at the Lupine Meadows Trailhead.

POSSIBLE ITINERARY

	CAMPS & SIDE TRIP	MILES	ELEVATION GAIN
DAY 1	Upper Paintbrush Canyon	10.5	3300'
DAY 2	South Fork Cascade Creek	10.5	2950'
DAY 3	Alaska Basin, including side trips to Avalanche Divide, Icefloe Lake, and Buck Mountain Pass	12.0	3300'
DAY 4	Death Canyon, including a side trip to Marion Lake	12.4	1400'
DAY 5	Bradley Lake	12.8	600'
DAY 6	Out	2.8	250'

VARIATIONS

One enticing way to lengthen this trip, while maintaining the basic loop, is to skip Death Canyon and opt instead to go south from Fox Creek Pass on the Teton Crest Trail. A little past Marion Lake turn east and return via Mount Hunt Divide and Open Canyon to Phelps Lake. This option adds 6.9 miles to your trip and misses spectacular Death Canyon, but it also visits more of the great scenery that characterizes the high country of Grand Teton National Park. With a second car, another option is to forego the loop entirely and exit via the Teton Crest Trail at a trailhead along Wyoming Highway 22 west of Jackson.

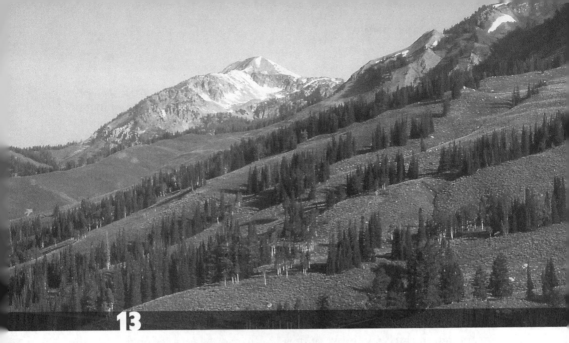

13

GRANITE CREEK
& GRANITE HIGHLINE LOOP

RATINGS: Scenery 8   Solitude 6   Difficulty 7

MILES: 32.5

ELEVATION GAIN: 6400´

DAYS: 3–5

MAPS: USGS *Bull Creek, Crystal Peak, Granite Falls,* and *Turquoise Lake*

USUALLY OPEN: July to mid-October

BEST: Mid-July and early August

CONTACT: Jackson Ranger District, Bridger-Teton National Forest

SPECIAL ATTRACTIONS: Miles of high meadows covered with wildflowers; excellent views; plenty of wildlife

PERMIT: None required.

RULES ·

Groups are limited to 15 people.

CHALLENGES ·

The area has a few grizzly bears—camp and act accordingly. The Granite Highline Trail frequently disappears, so patience and route-finding skills are required. Turquoise Lake is often crowded on weekends. Parts of the Granite Highline Trail have lots of cattle.

Photo: Pinnacle Peak from Granite Highline Trail

HOW TO GET THERE ·

From Hoback Junction where U.S. Highways 26 and 191/189 converge about 12 miles south of Jackson, drive 11.8 miles east on Highway 191/189 to a junction with Granite Creek Road (Forest Service Road 30500). Turn left (north) on this bumpy but good gravel road, and go 7.8 miles to a signed junction. The Granite Highline Trail, your return route, meets the road here, coming in from the left (west). To find the starting point and trailhead parking lot, turn right at the junction, drive 0.2 mile, crossing a bridge over Granite Creek, then turn left where the road forks and go 100 yards to the trailhead parking area.

DESCRIPTION ·

From the trailhead head north up the wide canyon of Granite Creek on a gated jeep track that wanders very gradually uphill through a land of sagebrush, wildflowers, and open views of the towering peaks of the Gros Ventre Range. After just 75 yards the jeep road curves to the right, but you veer left on a trail that soon takes you past a series of active beaver ponds. Early in the morning you may be lucky enough to catch a glimpse of these industrious large rodents. After the ponds the trail passes a pair of large springs and at 1.6 miles crosses the hillside above loud, impressive Granite Falls. Since the view from the trail is a bit restricted, the best place to get a good look at this falls is from a roadside viewpoint on the other side of the canyon. This spot is worth driving to and checking out either before or after your hike. At 1.9 miles is Granite Hot Springs, where there is a developed resort complete with picnic tables, soaking pools, and a footbridge linking the hot spring with a resort complex on the west side of the creek.

TAKE THIS TRIP

The Gros Ventre Range is always a delightful area to hike because of its grand scenery and surprising solitude. Except for around Turquoise Lake, where solitude is a rarity, this trip has plenty of both features. It also includes some of the best high-elevation meadow hiking in Wyoming, with mile after mile of lush, wildflower-covered meadows and extensive views along the magnificent Granite Highline Trail. Wildlife is abundant as well, so it is the rare hiker who completes this loop without seeing at least a few moose and elk.

But the truth is that it is the rare hiker who completes this loop *at all*, a fact attested to by the frustratingly large number of times that the Granite Highline Trail simply disappears amid steeply sloping meadows leaving the confused backpacker to pull out her contour map and search in vain for a tread that lies hidden beneath the wildflowers and lost amid a maze of livestock trails. Good map-reading skills and plenty of patience are required, but the loop's magnificent scenery, and especially its miles of outstanding meadows, are worth the aggravation.

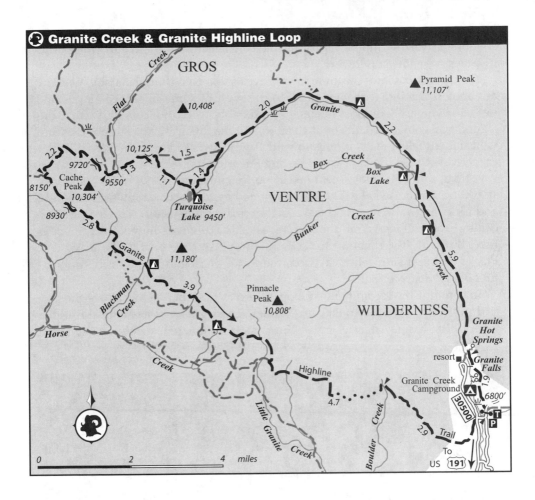

Granite Creek & Granite Highline Loop

GROS

VENTRE

WILDERNESS

Pyramid Peak
11,107'

10,408'

2.0

Granite

2.2

10,125'

1.5

Box   Creek

Box
Lake

2.2

9720'

1.3

1.4

Cache

9550'

1.1

8150'   Peak

10,304'

Turquoise
Lake 9450'

Creek

8930'

2.8

Bunker

Granite

5.9

11,180'

Creek

Granite

3.9

Pinnacle
Peak

10,808'

Granite
Hot
Springs

Blackman

resort

Granite
Falls

Horse

Creek

Highline

Granite Creek
Campground

6800'

4.7

30500

Little Granite

Creek

2.9   Trail

Boulder   Creek

To
US 191

0   2   4   miles

Your trail continues straight on a sometimes rugged up-and-down route through meadows and forest. At about 4 miles you enter a large burn area where you have a good chance of seeing several different species of woodpeckers; they feed on the insects that burrow into the decaying wood of the burned snags. At a little more than 5 miles the canyon starts to open up as the valley widens, and views of the surrounding peaks and ridges become more impressive. Also here are the first of numerous good campsites, which are scattered over the next several miles. Arguing in favor of a night in this area is the fact that Granite Creek offers good wildlife watching, especially for moose in the willow flats along the creek, and good fishing. As for views, red-tinged Pyramid Peak looms impressively over the eastern wall of the valley.

At 7.8 miles is a confusing and unsigned fork. The well-traveled trail to the left leads to a creek ford and an outfitter's camp below Box Lake. Go right on what looks like the lesser-used trail, and begin a gradual but unrelenting climb. As the canyon curves west you pass through a series of lush, sloping meadows filled with tall wildflowers that often crowd the path and will soak your lower body if it has rained recently. The most abundant flowers are monument plant, coneflower, yarrow, lupine, larkspur, wild carrot, geranium, and particularly fine displays of yellow sunflowers.

The mountain views continue to improve as you pass a large marshy meadow at about 10.5 miles with fine vistas to the west of some unnamed ridges and peaks. If you are like most hikers, you probably won't notice a very faint, unsigned trail going north at about 10 miles, but the fork at 12 miles is obvious and well signed. Take the left branch toward Turquoise Lake and soon cross hillsides carpeted with wildflowers and featuring fine mountain views.

A final, tiring 500-foot ascent takes you to a junction at 13.4 miles just above sparkling Turquoise Lake. The lake is rimmed by heather meadows, open forest, and rocky areas and has good views of the surrounding peaks. A pretty little cascading waterfall feeds into the lake's west side. There are numerous campsites here, but with its proximity to Jackson, Turquoise Lake gets fairly heavy use. Please choose a site well away from the water and be especially careful about following "no trace" rules.

To continue the recommended loop, return to the junction just above the lake and go northwest on a trail that contours across grassy slopes and through a lovely little basin. After 1.1 miles you come to a junction where you turn left

Cache Peak

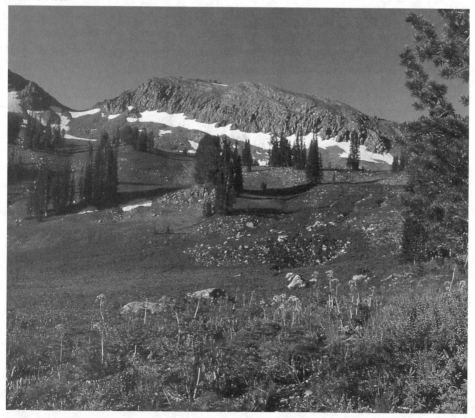

and climb to a 10,125-foot pass. From here there are fine views of Cache Peak to the west-southwest and the distant Teton Range to the northwest. The trail now gradually descends across gentle slopes on the north side of a ridge for 0.8 mile to where you splash across the cascading headwaters of Flat Creek and come to a junction. Keep straight and walk 0.2 mile to a second junction, this one situated in a scenic basin beneath the rounded hump of Cache Peak.

The Goodwin Lake Trail goes straight at this junction, but you turn left, following signs to Cache Creek, and make a very brief climb to another pass. Now you must negotiate a long downhill, first steeply on rocky tread, then down a series of lazy switchbacks over wildflower-covered slopes. As you descend, you will enjoy fine views of the Teton Range, Jackson Hole, and the Snake River Range. At just a little more than 2 miles from the pass look carefully for the junction with the faint Granite Highline Trail, which goes to the left.

Turn onto the Granite Highline Trail and almost immediately discover what will be the dominant feature of this path for the next several miles: lush and overgrown meadows filled with tall wildflowers. The trail begins with an 800-foot climb to an open grassy pass. Here the trail pulls the first of several disappearing acts (get used to it) amid a confusion of wildflowers and game trails. You will need a good contour map, plenty of patience, and good navigation instincts to stay on course. Whenever possible, try to avoid traveling off-trail on the steepest slopes in this area since the lush vegetation makes for tiring, treacherous footing. The terrain is generally open, making navigation pretty easy.

From the pass the proper course goes slightly uphill for about 0.2 mile, and then heads east-southeast, contouring for about 1.5 miles before you cross a creek and climb to the next grassy ridgetop. The Forest Service map confidently shows a trail junction here, but no sign of it exists on the ground. In any event, your trail stays high, still crossing steep slopes covered with wildflowers and with views that seem to extend forever. Gradually gain elevation on a reasonably distinct path that dips into gullies and goes over or around little spur ridges. Shade is almost impossible to find so the hiking can be hot, but it is always inspiring. Established campsites are rare to nonexistent, but the terrain flattens out enough for camping at the crossing of Blackman Creek near 21.5 miles and again near 24 miles in the trees near a small creek and marshy area just below the trail. Anywhere you choose to camp will be extremely scenic.

Just after the camp near the small creek and marshy area, you pass below a tiny unseen pond, then another phantom Forest Service junction before coming to the top of a grassy ridge. Immediately on the other side of this ridge is an unsigned but obvious junction with a trail going to the right. You go straight and descend to a step-over crossing of Little Granite Creek. Soon after this crossing you descend again, still on the glorious wildflower-covered slopes that typify this trail. After losing about 400 feet from the creek crossing you may see a faint trail going to the right, which continues down Little Granite Creek. You go left, sticking with the Highline Trail, picking it out as best you can from a confusion of livestock paths. The proper trail soon rounds another little ridge and heads almost due east generally contouring or going slightly uphill. Do not be fooled by an official-looking livestock trail that goes gradually downhill toward a large flat meadow. (Don't ask me how I know this, just believe me.) The correct trail climbs to the top of yet another ridge from which you can look back to the northwest for fine views of Pinnacle Peak.

Unless you are super-human you are bound to lose the trail in the next mile or so. Cattle are the main problem, as they merrily create new trails all over the place. Check your contour map frequently to remain more or less on course, if not on the actual tread. Once (re)located the official trail stays fairly high as it goes over a couple more small ridges and enters a 2007 burn area. After crossing Boulder Creek, you climb a bit on a more distinct path following a hillside to the southeast. Eventually the trail loses elevation, then curves back to the northeast and gradually descends to the Granite Creek Road (Forest Service Road 30500) directly opposite where the spur road to the trailhead goes to the east. It is an easy 0.2-mile roadwalk from here to the trailhead.

POSSIBLE ITINERARY

	CAMPS & SIDE TRIPS	MILES	ELEVATION GAIN
DAY 1	Turquoise Lake	13.4	2800′
DAY 2	Granite Highline (plus a number of wandering-around-in-search-of-the-tread miles)	10.6	2700′
DAY 3	Out, with a 0.2-mile roadwalk back to the trailhead	8.5	900′

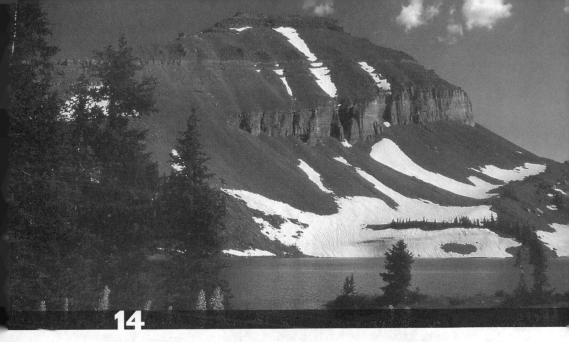

14

BREWSTER LAKE
& GROS VENTRE RIVER LOOP

RATINGS: Scenery 10   Solitude 8   Difficulty 8
MILES: 37.2
ELEVATION GAIN: 9200´
DAYS: 4–7
MAPS: USGS *Crystal Peak, Darwin Peak, Doubletop Peak,* and *Granite Falls*
USUALLY OPEN: Mid-July to mid-October
BEST: Late July and August
CONTACT: Big Piney and Jackson ranger districts, Bridger-Teton National Forest
SPECIAL ATTRACTIONS: Outstanding mountain scenery; the chance to visit spectacular Brewster Lake ("Wow" simply doesn't cover it); plenty of solitude
PERMIT: None required

RULES ·

Groups are limited to 15 people.

CHALLENGES ·

The area has a few grizzly bears—camp and act accordingly. The route has an extended but mostly easy cross-country section (with one short but quite challenging segment) and sketchy trails in places.

Photo: Triangle Peak over Brewster Lake

TAKE THIS TRIP

This magnificent loop includes arguably the best scenery in the Gros Ventre Wilderness, which anyone who has traveled in this vast preserve will realize is an extremely high recommendation. From towering waterfalls to huge wildflower-sprinkled meadows to cliff-edged peaks to amazingly beautiful Brewster Lake, this loop has so much mountain scenery it is positively overwhelming. Amazingly, the loop also has so few people the trail occasionally disappears amid the wildflowers. Other than a concerted effort by locals to keep this range a secret (to which they readily admit), I have no adequate explanation for the lack of crowds. But don't complain, just enjoy the solitude amidst some of the best mountain scenery in the continental U.S.

Completing the recommended loop requires an extended cross-country section that is entirely above treeline and should not be attempted in questionable weather. In good weather, however, almost the entire off-trail portion is relatively easy rambling over tundra and snowfields, which is well within the abilities of any hiker with reasonably good navigation and map-reading skills. There is, however, one 0.2-mile segment that is very challenging and requires some steep scrambling on a rocky track. Experienced hikers should have no problems, but novice hikers and anyone who is afraid of heights should take the long way around to Brewster Lake.

HOW TO GET THERE

From Hoback Junction where U.S. Highways 26 and 191/189 converge about 12 miles south of Jackson, drive 11.8 miles east on Highway 191/189 to a junction with Granite Creek Road (Forest Service Road 30500). Turn left (north) on this bumpy but good gravel road and go 7.8 miles to a signed junction. Turn right, drive 0.2 mile, crossing a bridge over Granite Creek, then turn left where the road forks and go 100 yards to the trailhead parking area.

DESCRIPTION

Several trails meet at or near this popular trailhead. The most heavily traveled route goes north up the canyon of Granite Creek (see Trip 13, page 113). For this trip, however, you go east on a trail that begins at the northeast corner of the parking area beside a small sign saying SHOAL FALLS.

Right from the start the scenery on this hike is impressive. Tall peaks of the Gros Ventre Range rise above you, while open forests, meadows, and rolling sagebrush flats allow almost unlimited views. Beginning in one of those sagebrush flats, the trail gradually ascends into forest and settles in for a slow, steady climb. The route follows Swift Creek for almost 0.5 mile, and then turns right where a spur trail goes left to the creek and a junction with your return trail.

From here you gradually lose elevation for 0.1 mile to a second junction. The trail going straight (downhill) leads to a horse facility.

Turn left and ascend a dozen or so curving switchbacks to the top of a rounded ridge. The summit area rewards your efforts with a glory of rolling meadows featuring fine views of an unnamed 11,086-foot mountain to the northeast and the distant Wyoming Range to the southwest. The meadows are also carpeted with wildflowers in early to mid-July; look for geranium, arrowleaf balsamroot, phlox, buckwheat, monument plant, flax, aster, lupine, horsemint, groundsel, vetch, larkspur, wild carrot, coneflower, and dozens more. The meadows are rimmed with a varied forest of aspens, firs, lodgepole pines, and Douglas firs.

The trail eventually tops an indistinct high point on the ridge and then descends about 400 feet to cross small West Shoal Creek. From there more uphill, first in forest then in meadows, leads to a pass on Deer Ridge. From this pass there are thrilling views to the northeast of Palmer Peak and the deep meadow-filled valley of Shoal Creek. Over the next mile you descend fairly steeply into that valley to a campsite a bit before the easy calf-deep ford of Shoal Creek. Just upstream from this crossing are some active beaver dams, and above those you can see and hear the thunderous cataract of Shoal Falls.

Just 100 yards after the crossing of Shoal Creek is a junction. If you want to visit Shoal Falls, turn left, pass a fine campsite after 0.1 mile, and continue through forest and flood-damaged areas for 0.3 mile to the base of the impressive cataract, which tumbles down a cliff-edged chute.

The main trail veers right (uphill) from the junction above the ford and takes you to a junction with a trail that continues downstream. You keep left and climb, often steeply, on a rocky tread through lovely meadows and across partly forested hillsides to a second ford of Shoal Creek at about 7.5 miles. Above this crossing you climb very steeply for about 1 mile before things get easier where you pass some wet meadows and reach a possible campsite near the third crossing of Shoal Creek. The next 0.6 mile includes a fourth and final crossing of Shoal Creek but is otherwise an easy climb in meadows and rocky areas to the shores of Shoal Lake. In a word, the lake is beautiful. Rimmed by sloping meadows and rocky cliffs, and with plenty of potential campsites, Shoal Lake invites hikers to spend some time taking in its beauty and may even convince them to spend an extra day.

The trail crosses the outlet creek of Shoal Lake and then ascends rocky slopes to a 10,300-foot pass. Make room on your list of the best viewpoints you have ever seen, because this spot is a candidate. Most striking are the views to the north of Black Peak and east of Darwin Peak, both rimmed with towering cliffs.

From this pass you have a choice. For a shorter loop, continue down the trail 1.9 miles to its junction with the Gros Ventre River Trail and turn left. (See the later description in this trip, p. 125, for a continuation of this shorter loop.) Unfortunately, without a very long side trip, this loop misses spectacular Brewster Lake. So, if you don't mind a rather long but for the most part fairly easy cross-country section, turn right (east-southeast) leaving the trail and heading over alpine terrain toward Darwin Peak.

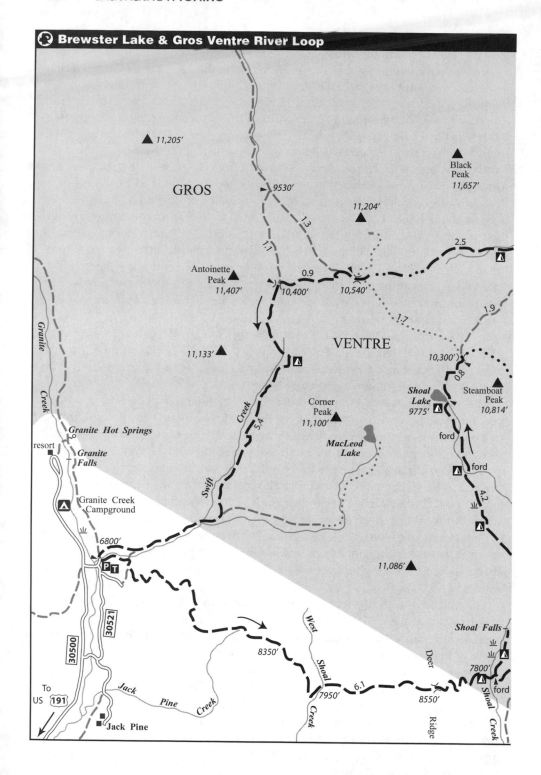

Brewster Lake & Gros Ventre River Loop

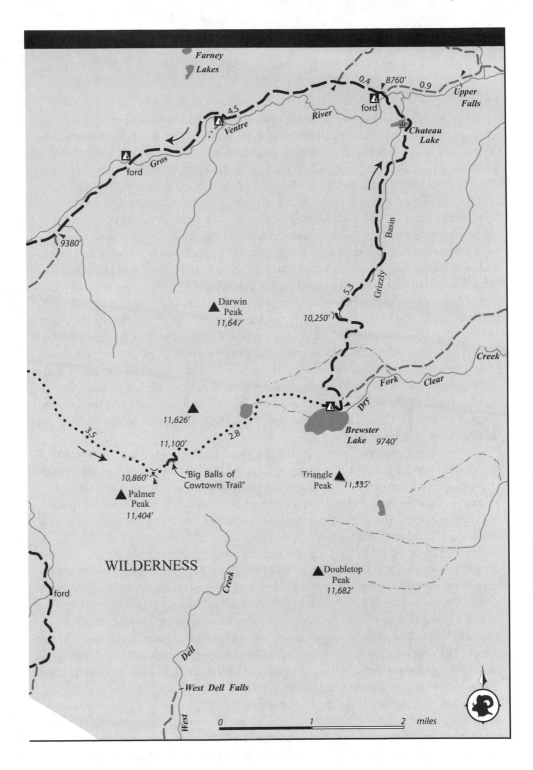

Farney
Lakes

0.4   8760'   0.9

ford

Upper
Falls

4.5

River

Ventre

Chateau
Lake

ford   Gros

9380'

Basin

Grizzly

5.3

Darwin
Peak
11,641'

10,250'

Creek

Fork   Clear

Dry

11,626'

2.8

Brewster
Lake   9740'

3.5

11,100'

"Big Balls of
Cowtown Trail"

Triangle
Peak   11,335'

10,860'

Palmer
Peak
11,404'

WILDERNESS

Creek

Doubletop
Peak
11,682'

ford

Dell

West Dell Falls

West

0   1   2   miles

WARNINGS: Although generally easy, this cross-country section eventually includes one short but very challenging section that requires some very steep scrambling on a rocky and slippery tread. Novice hikers should not attempt it. In addition, *no one* should begin this cross-country section if the weather is iffy at all, as the entire way is exposed and above treeline.

If the above warnings don't scare you off, wander off-trail along a gentle alpine plateau, staying level or climbing very gradually over rocks, tundra, and snowfields as you round the northeast side of Steamboat Peak. You then continue southeast past Palmer Peak and climb to a wide, obvious pass north of Darwin Peak's impressive cliffs and about 3.5 miles from the pass above Shoal Lake.

Once at this pass you will see a long sloping bench heading southeast toward Doubletop Peak. This bench is lined with several unbroken miles of tall cliffs on its left (northeast) side, which seem to completely block your access north toward Brewster Lake. But there is a way around them. Look up to your left on the ridge coming off Darwin Peak and you will see a very rugged and faint trail that goes steeply up through the jagged rocks. Take this short, steep, rocky trail—reasonable for experienced hikers who are strong and careful. After a tough 0.2 mile you reach the top of the rugged cliffs and the gentler upper plateau of the ridge. At the top of the route you may find a small flat rock with a message etched into it saying BIG BALLS OF COWTOWN TRAIL—ROBERTSON TRAIL CREW; JULY 2001. (Actually good balance, steady nerves, strong lungs, and strong legs are the trail's only anatomical requirements.) Now on much gentler, rolling, alpine terrain, you go northeast down to an unnamed turquoise lake on the east side of an unnamed peak. Cross the lake's outlet creek and then angle downhill to the east to the north shore of Brewster Lake.

Large, deep Brewster Lake is one of the great undiscovered wonders of Wyoming, and *that's* a competitive category. The lake is rimmed by trees and meadows, has fine views of snowy ridges all around, and sits directly at the base of massive Triangle Peak, which towers almost 2000 feet above the tranquil waters. It is quite a spot. The best campsites—and you will definitely want to spend *at least* one night here—are on the north shore.

To continue the loop, pick up the maintained trail that goes uphill starting about 160 yards west of the lake's outlet creek and follow it as it climbs for 0.1 mile to a fork. Go left to the top of a low ridge, descend a wide gully to cross a small seasonal creek, and then climb over a 10,250-foot pass. From here you make a long descent of wide Grizzly Basin, whose name should remind you that at least a few of those large bruins live in this area. Near the bottom of the gently sloping basin you pass through rolling sagebrush-covered terrain before descending more steeply in forest to small, marshy Chateau Lake, which features a nice reflection of distant Black Peak to the west.

Just below Chateau Lake the trail disappears as it enters the wide, grass- and willow-choked valley of the Gros Ventre River. To relocate the route simply walk northwest near the edge of the big meadow until you come to a ford of the slow-moving, knee-deep river. This ford is almost directly opposite a large hunter's camp. A little east of this camp is a signed junction with the Gros Ventre River

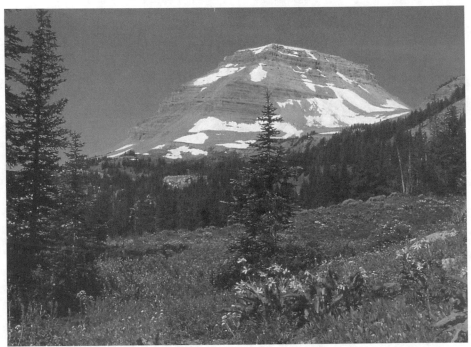

Black Peak over meadow to the east

Trail. If you have some extra time, consider making a side trip 0.9 mile down-stream to Upper Falls, a fairly low but photogenic drop in the river.

The recommended loop trail goes upstream and climbs gradually through forest for 0.4 mile to an unsigned fork. Go left and soon pass along the edge of another huge meadow, this one with particularly fine views of Black and Darwin peaks. After more than a mile of walking beside and through this remarkably flat meadow, the trail forks again. Straight ahead, what looks like the main trail leads 50 yards to a campsite and a ford of the river. The official trail, however, goes right at the fork, avoiding the ford, and climbs in forest to two more large meadows, the last offering exceptional views of blocky, misnamed Black Peak. At the head of the fourth meadow are some possible campsites and another, this time unavoidable, ford of the Gros Ventre River.

After passing above a fifth meadow, you ford a good-sized but unnamed trib-utary creek and almost immediately reach a junction marked with a post. The trail to the left goes up to the pass above Shoal Lake and is part of the shorter loop alternative mentioned previously. You go straight, on what appears to be the lesser-used trail and gradually climb through increasingly alpine meadows with fine views of the surrounding cliffs, peaks, and ridges. Although there are no established sites, wonderfully scenic camping is available almost anywhere in this area.

In the middle of these gorgeous alpine meadows you ford the now-much-smaller Gros Ventre River a final time and continue hiking west as the trail grad-ually disappears. To relocate it, wander west to the head of the meadows where

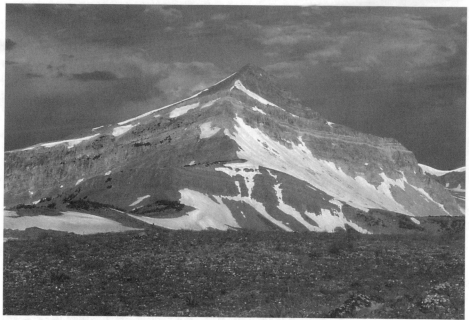

Antoinette Peak from pass to the east

the tread can be found again, but it is at best intermittent for the next couple of miles. What can be found of the trail leads you uphill to the west back into the realm of rocks, snow, and tundra. You eventually top out at a 10,540-foot pass marked with a prominent tall signpost, a good landmark for those who lost the tread below. The views from this pass are outstanding, including not only most of the terrain you have already passed through, but towering Antoinette Peak to the west and the tops of the Teton Range in the distance to the northwest. A worthwhile cross-country exploration from the pass goes north to a small lake tucked in a deep bowl beneath the cliffs of nearby Black Peak.

From the pass, follow the now-obvious trail as it goes downhill for 0.15 mile to a fork. You turn left on a relatively new trail (not shown on the USGS map) and follow bits of tread and strategically placed cairns for 0.8 mile to an unsigned junction at a pass on the east shoulder of Antoinette Peak.

Turn left (south) at the pass and descend a steep but easy-to-follow trail into the canyon of Swift Creek. After 0.9 mile you reach a meadow-covered bench beneath Corner Peak that would make a fine campsite. Another 2 miles of often very steep, rocky downhill takes you past steep canyon walls and fine viewpoints back into forest and an unsigned but obvious junction with an unofficial trail that goes left toward the basin holding MacLeod Lake. Keep straight, soon cross Swift Creek on rickety logs, and wander gradually downhill to a signed junction with the spur trail to the Shoal Falls Trail you passed early on your first day of hiking. Go straight and descend in meadows another 0.4 mile to a junction with a closed jeep track. Turn left and in only 60 yards finish your grand adventure at the Granite Creek Trailhead.

POSSIBLE ITINERARY

	CAMPS & SIDE TRIPS	MILES	ELEVATION GAIN
DAY 1	Shoal Creek	6.0	2250'
DAY 2	Shoal Lake, with a side trip to Shoal Falls	5.1	2200'
DAY 3	Brewster Lake	7.1	1750'
DAY 4	Upper meadows along the Gros Ventre River	10.5	1550'
DAY 5	Out	8.5	1450'

VARIATIONS

Those hikers who prefer to skip the long cross-country section can hike over the pass north of Shoal Lake, take the trail that goes downhill (northeast) from there, and camp in one of the lower meadows along the Gros Ventre River. From there it is a long but reasonable dayhike up to Brewster Lake, although packing in your overnight gear and spending the night at that gorgeous lake is a better plan.

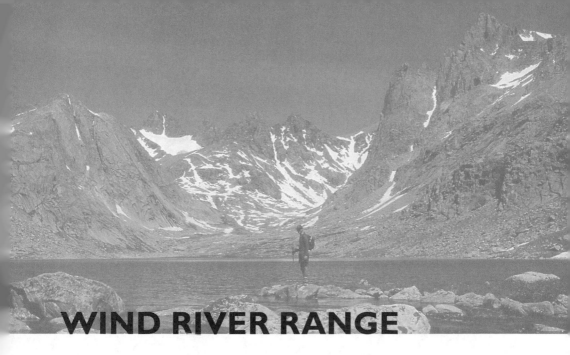

WIND RIVER RANGE

With somewhere between 1,200 and 2,000 lakes (depending on when you start to define a small glacial pond or tarn as a "lake"), the largest glaciers in the American Rockies, the highest peaks in Wyoming, and some of the most scenic terrain *anywhere*, the Wind River Range is defined by superlatives. It also happens to be one of my all-time favorite hiking areas on the continent. And I am certainly not alone. For decades this range has drawn legions of admiring pedestrians, as well as thousands of climbers looking to ascend the solid granite walls and spires that abound in these mountains.

But even with their wide fame, the enormity of the Wind River Range ensures that there is plenty of elbow room for visitors. In fact, in parts of the less popular (but no less beautiful) central portion of the range you can often hike for days in almost perfect solitude. The range's large size and its web of hiking trails make these mountains ideal for the long-distance backpacker, with enough options for dozens of magnificent weeklong adventures. And for hikers who are willing to go off-trail, the possibilities are literally endless, with lakes, meadows, and viewpoints around every corner and each more beautiful than the last. Even if you couldn't care less about the scenery, you might want to visit just to see the unique granite exposed in the central Wind River Range. Scientists have dated some of these rocks as being among the oldest on Earth, more than 3.4 billion years.

This book describes six long backpacking trips in the Wind River Range, and touches on all of the area's most famous attractions. Be aware, however, that there is infinitely more to see; you may fall so in love with these mountains that you find yourself immediately planning more trips here. And more than one person has found that they never want to hike anywhere else for the rest of their lives. Few, if any, of these dedicated souls regret that decision. So don't say I didn't warn you.

Photo: *Upper Titcomb Lake (Trip 15)*

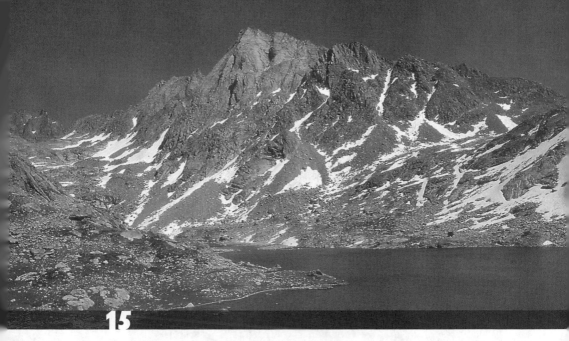

15

GREEN RIVER LAKES
& TITCOMB BASIN LOOP

RATINGS: Scenery 10   Solitude 5   Difficulty 6
MILES: 70.9
ELEVATION GAIN: 10,100´
DAYS: 6–14
MAP: Earthwalk Press *Northern Wind River Range*
USUALLY OPEN: Mid-July to early October
BEST: Late July and August
CONTACT: Pinedale Ranger District, Bridger-Teton National Forest
SPECIAL ATTRACTIONS: Just plain spectacular mountain scenery, and plenty of it
PERMIT: None required—sign in at the trailhead.

RULES ·

Fires are prohibited above treeline. Groups are limited to 15 people and 25 stock. Camping is prohibited within 100 feet of streams and 200 feet of lakes or trails.

CHALLENGES ·

The trail can be quite crowded, especially around Island Lake and Titcomb Basin. Expect mosquitoes in July and early August as well as frequent thunderstorms. A few stream crossings are potentially difficult, if the bridges are not in place.

Photo: Ellingwood Peak over Indian Basin

TAKE THIS TRIP

This is the hike that made me fall in love with the Wind River Range, so fair warning that, after taking this trip, you may never want to hike anywhere else again. Simply put, backpacking trips in the Lower 48 don't get much (possibly *any*) more scenic than this. Long, beautiful, lower-elevation lakes and meadows with views up to cliff-edged mountains; dozens (perhaps hundreds) of sparkling alpine lakes filled with hungry trout; an absolutely stunning mountain basin rimmed with glaciers and 13,000-foot granite spires; high mountain passes with views that encompass peaks and valleys in every direction; glorious sunsets and sunrises highlighted by jagged ridgelines; wildflower-covered alpine rock gardens and meadows; deep mountain valleys bordered by impossibly steep cliffs and ridges; mile after mile of above-treeline rambling with nothing to obstruct the view. All these wonders and more are here in embarrassing abundance.

Of course it's not *all* sweetness and light. Hikers must be prepared to camp at above-treeline lakes while frighteningly strong thunderstorms lash at their tent keeping them up all night; to gasp for oxygen while trudging slowly over passes well over 11,000 feet in elevation; to search (possibly in vain) for a secluded campsite at one of the most crowded spots in the entire Wind River Range; and to swat at hordes of mosquitoes in July that may make you hide in the tent all evening and possibly miss that aforementioned glorious sunset. But nothing worthwhile in life comes easy, so get in shape, become acclimated, have a tent with plenty of guylines, bring an extra gallon of insect repellent, and enjoy.

HOW TO GET THERE

From Pinedale, drive 5.3 miles west on U.S. Highway 191 then turn right (north) on Wyoming Highway 352, following signs to Cora and Green River lakes. The road remains paved for the first 25.7 miles, then enters national forest land, turns to gravel, and deteriorates into a sometimes ugly affair full of washboards, potholes, and ruts. The road is supposedly maintained for passenger cars and is usually reasonable, but can become difficult or even impassable after heavy rains. Remain on the main road at all intersections until you reach a fork about 45 miles from U.S. Highway 191 and shortly before you enter the Green River Lakes Campground. Bear left and proceed 0.4 mile to the signed hiker's trailhead.

DESCRIPTION

Beginning from the southwest corner of the parking lot, the trail goes briefly down a draw and comes to a fork, where the Lakeside Trail goes to the right. If the bridge over Clear Creek is in place (something you know because you called the Pinedale Ranger Station to check before you left, right?), then this is the start of the recommended loop. Bear left and walk 0.3 mile slightly downhill to a large metal bridge spanning the Green River a little below where that stream flows out of Lower Green River Lake. On the other side of the bridge is a junction. Keep right on the Highline Trail and spend the next 1.7 miles wandering along on a gentle up-and-down path through the meadows, open forests, and sagebrush on the hillside above large Lower Green River Lake. The views across the water are very pleasant and the country is both open and attractive. The large mountain that rises in a series of steep ridges and forested hills southwest of the lake is Big Sheep Mountain.

At 2 miles is a junction. The Clear Creek Trail goes left on its way to Clear and Slide lakes. If you have the time, this is the start of a fine 4.6-mile round-trip side trip that passes some nice views of Clear Creek Falls and large Flat Top Mountain on its way to Clear Creek Natural Bridge. Although hard to photograph, this bridge is very impressive as the waters of Clear Creek have dug a hole through the bottom of an enormous wall of dark limestone.

Back at the Clear Creek junction, the Highline Trail goes straight and soon reaches the crossing of Clear Creek. The Forest Service has replaced this bridge numerous times over the years and it will probably be there when you arrive, but if Mother Nature has washed it out again, you face a tricky ford that can be difficult before midsummer. Once across, the gentle trail wanders beside a large, willow-choked meadow at the southeast end of Lower Green River Lake with good views of the surrounding peaks and ridges and the possibility of spotting moose. Near the south end of the meadow is a junction. The trail to the right crosses the Green River on a bridge and then goes 0.3 mile to a junction with Lakeside Trail, which turns north back to the trailhead. The Lakeside Trail is an alternate route if the bridge over Clear Creek is gone and is the return route of the recommended loop.

The Highline Trail continues south from the junction above Lower Green River Lake, climbs over a forested knoll, and then descends a bit to the meadow-fringed north end of Upper Green River Lake. Anyone who has seen a travel brochure or calendar of Wyoming will recognize this location, one of the most photographed spots in the state. The main subject is distant, remarkably well-named Squaretop Mountain, a massive, sheer-sided block of granite that looms above the west side of the valley to the south-southeast. For those who want extra time to enjoy this scene, there are campsites near Upper Green River Lake, but don't expect to be alone.

The trail now wends its way south along the east side of Upper Green River Lake through a mix of meadows and forest and with fine views around almost every bend. After about 1.5 miles you pass the south end of the lake and continue on a very gentle trail that goes through or beside a nearly continuous meadow bisected by the meandering Green River. Unfortunately for anglers, the river's waters are full of glacial silt and have few, if any, fish. Across the valley to the south and west Squaretop Mountain gets closer with every step, eventually towering over the valley bottom and causing you to crane your neck upward to get a

Green River Lakes & Titcomb Basin Loop

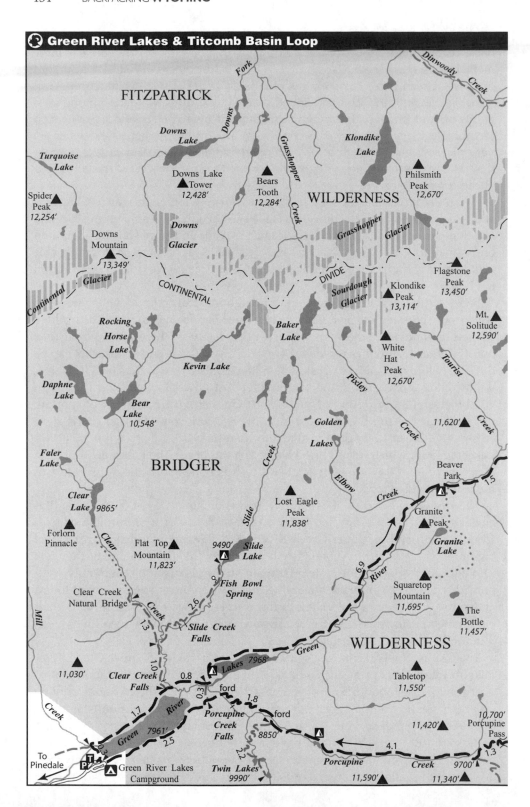

FITZPATRICK

Downs
Fork

Downs
Lake

Grasshopper
Creek

Klondike
Lake

Philsmith
Peak
12,670'

Turquoise
Lake

Downs Lake
▲ Tower
12,428'

Bears
Tooth
12,284'

WILDERNESS

Spider
Peak
12,254'

Downs
Mountain
▲ 13,349'

Downs
Glacier

Grasshopper   Glacier

DIVIDE

Flagstone
Peak
13,450'

Continental Glacier

CONTINENTAL

Sourdough
Glacier

Klondike
Peak
13,114'

Mt.
Solitude
12,590'

Rocking
Horse
Lake

Baker
Lake

White
Hat
Peak
12,670'

Tourist

Kevin Lake

Pixley

Daphne
Lake

Bear
Lake
10,548'

Golden

Lakes

Creek

11,620' ▲

Creek

Faler
Lake

BRIDGER

Slide

Beaver
Park

1.5

Clear
Lake 9865'

Lost Eagle
Peak
11,838'

Elbow   Creek

Granite
▲ Peak

Forlorn
Pinnacle

Clear

Flat Top ▲
Mountain
11,823'

9490' ▲
Slide
Lake

Granite
Lake

Clear Creek
Natural Bridge

Creek

2.6

Fish Bowl
Spring

6.9   River

Squaretop
Mountain
11,695'

Mill

1.3

Slide Creek
Falls

▲ The
Bottle
11,457'

11,030' ▲

Clear Creek
Falls

1.0

0.8

Lakes 7968

Green

WILDERNESS

Tabletop
11,550'

0.3
ford

Creek

1.7

River   7961'

2.5

Porcupine
Creek
Falls

1.8
ford

8850'

2.2

4.1

11,420' ▲

10,700'
Porcupine
Pass

1.3

To
Pinedale

Green River Lakes
Campground

Twin Lakes
9990'

Porcupine   Creek   9700' ▲

11,590' ▲

11,340' ▲

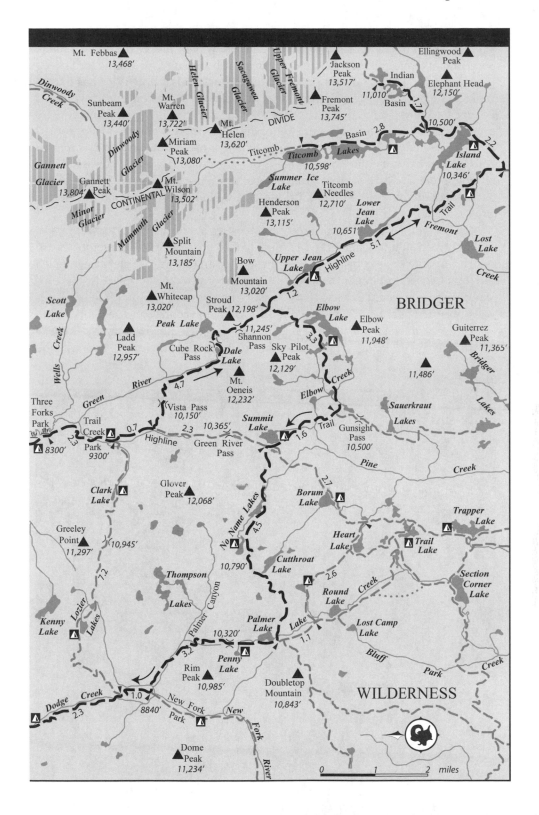

full view of the peak. At about 6.5 miles the meadows finally end as you continue up the valley amid a dense forest with fewer views but plenty of cooling shade. Side streams cross the route at several locations, but bridges or simple fords keep these from being a significant problem. However, the Forest Service has had to replace the bridge crossing Green River at 9.7 miles in a small meadow called Beaver Park a few times over the years, so it may or may not exist when you are there. Typically a large, very sturdy-looking structure ushers hikers dry-footed to the other side, but the river doesn't always agree about the bridge's sturdiness, so don't count on it. If the bridge is out, the crossing may be impossible for hikers before late July or early August—call the Pinedale Ranger Station about current conditions before hiking. Bridge or not, there are some good and scenic campsites at Beaver Park.

Not far on the other side of the river crossing is an unsigned, easily missed junction with an unofficial scramble route to Granite Lake and Squaretop Mountain, a fun but very steep side trip for those with an uncontrollable urge to reach the top of such a prominent landmark. The view from the summit is just as outstanding as you might expect.

Continuing upstream from Beaver Park, you reenter forest and keep hiking up the valley another 1.5 miles before reaching the large, somewhat marshy expanse of Three Forks Park. Jagged pinnacles and massive cliffs rise above the east side

Three Forks Park

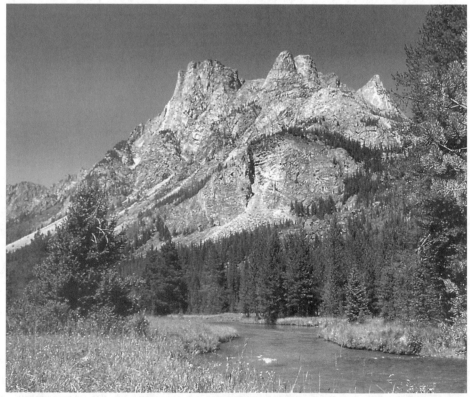

of this mile-long meadow, making for dramatic backdrops for the photographer. Unfortunately, the meadow hosts lots of mosquitoes and only a few rather mediocre campsites, so for better overnight options put your pack back on and follow the trail as it leaves the valley bottom and switchbacks fairly steeply up the west wall of the canyon following cascading Trail Creek. Almost 2 tiring miles later you cross the creek and reach the excellent campsites at Trail Creek Park. Given the scenery and the convenient location—don't expect to be alone.

Just past the south end of Trail Creek Park is a junction. Go straight, still on the Highline Trail, and keep climbing for another 0.7 mile to a second junction. The Highline Trail goes straight, follows Trail Creek to its source, and then descends a short distance through gentle alpine meadows to a junction and campsites around dramatically scenic Summit Lake. This trail is an option for those hikers who want a shorter loop, but it skips the magnificent side trip to the otherworldly scenery of Titcomb Basin.

Since only the most time-crunched backpackers would choose to miss Titcomb Basin, it is better to turn left at the junction above Trail Creek Park and climb on an irregularly maintained, sometimes rough trail that travels through open forest and small meadows to Vista Pass, where this trip's truly grand scenery begins. Although not yet above treeline, this 10,150-foot pass offers photographers and other admirers a foreground of meadows and small ponds with stunning views of rugged summits in every direction. From the pass the trail descends slightly and then turns south and climbs beside a creek to tiny and above-treeline Dale Lake. You then climb a rocky defile to Cube Rock Pass and marvel at the view down to gorgeous Peak Lake. Several rocky peaks, all approaching or higher than 12,000 feet, surround this deep lake, making it superbly scenic.

From Peak Lake the trail switchbacks up a rocky slope to 11,245-foot Shannon Pass, high on the slopes of Stroud Peak. This section of trail is particularly prone to landslides, which often block the trail. Call the ranger station before your trip about the latest conditions. Views from Shannon Pass are absolutely gorgeous with alpine rock gardens at your feet, several nearby ponds and lakes, and tall peaks all around. A gentle stretch of alpine meadow rambling now leads to a junction where you reunite with the Highline Trail.

This junction is where the recommended return loop back to Green River Lakes begins. But first, you simply *must* make the long side trip to Titcomb Basin. Keep left at the junction and go southbound on the Highline Trail as it travels up and down through a rocky alpine paradise, over a minor rise, then past a small unnamed lake to much larger Upper Jean Lake. What's to say here without running out of superlatives? It's simply wonderful, with the best views to the north of jagged Bow Mountain and Mt. Arrowhead. There are good campsites here, although like many others in the Wind River Range they are quite exposed should thunderstorms roll through in the afternoon and evening.

The glories continue as you wander downstream, fording a creek twice before you reach larger but not quite as scenic Lower Jean Lake, where sloping ground and lots of rocks make camping unattractive. You then descend through wildflower gardens for another mile or so back into the land of scraggly trees to a bridged crossing of Fremont Creek at a place known, rather unimaginatively, as Fremont Crossing. From here you do more up-and-down hiking for 1.5 miles past small tarns with possible campsites (much less crowded than those near Island Lake) and over rocky terrain to a junction.

To reach Titcomb Basin, turn left on a very busy trail, which goes up a bit to a minor saddle, then descends to extremely popular Island Lake. The views across the waters of this large alpine gem are exceptional, but camping here means sharing those views with dozens of other people, most of whom approached this lake by a somewhat shorter trail from the west. Campsites are plentiful, but follow "no trace" principles scrupulously at this fragile location.

The trail loops around the southeast shore of long Island Lake then pulls away from the water and climbs to a junction near a fairly good-sized but apparently unnamed lake. A steep but superb side trip from here goes right and climbs to the ruggedly scenic alpine grandeur of Indian Basin, well worth every extra calorie of effort to get there.

The main trail, however, goes straight at the Indian Basin junction, almost immediately fords the creek that tumbles down from Indian Basin, and then takes you through more alpine rock gardens of hardy little wildflowers to the lower end of stupendous Titcomb Basin. A string of sparkling, unusually large lakes fills the bottom of this glacially carved wonderland with towering granite pinnacles and 13,000-foot peaks lining both sides. Giddy with joy at the incredible scenery, you follow the gentle trail as it wanders northward along the east side of the Titcomb Lakes as far as you want to go. The recommended turnaround point is beside incredibly dramatic Upper Titcomb Lake, almost directly under the spires of the Continental Divide. Adventurous hikers, however, could continue beyond this lake on boot-beaten climber's routes all the way to the base of the peaks and glaciers at the head of the basin. For those with less ambition, an enjoyable way to spend your time is fishing for golden trout, which thrive in the lakes of Titcomb Basin.

Back at the junction northwest of Upper Jean Lake, turn left (southwest) and follow a circuitous alpine route that snakes around rocky areas and past small lakes to a ford of Elbow Creek and a nice viewpoint above Elbow Lake. Enclosed in an impressive basin beneath a peak with the same name, this large lake is very scenic. There are possible campsites above Elbow Lake's northwest shore.

Several smaller but just as stunning alpine lakes highlight your route as you keep hiking west from Elbow Lake, enjoying some fine views along the way to the north of the steep-sided pyramid of Sky Pilot Peak. After fording or hopping over Elbow Creek you come to a minor junction, where you keep right, descend to a second crossing of Elbow Creek (this time on a bridge) and then reach a junction near the southwest corner of beautiful Summit Lake. There is plenty of flat ground and many excellent campsites at this fairly large meadow-rimmed jewel, although the lake is heavily used by horse parties, with the usual aromatic, dusty consequences.

Keep right at the first junction beside Summit Lake and walk north along the shoreline for 0.1 mile to a second junction. You turn left this time, onto the

Doubletop Mountain Trail, and continue with the glorious high-elevation wandering you began some days ago. More pretty creeks, more sparkling tarns and lakes, and lots more wildflower-covered meadows greet your enchanted eyes as you walk west to the two No Name Lakes. This widely separated pair of lakes sits above treeline in a scenic basin and host lots of hungry cutthroat trout. I don't know for sure, but I suspect that the uninspired name for these lakes was probably bestowed by someone who had seen too many other nearby wonders to come up with anything more original. Some very scenic campsites are available north of the lakes, but the only shelter from those famous Wind River thunderstorms is from large boulders and rocky outcroppings.

The trail now goes over a minor divide and then descends on a rocky track to a corner of Cutthroat Lake, which offers very good fishing for, what else, cutthroat trout. From here you descend back below treeline to a hop-over crossing of Lake Creek and a junction.

Turn right (north) at this junction, soon walk past lovely Palmer Lake, then cross a grassy slope to a small creek feeding out of Penny Lake. That small lake is about 200 yards to the west and offers decent camping. The main trail goes straight, soon reaches a meadow-covered pass, and then tackles a long, switchbacking descent into the depths of steep-sided Palmer Canyon. Like everywhere else on this loop, the scenery here is grand, although the long, rocky downhill can be tough on your knees. At the bottom of the canyon you cross first Palmer Creek then fairly small New Fork River before reaching a junction.

The large expanse of lovely New Fork Park lies a little less than 1 mile down the trail to the left, but you turn right and begin the long climb to Porcupine Pass. After gaining some 600 feet in several short switchbacks you come to a junction above rushing Dodge Creek. The trail to Lozier Lakes goes right, but you keep straight, soon cross Dodge Creek, and then resume your ascent. The trail generally stays on the partly forested and brushy hillside above Dodge Creek for almost a mile, then it crosses a gully and switchbacks up into higher, more open terrain. Eventually the occasionally faint trail climbs past a few possible campsites to 10,700-foot Porcupine Pass. The best view from this narrow grandstand is to the north down the impressive U-shaped canyon of Porcupine Creek.

The aforementioned canyon is your next goal, so walk down a series of tightly spaced switchbacks, rapidly losing 1000 feet to where you reenter forest, cross a tiny creek, and come to a junction with an abandoned trail. Elk are common in the high meadows of this area. Keep right on the main trail, soon hop over a small creek, and then continue downstream, staying on the east side of ever-growing Porcupine Creek. Avalanche chutes cross the trail in several places along this section, which means that downed trees and leftover snowdrifts can be a problem. The upper part of the canyon is mostly forested, but the farther down you go, the more open and dramatic it becomes. About 5 miles from Porcupine Pass is a particularly impressive area where you walk around a couple of lovely creekside meadows with neck-craning views up to the dark, imposing ramparts of the canyon's western wall. There are possible campsites near here, and the willow thickets beside the creek are a good place to look for moose. Not far below this area you cross Porcupine Creek (on a log, if you're lucky) and come to a junction. The trail to the left climbs a series of fairly steep switchbacks to the tiny Twin Lakes, a worthwhile side trip if you have the energy.

The main trail goes straight at the junction, almost immediately crosses Porcupine Creek again (expect wet feet this time), and then wanders through an increasingly dense, viewless lodgepole pine forest. After about 0.4 mile the trail begins a series of steep downhill switchbacks, allowing you to hear, but generally not see, Porcupine Creek Falls in the wooded canyon on your left. At the bottom of the switchbacks you reach the edge of the meadow above Lower Green River Lake and face a third crossing of Porcupine Creek. There might be some logs across the flow a bit upstream from the official crossing, but more than likely you will have to make a knee-deep ford.

About 0.2 mile of level walking past the ford is a junction. The trail to the right is the 0.3-mile shortcut to the Highline Trail mentioned earlier in the text. To close out this loop, however, you go straight and hike the gentle up-and-down Lakeside Trail along the mostly forested west side of Lower Green River Lake to a trailhead in Green River Campground. Follow the campground road for about 0.2 mile, then bear right on a trail that soon reaches the junction just below the hiker's trailhead and, sadly, the close of what may be the trip of a lifetime.

POSSIBLE ITINERARY

	CAMPS & SIDE TRIPS	MILES	ELEVATION GAIN
DAY 1	Beaver Park	9.7	500′
DAY 2	South of Fremont Creek	14.3	3500′
DAY 3	South of Fremont Creek (dayhike to Indian and Titcomb basins)	15.8	1300′
DAY 4	Summit Lake	9.9	1000′
DAY 5	Penny Lake	5.2	1200′
DAY 6	Porcupine Creek	10.9	2300′
DAY 7	Out	5.1	300′

VARIATIONS

You could easily spend a month in this country exploring the dozens of worthwhile off-trail lakes, peaks, and meadows. No guidebook could possibly list all of the options, but a good map allows you to make up your own itinerary and secret discoveries. The best way to enjoy it is to bring several extra days of food and have a boss who will look the other way at some unscheduled "sick" days.

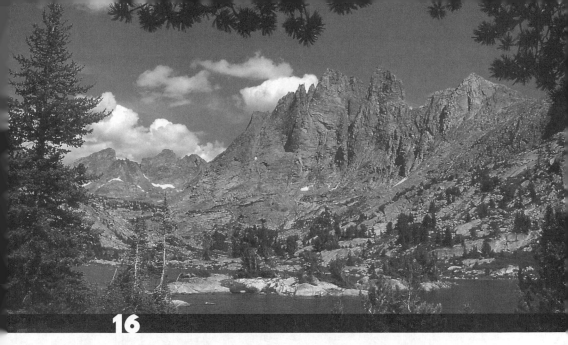

16

CENTRAL WIND RIVERS LOOP

RATINGS: Scenery 10   Solitude 6   Difficulty 7
MILES: 61.7 (79.9)
ELEVATION GAIN: 7700´ (10,100´)
DAYS: 6–10
MAP: Earthwalk Press *Southern Wind River Range*
USUALLY OPEN: July to October
BEST: Mid-July through August
CONTACT: Pinedale Ranger District, Bridger-Teton National Forest
SPECIAL ATTRACTIONS: Relative solitude amid some of the most dramatic mountain scenery in North America
PERMIT: None required—sign in at the trailhead.

RULES

Fires are prohibited above treeline. Groups are limited to 15 people and 25 stock. Camping is prohibited within 100 feet of streams and 200 feet of lakes or trails.

CHALLENGES

This long, rugged trip has several relatively long cross-country sections, most of which are fairly easy and have sketchy use paths for much of the distance. The area frequently has thunderstorms. The route involves some relatively easy stream crossings.

Photo: Mt. Bonneville over Little Bonneville Lake

TAKE THIS TRIP

The Wind River Range is ideal for extended backpacking adventures, and many of the best of these hikes are off-trail. Unfortunately, many involve difficult scrambling or glacier travel beyond the abilities of the average backpacker. Still, you can't really get the full experience of what the Wind Rivers have to offer without occasionally leaving the trails.

In the course of visiting almost all the most outstanding attractions in the lesser-visited central part of the range, this hike takes you on long sections off the official trails. Unlike other such cross-country trips, however, almost all this hike's off-trail miles follow abandoned routes or established boot paths that, while unsigned and unmaintained, are relatively easy to follow. Best of all, the rewards for your efforts are tremendous, including high alpine passes with far-ranging views, sparkling lakes set in classic cirques beneath towering peaks, stupendous looks at sheer granite cliffs thousands of feet high, great fishing in little-visited lakes with lots of hungry trout, huge meadows with wildflowers and days worth of fun exploring, and incredibly scenic campsites that will leave you wanting to spend far more days than any company vacation plan will allow. Bring a good contour map and reasonably good navigation skills and savor the delights.

HOW TO GET THERE

From U.S. Highway 191 just south of the community of Boulder (about 12 miles south of Pinedale) go east on Wyoming Highway 353, following signs to Big Sandy. After 6.7 miles turn left on gravel County Road 122, signed as SCAB CREEK ACCESS, and drive 1.5 miles to a fork. Go left and continue 6.6 miles on this reasonably good gravel road to the turnoff to the designated equestrian trailhead. Go straight and drive 0.4 mile to the hiker's trailhead parking lot on the right. The road continues another 0.4 mile to a nice (but waterless) BLM campground for those looking to spend the night before starting their hike in the morning.

DESCRIPTION

The trail leaves from the north side of the road directly across from the parking lot and, after uniting with the separate horse access trail, ascends a slope partly forested with lodgepole pines, Douglas firs, limber pines, and quaking aspens and partly covered with grasses, sagebrush, bitterbrush, and various wildflowers.

After gaining about 1200 feet in 2.1 miles on a somewhat rocky trail you pass marshy little Boundary Lake just before reaching a sign announcing your entry into the Bridger Wilderness. From here the pace of the ascent is less evident as you go up and down in forest and past frequent granite outcroppings. You also pass a series of marshy lily-pad-filled lakes in the Toboggan Lakes area. At 6.2

miles is a signed junction beside attractive Little Divide Lake, where you'll find the trip's first good campsites a short way down the trail to the right. For even better campsites continue down the trail another 0.5 mile to larger Divide Lake.

The main trail goes left at the junction beside Little Divide Lake, rounds the north end of that lake, then goes up and down through pleasant but viewless subalpine terrain. A little more than 1 mile from Little Divide Lake you pass one of the Lightning Lakes and soon thereafter start to catch enticing glimpses of the high peaks to the east. More frequent and more impressive as you continue east, those glimpses open up with a bang when you break out of the forest into the vast rolling meadows around South Fork Boulder Creek. The view encompasses a dazzling array of tall peaks from Mt. Victor in the north to Mt. Geikie to the south and dozens of peaks and canyons in between. This awe-inspiring scene is made more intriguing by the knowledge that you will be exploring all this scenic country over the next several days.

Near the beginning of the meadows is a signed fork in the trail. Bear left on the Dream Lake Trail and walk through meadows for 0.3 mile to a shin-deep ford of South Fork Boulder Creek. About 0.2 mile after this ford is an unsigned but obvious junction.

The official trail goes straight and is the trail on which you will return at the end of the recommended loop. For now, though, turn left on a good outfitter's trail that soon loops around Crescent Lake and then climbs to a higher plateau where you cross the route of the very faint, unsigned, and easy-to-miss Highline Trail. Stay straight on the unofficial but more distinct outfitter's trail, which winds through lovely meadows with views down to Dream Lake and the countless peaks beyond. As the trail starts to fade, you reach a well-traveled older section of the Fremont Trail at the northwest end of Bobs Lake.

WARNING: If you try to do this loop in the opposite direction it is very hard to find this junction.

Go left on the old Fremont Trail and walk downhill beside a tiny creek to large, very attractive Sandpoint Lake. There are good campsites near this lake's southeast and north ends and plenty of good-sized brook trout to entice the angler.

The trail goes around the east side of Sandpoint Lake, meeting the new course of the Fremont Trail along the way, and then comes to a crossing of Middle Fork Boulder Creek. This crossing typically involves a calf-deep ford, but it's easy because the water is not swift. Immediately afterward is an unsigned but very apparent fork in the trail. The trail to the right goes up to huge, very scenic Middle Fork Lake, a destination you will pass along the recommended loop in two or three days.

For now veer left at the fork and walk past a pretty meadow. At the northwest end of this meadow is an unsigned, easily missed junction with an obscure trail that goes left toward Junction Lake. You stay straight on the main trail passing small meadows and unnamed lakes for another mile to a junction marked with a cairn immediately before the trail crosses Halls Creek.

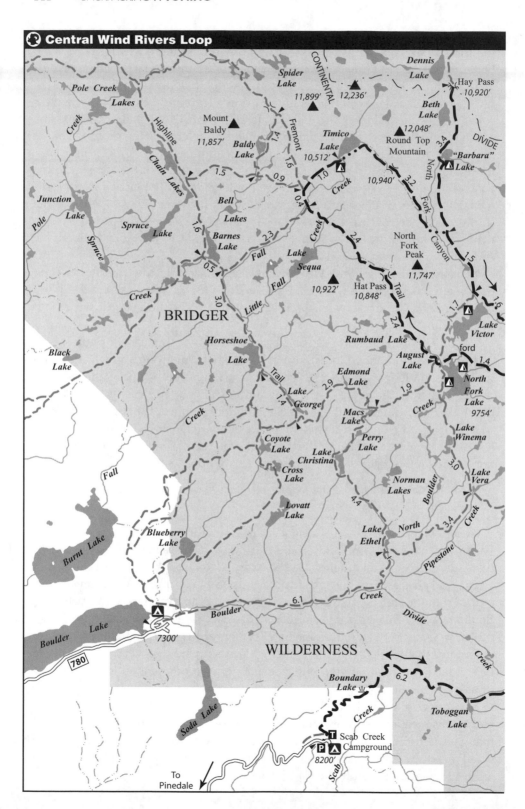

Central Wind Rivers Loop

Pole Creek Lakes

Pole Creek

Highline

Chain Lakes

Junction Lake

Pole

Spruce

Spruce Lake

Black Lake

Mount Baldy 11,857'

Baldy Lake

1.4

1.6

1.5

0.9

Bell Lakes

1.6

Barnes Lake

0.4

2.3

Fall

0.5

3.0

Little

Fall

BRIDGER

Fremont

Spider Lake 11,899'

CONTINENTAL

12,236'

Timico Lake 10,512'

Creek

1.0

Creek

2.4

Lake Sequa 10,922'

Dennis Lake

Hay Pass 10,920'

Beth Lake

Round Top Mountain 12,048'

10,940'

3.2

North

"Barbara" Lake

3.4

DIVIDE

1.5

Fork

North Fork Peak 11,747'

Canyon

1.7

1.6

Hat Pass 10,848'

2.4

Trail

2.4

Lake Victor

Horseshoe Lake

Trail

1.4

Rumbaud Lake

August Lake

ford

1.4

Lake George

2.9

Edmond Lake

1.9

North Fork Lake 9754'

Creek

Black Lake

Creek

Fall

Coyote Lake

Cross Lake

Lovatt Lake

Lake Christina

Macs Lake

Perry Lake

Norman Lakes

4.4

Lake Ethel

North

Boulder

Lake Winema

3.0

Lake Vera

3.4

Creek

Pipestone

Burnt Lake

Blueberry Lake

Boulder Lake

7300'

780

Boulder

6.1

Creek

Divide

WILDERNESS

6.2

Creek

Soda Lake

Boundary Lake

Creek

Toboggan Lake

Scab Creek Campground

8200'

Scab

To Pinedale

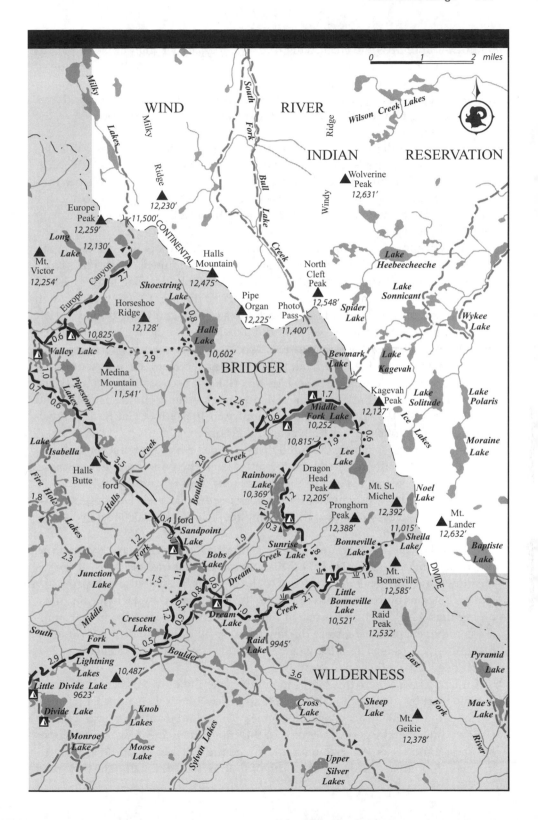

WIND   RIVER   INDIAN   RESERVATION

Milky

Lakes

Milky

Ridge

South

Fork

Bull

Lake

Creek

Windy

Ridge

Wilson Creek Lakes

Wolverine
Peak
12,631'

Europe
Peak
12,259'

Long
Lake

12,130'

Mt.
Victor
12,254'

11,500'

CONTINENTAL

Europe

Canyon

2.7

Halls
Mountain
12,475'

Shoestring
Lake

Horseshoe
Ridge
12,128'

0.8

Halls
Lake

10,602'

Pipe
Organ
12,225'

Photo
Pass
11,400'

North
Cleft
Peak
12,548'

Spider
Lake

Lake
Heebeecheeche

Lake
Sonnicant

Wykee
Lake

0.6

10,825'

Valley Lake

1.0

0.7

Pipestone

Lakes

0.6

Medina
Mountain
11,541'

2.9

BRIDGER

Bewmark
Lake

Lake
Kagevah

Lake
Solitude

Lake
Polaris

Ice

Moraine
Lake

Lake
Isabella

Halls
Butte

Fire Hole

1.8

Creek

3.5

ford

Halls

Creek

2.8

Kagevah
Peak
12,127'

2.6

1.7

Middle
Fork Lake
10,252'

0.6

10,815'

1.9

0.9

Lee
Lake

Lakes

Lakes

Lake
Isabella

Rainbow
Lake
10,369'

Dragon
Head
Peak
12,205'

1.2

1.0

Mt. St.
Michel
12,392'

Pronghorn
Peak
12,388'

11,015'

Noel
Lake

Mt.
Lander
12,632'

0.4

ford

Sandpoint
Lake

1.2

0.7

1.9

Fork

Bobs
Lake

0.3

Sunrise
Creek Lake

1.8

Sheila
Lake

Bonneville
Lake

Baptiste
Lake

2.3

Junction
Lake

1.5

1.1

0.8 0.6

Dream

1.6

Little
Bonneville
Lake
10,521'

Mt.
Bonneville
12,585'

DIVIDE

Middle

Crescent
Lake

0.4

0.9

1.2

1.0

Dream
Lake

Creek

2.7

Raid
Peak
12,532'

South

Fork

0.5

Boulder

Raid
Lake 9945'

2.9

Lightning
Lakes

10,487'

Little Divide Lake
9623'

Divide Lake

Monroe
Lake

Knob
Lakes

Moose
Lake

Sylvan Lakes

3.6 WILDERNESS

Cross
Lake

Sheep
Lake

Mt.
Geikie
12,378'

East

Fork

Pyramid
Lake

Mae's
Lake

River

Upper
Silver
Lakes

0   1   2 *miles*

Since the trail to the right is an unofficial cross-country route, stick with the main trail and cross the creek. This ford is rarely higher than ankle deep, but count on wet feet. After the crossing you climb to a saddle on the east side of flat-topped Halls Butte. From here the trail descends, passes to the east of an un-named, irregularly shaped lake, and then goes through a partially burned area before coming to a junction with the Lake Isabella Trail beside the first of the Pipestone Lakes.

Keep right on the Fremont Trail and soon come to the next Pipestone Lake, which features an excellent view of bulky Mt. Victor to the north. The trail quick-ly pulls away from this lake and ascends for 0.2 mile to a junction marked with a post. Keep left on the Fremont Trail and go up and down for 0.7 mile to another junction, this time with a very faint trail that follows a line of cairns to the right (north-northeast).

Keep straight on the main trail and wind downhill in open forest to the rel-atively flat basin holding large, meadow- and rock-rimmed North Fork Lake. Several good campsites surround this understandably popular lake. The trail takes you to an easy calf-deep ford of North Fork Boulder Creek, then through meadows on the north side of North Fork Lake to a junction. The trail to the left goes along the west shore of North Fork Lake. You go straight and a little more than 0.1 mile later reach a four-way junction.

Go straight on the Fremont Trail, following signs to Hat Pass, and soon reach small but very scenic August Lake. North Fork Peak rises to the north-northeast and forms a dramatic backdrop. The trail now begins a long climb past Rumbaud Lake, then up into increasingly alpine country to 10,848-foot Hat Pass. Marvel-ous views of countless peaks both near and far open up.

The trail now goes mostly downhill through open country of first tundra, then meadows, and finally forest. About 1.9 miles from the pass you see portions of large but trailless Lake Sequa to the west. From here it's another 0.5 mile to a junction marked by a post just before the crossing of Fall Creek. Go straight, cross the stream via an easy ford or rock-hop, and then climb about 300 feet in 0.4 mile to a signed junction.

After following the Fremont Trail for more than 12 miles, leave that path as you turn right toward Timico Lake. This sometimes faint trail ascends a gorgeous meadow traveling generally northeast to the obvious basin holding Timico Lake, one of the gems of the Wind River Range. It is surrounded by rocky peaks, most higher than 12,000 feet, and is one of the more scenic lakes in Wyoming. Camp-ing is rather exposed here, since the few trees are all rather small, but it is highly recommended, especially if the weather is good. The fishing is excellent as well, if you need any further enticement.

Timico Lake is where this loop's long but generally easy cross-country travel begins. Start by fording the outlet creek and then follow the southeast shore of the lake for 0.5 mile to a seasonal inlet creek. Turn right (southeast) and follow a sketchy but generally good boot path up this intermittent creek over open slopes of grasses and rocks. After gaining a fairly gentle 430 feet in a little less than 1 mile you top out at a wide saddle south of Round Top Mountain. The boot path continues on the other side of the pass, descending fairly steeply on a rocky route that stays well to the left (east) of a small creek. The path leads all the way down to a beautiful lower-elevation meadow along North Fork Boulder Creek. Near the lower end of this meadow the path fades away. To continue the hike, simply turn east, cross the creek, and then walk uphill until you intersect the maintained Hay Pass Trail.

The side trip up to Hay Pass is highly recommended, so drop your heavy pack, grab your camera, and go left (north). The trail gradually climbs through meadows and thinning forest to a large lake, sometimes identified as Barbara Lake but more often given no name at all, that sits just below treeline in a wide basin. There is at least one rather austere but feasible campsite here. The trail then crosses the lake's outlet creek and climbs steadily in rocky meadows. The tread is sometimes faint but the route is generally obvious. You pass to the right (east) of spectacular, above-treeline Beth Lake, which offers outstanding views across its waters to Round Top Mountain. Another 240 feet of uphill from this lake takes you to wide, rocky Hay Pass. The view here takes in an indescribable number of tall peaks, deep lakes, and rugged canyons, the most impressive of large, very deep Dennis Lake well below you to the north-northwest.

After your side trip, go south along the trail generally staying level or traveling gently downhill in forest and meadows. About 1.5 miles of easy hiking takes you to a point about 50 yards before the trail crosses North Fork Boulder Creek. If you need a campsite, stick with the main trail, cross the creek, and soon pass some possible campsites not far from the northwest shore of Lake Victor.

To continue the loop hike, veer left before the creek crossing onto a faint boot path and follow it through the meadows a little north of island-dotted Lake Victor. After hiking for about 0.15 mile, look for a well-worn boot path going up a grassy slope to the left. Follow this unofficial but good trail as it climbs steeply for about 0.3 mile, then goes up and down in forest. The trail disappears briefly after the climb, but if you head generally southeast you will relocate it. You soon come to a small meadow where you rock-hop a creek that feeds out of distant Long Lake. About 0.1 mile later, hop over the creek from Europe Canyon and then follow this stream past a series of pretty little ponds. The trail then pulls away from the creek and goes south through forest to an unsigned junction in the meadow at the north tip of Valley Lake. Campsites are available on this lake's east and west shores.

Keep left (southeast), walk about 0.15 mile, and then look for a sign about 20 yards to the left saying TRAIL ABANDONED—NOT MAINTAINED. This is the old trail up Europe Canyon and the start of the unofficial off-trail route to Halls Lake. Turn left onto this trail, which despite being abandoned is still easy to follow, and climb steeply up a ridge. After 0.4 mile the trail levels off then comes near a creek and follows it upstream for 0.3 mile to a small but very scenic unnamed lake with a few mediocre campsites.

For the highly recommended side trip up Europe Canyon, backtrack from the lake about 200 yards and turn onto a faint abandoned trail to the right (north). The trail becomes more obvious as it slowly makes its way up the narrow and

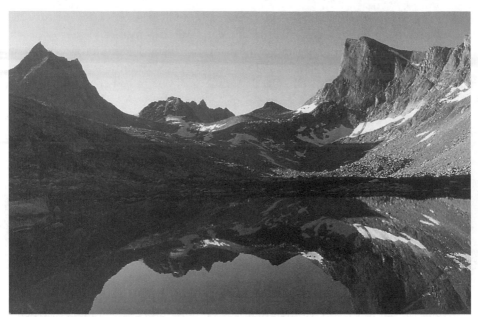

Mt. St. Michel "Nylon Peak" and Pronghorn Peak over Lee Lake

rocky depths of the lower reaches of Europe Canyon. In a few places it crosses small meadows and becomes faint, but is still fairly easy to follow. After passing a small lake on the left, you enter above-treeline meadows from which you can see a much larger, but still unnamed, lake a bit below you to the right. Keep ascending into increasingly stark, rocky terrain circling around the right (southeast) side of a long lake that sits beneath a huge rocky buttress. Then climb to a second, equally scenic lake where the tread disappears. To reach the last and most spectacular lake in Europe Canyon, climb the steep, open, and rocky slope to the northwest for a final 0.3 mile to Lake 11,023, a grandly scenic location directly beneath huge, craggy Europe Peak. From this lake you can see a trail going up the slope to the northeast toward an unnamed pass. A faint path goes down the other side of that pass to the Milky Lakes, but these are in the Wind River Indian Reservation and you must have a permit to visit.

Back at the base of Europe Canyon on the trail beside the small lake 0.7 mile above Valley Lake, go east on an unofficial but good trail for 0.1 mile to a fork. The left branch crosses a creek and climbs to a large lake (the same unnamed lake you saw below you on the Europe Canyon Trail). Bear right (east) and follow a faint, intermittent boot path. You will probably lose the tread occasionally, but if you stick close to a tiny creek and keep prominent Medina Mountain on your right you can't get lost. After some steep climbing you reach a windswept pass just above a large unnamed lake sitting beneath the bulk of Horseshoe Ridge.

The faint trail continues east, rounding the south side of the unnamed lake, and then it fades as you descend about 200 feet to cross just north of a pair of small lakes. From here continue east through open terrain that provides generally easy hiking and simple navigation, even though the trail is often nowhere to be found. The next 1.5 miles are mostly gentle but also include some rugged up-and-down hiking in brushy areas, over grasslands, and around rocks until you can see Halls Lake to the east-northeast. Make your way down to Halls Creek and follow that stream up to the south end of the lake it drains. The views across the waters of this large alpine lake up to Halls Mountain and Pipe Organ are magnificent. For a great side trip, follow the inlet creek from the southwest side of Halls Lake up to awe-inspiring Shoestring Lake, which is almost completely surrounded by the cliffs of Horseshoe Ridge.

To continue from Halls Lake, go cross-country south-southeast through open above-treeline terrain past a narrow unnamed lake. From time to time you will find sections of an obscure horse and boot path, but most of the travel is off-trail hiking over rocks, alpine grasses, and patches of low brush. The easiest route is to stay close to some rocky cliffs on your left as you climb to a minor saddle, where you gain a fine view down to your next destination at Middle Fork Lake. To reach it, pick your way steeply down through meadow basins and past a pretty little unnamed lake until you intersect the sketchy official trail that goes up toward Bewmark Lake.

Turn right on this trail and go slightly downhill to a junction with the well-defined Middle Fork Trail, then turn sharply left and in an easy 0.6 mile come to the southwest tip of Middle Fork Lake. This huge lake, which is more than 1.5 miles long, features terrific views of hulking Kagevah Peak to the east, Dragon Head Peak to the southeast, and various other unnamed summits all around. The fishing for brook trout is excellent. There are a couple of mediocre campsites near the outlet and another one in a small meadow basin about 0.8 mile from the outlet along the north shore.

To continue the loop, take the often faint trail around the mostly open north shore of Middle Fork Lake for 1.7 miles. Although this trail has a disturbing habit of disappearing, it provides fine views across the lake of Dragon Head Peak and the towering cliffs on that mountain's east face. When you reach the inlet creek at the east end of Middle Fork Lake, set aside an hour for an easy, very scenic side trip. To make the side trip, go south (upstream) over trailless but open terrain of grass and rocks for 0.6 mile until you reach large Lee Lake. The view here across the lake to the awesome nearby cliffs of Dragon Head and Pronghorn peaks is tremendous.

Your next goal is a pass on the north side of Dragon Head Peak. Most maps show a trail climbing west-southwest to this pass, but finding this tread is next to impossible. Fortunately, making your way up the open, grassy slopes to the obvious pass, although steep, is otherwise fairly easy. From the pass you can look south down to a portion of Rainbow Lake, your next destination.

On the south side of the pass a rocky but reasonably good trail leads you fairly steeply past a medium-sized tarn with a nice view of Dragon Head Peak, then descends less steeply to an unsigned junction at the north end of large Rainbow Lake. Take the left fork around the east side of the lake for 1.2 miles until you reach a good campsite near an inlet creek at the southeast tip of the lake.

From the campsite on Rainbow Lake you follow a good use trail southeast up a tiny inlet creek. After 0.1 mile you leave the main trail and go left on a sketchy route around the north side of a small lake and then descend to pretty Sunrise Lake. Still following intermittent tread, go around the north and east sides of Sunrise Lake, then go southeast up a wide, grassy, gently sloping swale. The tread disappears in this area so it is pretty much all cross-country from here. After going through an imperceptible saddle, boulder hop and then descend rather steeply to a pond in a meadow. From here, climb very steeply up a small gully almost straight across from where you entered the meadow, following a faint use path and game trail whenever possible. After almost 300 feet of tough climbing you level off and reach a small but very scenic pond. Wander through a low gap just above the pond's southeast shore, and almost immediately intersect an unofficial but perfectly good trail next to gorgeous Little Bonneville Lake, with an excellent, very scenic campsite a little to your right.

Little Bonneville Lake is a spectacularly beautiful spot, with outstanding views across its waters of extremely jagged Mt. Bonneville, as well as other unnamed peaks. For adventurous types a rugged, faint use trail goes gently upstream from Little Bonneville Lake for 0.4 mile, then crosses a creek and charges up an extremely steep route on the east side of a sliding waterfall. At the top of the falls is Bonneville Lake, beneath the awe-inspiring crags of Mt. Bonneville. From here you can round this lake's west shore and make an easy climb to Sheila Lake, which is surrounded by a host of towering peaks, including pointed Mt. St. Michel (Nylon Peak). Unfortunately, there are no decent campsites at either Bonneville or Sheila lakes, so they are best visited from a base camp at Little Bonneville Lake.

To exit from Little Bonneville Lake, follow the unofficial but good trail that goes downstream and in 0.2 mile passes an unnamed smaller lake. You then steeply lose about 250 feet before the trail's grade eases off in the meadows along South Fork Boulder Creek. Stick with the north side of that stream for the next mile before easily fording or rock-hopping the flow in a large meadow near a marshy pond. The trail then stays on the south side of the creek for 0.5 mile to a second easy crossing just 100 yards from the tip of Raid Lake's northern arm. Just 30 yards after the crossing is an unsigned junction with the Fremont Trail.

Turn right, wander past a small, shallow lake, and then hike northwest along the edge of the expansive rolling meadows that characterize this scenic area. The rocky meadows extend over several thousand acres and are dotted with lakes of various shapes and sizes. Exploring these meadows, and enjoying the views of the high peaks to the east that they afford, is very rewarding and could easily keep you busy for days.

The trail explores the rolling terrain on the east side of large Dream Lake and then comes to a junction with the Middle Fork Trail to Rainbow Lake. Veer left, pass a couple of faint paths leading left to campsites on Dream Lake, and then either rock-hop or splash across shallow Dream Creek. Still in meadows, you climb a bit to a narrow, little unnamed lake and reach a signed junction at its north end.

Turn left, following signs to the Scab Creek Trailhead, and follow a faint trail marked with cairns topped with tall posts. After 0.2 mile the tread becomes more distinct near Dream Lake as you round the northwest side of this meadow-rimmed gem with its views of Dragon Head Peak, Mt. Bonneville, Mt. Geikie, and a host of other summits. About 0.8 mile from the last junction is a four-way junction with the Highline Trail.

The tread to the right is so faint it is difficult to see. The trail to the left goes back to Raid Lake. You go straight and follow meandering Dream Creek then South Fork Boulder Creek for 0.9 mile back to the unsigned junction with the outfitter's trail past Crescent Lake you took earlier in the trip. Go straight and retrace your route 9.6 miles, over South Fork Boulder Creek and past Lightning and Little Divide lakes to the trailhead.

POSSIBLE ITINERARY

NOTE: As with any trip that includes significant off-trail travel, some of the mileages shown here are approximations.

	CAMPS & SIDE TRIPS	MILES	ELEVATION GAIN
DAY 1	Sandpoint Lake	12.1	1800'
DAY 2	Timico Lake	13.3	1700'
DAY 3	Lake Victor, including a side trip to Hay Pass	11.8	1300'
DAY 4	Lake above Valley Lake, including a side trip up Europe Canyon	8.0	1600'
DAY 5	Middle Fork Lake, including a side trip to Shoestring Lake	7.6	1000'
DAY 6	Little Bonneville Lake, including a side trip to Lee Lake	7.8	1600'
DAY 7	Dream Lake, including a side trip to Sheila Lake and some exploring in the meadows around Dream Lake	8.5	700'
DAY 8	Out	10.8	400'

VARIATIONS ·

For a slightly shorter trip, begin this loop at the Boulder Lake Trailhead (see map, pp. 144–145). This option involves less backtracking on the return trip, but it starts at a lower elevation, so more climbing is required. More important, completing that loop involves many miles of hiking through the charred, mostly shadeless landscape of the 38,507-acre Fayette Fire of 1988, which significantly diminishes the scenic appeal. By starting at the Scab Creek Trailhead, you miss almost all of the burn areas and enjoy a more attractive trip.

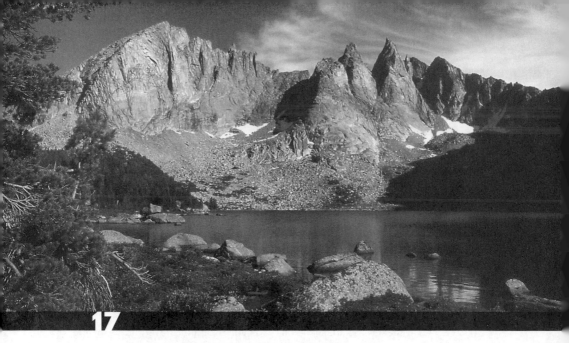

17

LONESOME & BAPTISTE LAKES LOOP

RATINGS: Scenery 10   Solitude 3   Difficulty 5
MILES: 39.3 (57.3)
ELEVATION GAIN: 7500´ (10,000´)
DAYS: 4–7
MAP: Earthwalk Press *Southern Wind River Range*
USUALLY OPEN: Mid-July to October
BEST: Late July through early September
CONTACT: Pinedale Ranger District, Bridger-Teton National Forest; Washakie Ranger District, Shoshone National Forest
SPECIAL ATTRACTIONS: The absolutely awesome peaks around Cirque of the Towers; generally outstanding mountain scenery
PERMIT: None required—sign in at the trailhead.

RULES ··

Fires are prohibited above treeline. Groups are limited to 15 people and 25 stock. Camping is prohibited within 100 feet of streams and 200 feet of lakes or trails and within 0.25 mile of Lonesome Lake.

Photo: Shadow Lake

CHALLENGES ·

The area can be quite crowded, especially around Lonesome and Big Sandy lakes, frequently has thunderstorms, and has mosquitoes in July. Camp-raiding black bears are a problem, particularly near Big Sandy and Lonesome lakes. There's a short but steep off-trail section over Texas Pass.

HOW TO GET THERE ·

There are several ways to access this popular trailhead. Coming from the east, drive 46 miles southwest from Lander on Wyoming Highway 28 to a junction 0.6 mile past a rest area and just before South Pass. Turn right (north) at a brown sign saying BIG SANDY ENTRANCE and follow this good gravel county road through a rolling sagebrush landscape for 19.8 miles to a T-junction. Go right and drive 5.5 miles to a junction signed BIG SANDY CAMPGROUND. This junction is the interim goal for all drivers, regardless of the route they use to reach it.

If you are coming from the north, the quickest way to reach this junction is to drive 12 miles south of Pinedale on U.S. Highway 191, then turn left (east) onto Wyoming Highway 353. Stay on this highway for 18 miles to the end of

TAKE THIS TRIP

The Big Sandy Entrance in the southern Wind River Range provides relatively short, easy access to some of the most outstandingly beautiful high country in the American Rockies. It's not surprising, then, that this is also one of Wyoming's most popular trailheads. Another reason for the crowded parking lot is that Big Sandy is the closest trailhead to the world-famous Cirque of the Towers. Although overcrowded, this spectacularly scenic mecca for both hikers and climbers is well worth a visit to marvel at the amazing views of the jagged granite peaks and towers that nearly encircle this basin. Camping near Lonesome Lake, which sits at the bottom of the cirque, is so gorgeous it is beyond my ability to describe, but even so it is usually better to avoid the crowds and camp elsewhere. Not only will doing so help protect the basin from overuse and allow you more solitude, it will also keep your food safe from the area's notorious black bears. These intelligent and hungry bruins have become a significant problem by regularly raiding the camps of backpackers and climbers.

The figure-eight recommended here not only visits Cirque of the Towers but takes you to large and almost equally beautiful Baptiste Lake, which is far more "lonesome" than misnamed Lonesome Lake. In addition, the loop passes Shadow Lake on the less visited west side of Cirque of the Towers, includes a side trip to the wonderful high country around Clear and Temple lakes, and visits countless other nearby peaks, lakes, and meadows. Completing the loop requires one steep, rocky cross-country section, but this should not be a problem for any reasonably fit, experienced hiker. Expect plenty of mosquitoes through the end of July.

Lonesome & Baptiste Lakes Loop

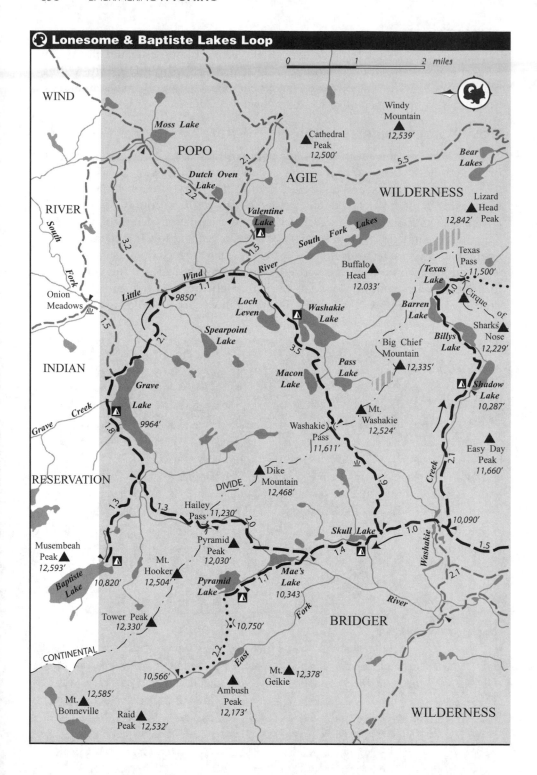

0   1   2 miles

WIND

POPO

Moss Lake

2.1

Dutch Oven
Lake

2.2

RIVER

South Fork

3.2

Valentine
Lake

1.5

Cathedral
Peak
12,500'

AGIE

Windy
Mountain
12,539'

5.5

Bear
Lakes

WILDERNESS

Lizard
Head
12,842' Peak

South Fork   Lakes

Wind

1.1

9850'

Buffalo
Head
12.033'

Texas
Pass
11,500'

Texas
Lake

4.0

Cirque

of

Little

1.5

Onion
Meadows

2.1

Loch
Leven

River

Washakie
Lake

3.5

Barren
Lake

Big Chief
Mountain
12,335'

Billys
Lake

Sharks
Nose
12,229'

INDIAN

Spearpoint
Lake

Macon
Lake

Pass
Lake

Shadow
Lake
10,287'

Grave
Lake

9964'

Grave   Creek

1.8

Washakie
Pass
11,611'

Mt.
Washakie
12,524'

Easy Day
Peak
11,660'

RESERVATION

1.3

DIVIDE

1.3

Hailey
Pass 11,230'

Dike
Mountain
12,468'

2.0

Skull Lake

1.4

1.9

1.0

Washakie Creek

2.1

10,090'

1.5

Musembeah
Peak
12,593'

Baptiste
Lake 10,820'

Mt.
Hooker
12,504'

Pyramid
Peak
12,030'

Pyramid
Lake

1.1

Mae's
Lake
10,343'

2.1

Tower Peak
12,330'

CONTINENTAL

10,566'

2.2

10,750'

East   Fork

River

BRIDGER

Mt. 12,378'
Geikie

Mt. 12,585'
Bonneville

Raid
Peak 12,532'

Ambush
Peak
12,173'

WILDERNESS

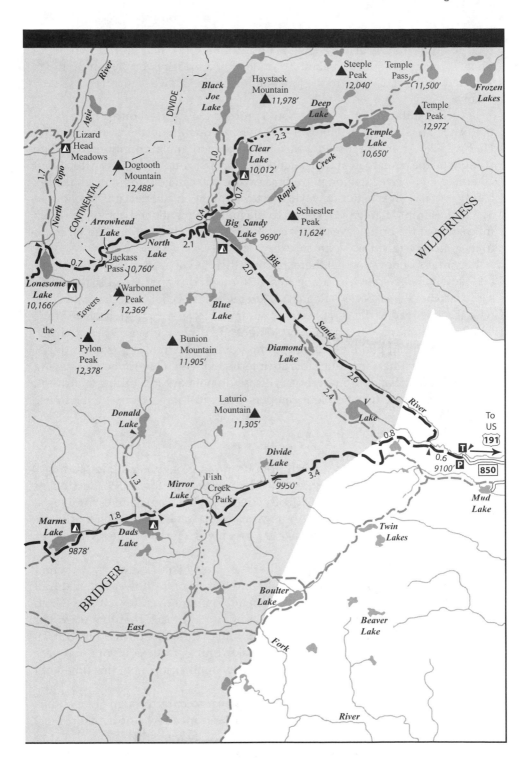

pavement, then proceed another 0.7 mile on a washboarded but decent gravel road to a junction. Bear left, drive 2.8 miles to a fork, then go right and continue 4.7 miles to a junction about 0.5 mile after a bridge over Big Sandy River. Turn left, and go 7.1 miles to the junction mentioned above signed for BIG SANDY CAMPGROUND.

Drivers coming from the south should proceed to Farson (about 40 miles north of Rock Springs along U.S. Highway 191) where you turn northeast on Wyoming Highway 28. After 4.6 miles you turn left on a good gravel county road and go straight on the main road at two junctions in the first couple of miles. After about 20 miles you reach a junction with signs saying you can go right to reach the Big Sandy entrance. It is better however, to stay straight on a better gravel road that at 33 miles from Highway 28 comes to the junction mentioned above about 0.5 mile south of the bridge over Big Sandy River. Turn right (east) and go 7.1 miles to the junction signed BIG SANDY CAMPGROUND.

Regardless of how you get there, turn north at the BIG SANDY CAMPGROUND sign and slowly make your way along this very rough dirt and gravel road, which soon becomes Forest Service Road 850. After 9.3 miles keep straight at a junction with the side road to the Temple Creek Summer Home Area, then drive 0.9 mile to a fork with the road to Mud Lake. Go right and drive another 0.8 mile to reach the huge trailhead parking area and campground. The trailhead is often full of cars, and the trailhead parking slots are intermixed with those for people staying overnight at Big Sandy Campground. Please do not park in a campground slot, as these are strictly for overnight campers who must pay a camping fee to use the facilities.

DESCRIPTION ·

The heavily used trail goes north from near a large signboard and gradually wanders slightly uphill through an open lodgepole pine forest. Meadow openings and the beautifully clear Big Sandy River provide scenic interest and highlights. After a little more than 0.1 mile your trail is joined by a horse trail from the equestrian corrals near Mud Lake. At 0.6 mile is a fork and the start of your loop.

The loop is equally good in either direction. Most hikers, however, veer right here on the direct trail to Big Sandy Lake and Cirque of the Towers, so that trail is very crowded. In addition, the recommended climb over Texas Pass, which comes later in the trip, is marginally easier if you approach from the west. For both solitude and easier hiking, bear left (uphill) at this junction and proceed 0.8 mile to a fork in the trail. The Diamond Lake Trail goes straight, but you veer left, cross a meadow for 0.2 mile, and reach yet another junction, this time with the Fremont Trail.

Turn right (north) and climb steadily, but never steeply, through an open forest. After about 1.5 miles the trail levels off in a large meadow atop a minor ridge. From here there are excellent views to the east of the fingerlike pinnacles atop nearby Laturio Mountain and north to distant Mt. Geikie, Pyramid Peak, Mt. Hooker, and other summits.

The trail now descends a bit before crossing the west side of the rolling, boulder-strewn meadow at Fish Creek Park. Just past the north end of this meadow walk around the west side of small Mirror Lake, then keep left at the junction with the trail to Donald Lake and descend about 100 feet to island-studded Dads Lake. This meadow-rimmed lake has good views of distant Mt. Geikie, a couple of pretty good campsites, and plenty of hungry trout.

The trail loops around the east side of Dads Lake and then ascends a little gully to lovely Marms Lake, which has more good campsites as well as lots of big trout. About 0.1 mile past the north end of Marms Lake is a junction. Veer right, following signs to Shadow Lake, and walk mostly uphill in forest and meadows for 1.5 miles to a signed junction with the trail to outstandingly scenic Shadow Lake. This is where the south half of the figure-eight begins.

For now, go straight (north) and descend for 0.2 mile to another signed junction just before the crossing of Washakie Creek. The trail to the left (west) is faint and little used. Go straight and almost immediately ford or, by late summer, rock-hop Washakie Creek. The trail then climbs fairly steeply for about 0.5 mile before it levels off and comes to a junction with the Washakie Pass Trail, which angles off to the right and is your return route.

For now, go straight and soon reach very scenic Skull Lake, which has excellent views of numerous distant peaks and some good campsites above its south and west shores. After rounding the west side of Skull Lake the up-and-down trail leads north 0.8 mile to a signed but easy-to-miss junction with the Hailey Pass Trail about 0.1 mile before you reach Mae's Lake, which is visible up ahead.

Before turning toward Hailey Pass, consider an outstanding side trip to Pyramid Lake and the lakes at the headwaters of East Fork River. To make this side trip, go straight at the Hailey Pass junction and walk around the west side of Mae's Lake, which sits beneath the twin giants of Mt. Hooker and aptly named Pyramid Peak. The trail then climbs steeply away from Mae's Lake, following the cascading inlet creek to the rocky shores of Pyramid Lake. Sitting in a bowl directly beneath the impressive ramparts of Mt. Hooker and Tower Peak, this lake is quite a spot. Camping is rather austere, but is possible amid some stunted whitebark pines above the southwest shore.

Adventurers should consider an outstanding addition to this side trip. Follow an angler's path to the northwest shore of Pyramid Lake, then go cross-country to the west over grassy areas and past two ponds to a low, rocky saddle. From here you can look west across the deep chasm of East Fork River to the stupendous towers and cliffs on the east side of (from north to south) Mt. Bonneville, Raid Peak, Ambush Peak, and Mt. Geikie. Some of these cliffs are nearly 2000 feet high. You can reach a string of narrow lakes at the base of these amazing ramparts quite easily by walking downhill over open terrain of grasses, low shrubs, and rocks. This is huge, neck-craning country, but the scenery is awesome and the hiking is memorable. The largest, highest lake in the chain is perhaps the most spectacular, but that's a tough call.

To do the north half of the recommended figure-eight, return to the junction just south of Mae's Lake and turn east on the trail to Hailey Pass. This route gradually ascends in an open forest of whitebark pines and Engelmann spruces, crossing and recrossing a small creek as it ascends. The path climbs around the steep slopes south and east of Pyramid Peak, soon making its way above treeline and coming to the high basin holding the two tiny Twin Lakes. Cross between the two scenic lakes here and then ascend tundra-covered slopes to 11,230-foot Hailey Pass.

The views from this pass are a bit restricted, but as you steeply descend the north side, things improve. Mt. Hooker fills the skyline to the west, while the welcoming expanse of the Baptiste Creek valley beckons below. The tread is often obscure during the descent, in part due to snowfields that linger on this cold north slope until late July, but the way down is generally obvious. Once you reach the lower meadows along Baptiste Creek you can look west to the incredible

Pingora Peak, Cirque of the Towers

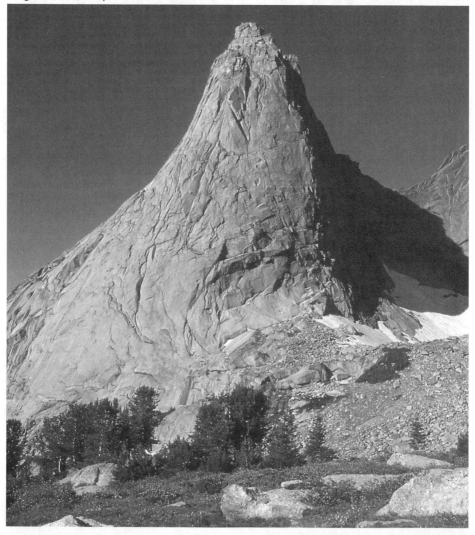

northeast wall of Mt. Hooker. The ramparts here are the highest unbroken cliffs in the Wind River Range—quite a statement given some of the scenery you have already seen on this trip.

Almost immediately after the trail crosses Baptiste Creek is a junction. To make the outstanding side trip to Baptiste Lake, turn left and climb through open forest then over view-packed grasslands and rocks for 1.3 miles to the southern shore of the large lake. All but the south shore of Baptiste Lake is in the Wind River Indian Reservation, so exploring to the north requires a tribal fishing permit. Even staying on the southern shoreline, however, is ample reward for your efforts with stunning views of Musembeah Peak, Mt. Lander, and a host of other jagged summits. Camping is possible at the lake, but the area is quite exposed, so only stay if the weather is good.

Back on the main loop trail, go east and drop into heavily forested terrain on the slopes above huge Grave Lake. You then go up and down well above that lake's north shore for a little less than a mile before making your way down to some excellent campsites near where Grave Creek feeds into the lake. Continuing east, keep right at the junction with the Onion Meadows Trail and then hike another 0.4 mile to a bridge over good-sized Grave Creek, filled to the brim by the waters of the 1.5-mile long lake it drains. From here follow the lakeshore a short distance farther and then cross a ridge and finally drop to a junction beside the clear waters of Little Wind River.

Keep straight (upstream) on the main trail and slowly gain elevation in forest and a lovely streamside meadow for 1.1 miles to a junction. The trail to the left climbs to Valentine Lake and the Bears Ears Loop (see Trip 19, p. 168). You keep right and gain almost 400 feet up to the slopes above large, irregularly shaped Washakie Lake. Huge Big Chief Mountain, with its long line of impressive cliffs, dominates the southwest shore of this lake. There are some good campsites on the gentle slopes north of Washakie Lake.

A moderately steep climb takes you away from Washakie Lake and up to smaller Macon Lake, a fine fishing spot and, like all the other lakes in this area, offering excellent scenery. To the southwest you can look upon rugged Mt. Washakie and the small glacier hidden in the shady basin between this mountain and nearby Big Chief Mountain.

From Macon Lake the trail goes steeply uphill over talus slopes and potentially dangerous lingering snowfields for a little less than 1 mile to Washakie Pass. The views from this rocky pass are excellent. Not only can you look east over much of the country you just traversed, but you can see west to the dramatic line of cliffs above East Fork River and on to the large meadows near Raid and Dream lakes. As it goes west from the pass, the trail steeply descends over talus and tundra to a marshy little alpine basin, then goes gradually downhill back into the land of scattered trees to the junction a little south of Skull Lake and the end of the north loop section.

Return to the junction with the Shadow Lake Trail about 0.2 mile south of the crossing of Washakie Creek, turn left (east), and gradually make your way up the wide valley of Washakie Creek. The encroaching mountains become higher and more spectacular with each step. At 1 mile from the junction cross Washakie Creek, via either an easy ford of a simple rock-hop depending on the time of year. From there it is another 1.1 miles of gradual uphill to the end of the official trail at Shadow Lake. Sitting right beneath the lesser-known back (west) side of the jagged peaks of Cirque of the Towers, Shadow Lake is an incredibly dramatic spot. Photo opportunities are unlimited and the sitting and gazing options are unparalleled. There are a few good campsites here, allowing overnighters to enjoy the view at leisure.

To continue the recommended loop, follow a good trail that takes you a little over halfway around the north side of Shadow Lake. Shortly before you cross the lake's main inlet creek, look for a cairn marking a boot path that goes uphill to the left. Follow this often faint path as it winds uphill and takes you to Billys Lake. While not as spectacular as Shadow Lake, this lake is very scenic, has lots of hungry trout, and features a few mediocre campsites amid stunted trees.

The easily followed boot path now leads you around the northwest side of Billys Lake, then uphill into increasingly alpine terrain to Barren Lake. Despite its name, this scenic lake has a good population of trout. The intermittent tread then goes around the south side of Barren Lake and up briefly to fishless Texas Lake and the end of easy walking.

Your next goal is Texas Pass, which lies southwest from Texas Lake and can be seen easily from the lakeshore. Reaching the pass is not technically difficult, but does involve some very steep uphill travel, partly over boulders and talus. Hikers with strong lungs and legs should have little difficulty. There is even a rough trail virtually all the way to the top. Still, if you are inexperienced or afraid of heights you probably shouldn't take this route.

Shortly after you reach narrow Texas Pass and begin to descend its south side, the tremendous array of granite peaks and spires of Cirque of the Towers come into view. With a scene like this it doesn't take long for you to understand why this place is so beloved by photographers, hikers, and mountain climbers. In fact, there is so much incredible scenery, it soon becomes hard to take it all in.

Even though there is no trail, the way down from Texas Pass is much easier than the way up, because it is less steep and the footing is more solid. Make your way down the east side of a wide, mostly grassy gully toward the base of a massive and unmistakable tower called Pingora Peak. When you get near the base of the peak you may want to watch the climbers who can frequently be seen slowly making their way up the almost sheer granite walls. Also from near the peak you will get your first views down to Lonesome Lake at the base of the cirque. Although no longer "lonesome," this lake is just as gorgeous as when it was first named. Your route soon picks up a steep but easy-to-follow boot path down to a wet meadow at the northwest corner of Lonesome Lake. The point where this trail leaves the forested hillside and enters the meadow is marked with a cairn.

If, despite my warnings about camp-raiding black bears and a lack of solitude, you still choose to camp near Lonesome Lake, keep in mind that the Forest Service requires that you set up at least 0.25 mile from the lake. Most climbers and backpackers choose to camp in the basin southwest of Lonesome Lake, although that area is now crowded and showing signs of overuse. A better alternative is to walk 1.7 miles downstream on the North Fork Trail to Lizard Head Meadows with its several comfortable and more private sites.

To continue the recommended loop, follow the wildly scenic angler's trail along the north shore of Lonesome Lake, then cross the outlet creek and walk uphill to the south through open forest and meadows until you intersect the official trail. Turn right and make a steep climb, mostly in view-packed meadows, to Jackass Pass (a.k.a. Big Sandy Pass) from which you enjoy wonderful views of Cirque of the Towers.

From Jackass Pass the trail becomes rough, rocky, and steep and is unsuitable for livestock. The trail goes steeply down about three-quarters of the way to small, very narrow Arrowhead Lake, which you can see below. Make a sharp left turn, hop over a tiny creek, and regain all of that elevation in order to skirt the cliffs on the east side of that tiny lake. After more rugged, rocky hiking down to narrow North Lake, make a tough up and down around the east side of this lake before finally hopping over a small creek and switchbacking down on a much better trail to a junction at the north end of Big Sandy Lake. This beautiful lake is a very popular destination and has many campsites. If you stay here, however, be aware that camp-raiding black bears pose a significant problem. Use the bear-resistant food containers at the southwest tip of the lake to protect your food and other odorous items.

For a great side trip from Big Sandy Lake, turn left (east) at the Jackass Pass junction and walk through meadows and over a couple of small creeks for 0.4 mile to a junction with the trail to Black Joe Lake. Go straight (staying level) and walk beside a beautiful meadow for 0.2 mile before you climb away from Big Sandy Lake. After about 0.5 mile of easy uphill you reach impressive Clear Lake, which is backed by the majestic granite mass of huge Haystack Mountain and has several good campsites on its north and west sides.

Nice as Clear Lake is, don't turn around here—there is plenty of spectacular terrain to explore nearby. To see it, follow the trail around the north side of the lake, then cross a creek and reach the beginning of a large expanse of gently sloping rock, which was polished smooth by ancient glaciers. The tread disappears here, but it isn't needed. Simply walk uphill over the smooth, open rock and past a few areas of grasses and trees; the walking is easy and you can't get lost. After gaining about 500 feet you reach Deep Lake, which sits at the base of both Steeple Peak and its side summit, Lost Temple Spire, both very impressive, aptly named pinnacles.

The trail's tread reappears at Deep Lake, making its way around the west shore and slowly climbing another 300 feet to a little ridge. From here you can look down on nearby Temple Lake and its amazing array of surrounding mountains. Most prominent among these is Temple Peak.

Those hikers with lots of extra energy can keep going on an often faint, quite steep trail that goes south-southeast up a talus slope to 11,500-foot Temple Pass. The views here of both nearby peaks and south down the valley of Little Sandy Creek to the distant deserts of southern Wyoming are terrific.

Returning to the junction with the Jackass Pass Trail beside Big Sandy Lake, follow the lake's northwest shore past excellent campsites and a signed trail to the bear boxes at the end of the lake. The gentle, heavily used trail then goes very gradually downhill through open forest for a little less than 2 miles to a junction.

The Diamond Lake Trail angles to the right, a somewhat longer, less crowded alternate return route that visits a couple of pleasant, if unspectacular, lakes. Most people stay on the shorter main trail, however, which goes straight at the Diamond Lake junction and continues its gentle downhill through mostly viewless forest. The scenery improves after 0.6 mile when you meet up with the (not very) Big (not in the least bit) Sandy (actually more of a creek than a) River. Follow this lovely stream through forest and along beautiful streamside meadows all the way back to the fork only 0.6 mile from the trailhead. Keep straight and retrace your steps to the trailhead.

POSSIBLE ITINERARY

	CAMPS & SIDE TRIPS	MILES	ELEVATION GAIN
DAY 1	Skull Lake	9.5	1500'
DAY 2	Skull Lake, with dayhike to Pyramid and East Fork Lakes	8.6	1000'
DAY 3	Grave Lake, including a side trip to Baptiste Lake	8.0	1600'
DAY 4	Shadow Lake	12.4	2200'
DAY 5	Clear Lake	7.9	2700'
DAY 6	Out, including a side trip to Temple Lake	10.9	1000'

VARIATIONS •

A shorter version of this trip skips the north half of the figure-eight and visits only Shadow Lake and Cirque of the Towers before returning via Big Sandy Lake.

Another popular option is a somewhat longer loop that stays entirely on maintained trails. To do this, go north to the junction just south of Skull Lake and turn northeast to climb over Washakie Pass. Go east past beautiful Valentine Lake and climb to a junction with the Bears Ears Trail. Turn south (see description in Trip 19, p. 168), hike the view-packed trail to Lizard Head Meadows, and then turn west to reach Cirque of the Towers. Return via Big Sandy Lake as described in the recommended trip above.

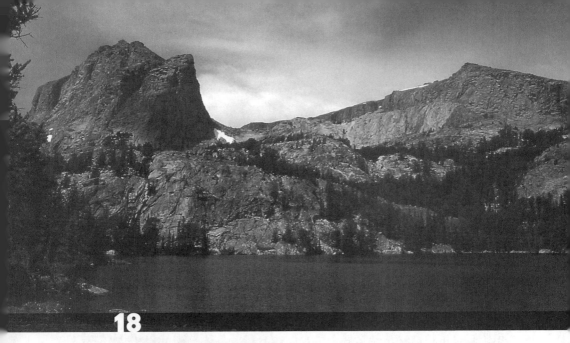

18

GLACIER TRAIL

RATINGS: Scenery 8   Solitude 3   Difficulty 6
MILES: 44.2
ELEVATION GAIN: 8000´
DAYS: 4–7
MAP: Earthwalk Press *Northern Wind River Range*
USUALLY OPEN: July to October
BEST: Mid-July to early September
CONTACT: Wind River Ranger District, Shoshone National Forest
SPECIAL ATTRACTIONS: Diverse and dramatic mountain scenery; access to Wyoming's highest peak and the largest glaciers in the American Rockies
PERMIT: None required—sign in at the trailhead.

RULES

Fires are prohibited above treeline. Groups are limited to 15 people and 25 stock. Camping is prohibited within 100 feet of streams and 200 feet of lakes or trails. All food and other odorous items must be stored away from bears.

CHALLENGES

The area can be quite crowded, especially around Double Lake and Floyd Wilson Meadows, frequently has thunderstorms, and has abundant mosquitoes in July.

Photo: Double Lake

HOW TO GET THERE ·

Despite this trail's importance and popularity, the turnoff to the trailhead is surprisingly unassuming and easy to miss. From Dubois, drive 3 miles east on U.S. Highway 26/287 to a junction with a gravel road to the right (south). The sign at this junction mentions only the Dubois Fish Hatchery and says nothing about the trailhead. Turn onto this road and just 10 yards later reach a fork. Take the left branch (Forest Service Road 411) and proceed 8.7 miles on an often washboarded, pothole-filled road past a series of large lakes to a fork. Keep right and drive 0.6 mile to the large trailhead turnaround and parking area.

DESCRIPTION ·

The wide, gravelly Glacier Trail takes off from the west end of the parking lot and switchbacks steadily up a semidesert hillside covered with grasses, sagebrush, junipers, and even a few prickly pear cacti. After 0.6 mile bear left at a junction with Whiskey Mountain Trail, soon enter the Fitzpatrick Wilderness, and at 0.8 mile come to a junction with the Lake Louise Trail. Go left and cross a sturdy wooden bridge over Torrey Creek, stopping first to admire the stream as it races down a narrow chasm in a roaring cataract.

Amid huge rounded buttresses of dark rock, the often rocky trail intermittently climbs into increasingly forested terrain, including many specimens of Douglas firs with their unusual cones. At a little more than 3 miles you reach Bomber Basin, a lovely subalpine meadow with a small campsite along East Torrey Creek. A little past this camp you reach a junction with the no-longer-maintained trail to Bomber Falls.

TAKE THIS TRIP

Situated in the northeastern Wind River Range, this very popular hike travels the entire length of the Glacier Trail, the main access route into the Fitzpatrick Wilderness. The trail provides the easiest access for climbers heading to Gannett Peak, the highest point in Wyoming, and while rugged, it's also very scenic, including a sampler of everything this part of the range offers. From desertlike sagebrush flats at the trailhead, you climb through a diverse evergreen forest to subalpine meadows, past imposing rock buttresses, over high alpine passes, past sparkling mountain lakes, then along a milky glacial stream to the base of the largest glaciers in the American Rockies. The variety of scenery ensures that at least part of the trail will appeal to every backpacker, and true wilderness lovers will enjoy every step.

Numerous potential side trips, mostly off-trail, allow you to escape the crowds and explore this magnificent country with a greater degree of solitude. Dedicated explorers could easily spend two or three weeks in the high country here and never run out of worthwhile destinations.

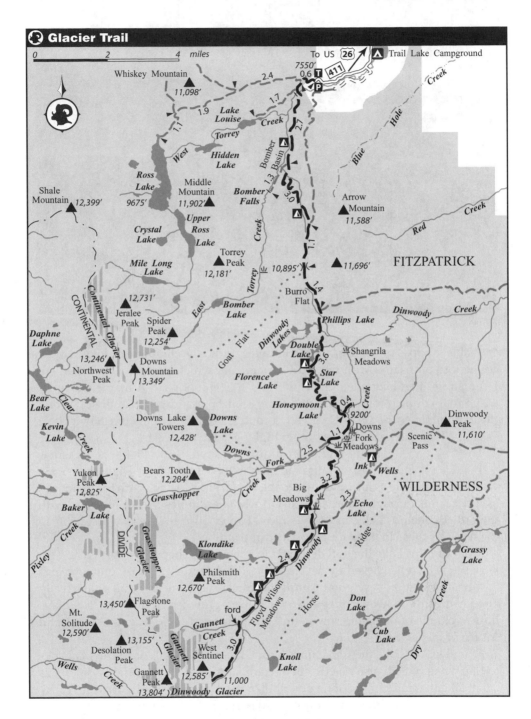

Glacier Trail

To US 26
Trail Lake Campground

0   2   4   miles

Whiskey Mountain
11,098'

7550'
0.6

2.4

1.7

1.9   Lake
Louise
Creek

1.7

Torrey

West   Hidden
Lake

Ross
Lake   Middle
Mountain   Bomber
Falls
Shale
Mountain   12,399'   9675'   11,902'

2.7

1.3   Bomber   Basin

Arrow
Mountain
11,588'

Blue   Hole
Creek

Red   Creek

Upper
Ross
Lake

Crystal
Lake

3.0

Mile Long
Lake

Torrey
Peak
12,181'

10,895'   1.1   11,696'   FITZPATRICK

12,731'

Jeralee
Peak   Spider
Peak
12,254'   East   Bomber
Lake   Torrey   Creek   Burro
Flat   1.4

Phillips Lake   Dinwoody   Creek

Daphne
Lake

Northwest
Peak   13,246'   Downs
Mountain
13,349'   Goat Flat   Dinwoody
Lakes   Double
Lake   3.6   Shangrila
Meadows

CONTINENTAL   Continental   Glacier

Bear
Lake

Kevin
Lake

Yukon
Peak
12,825'   Clear   Creek   Downs Lake
Towers
12,428'   Downs
Lake   Florence
Lake   Star
Lake

Honeymoon
Lake   9200'   0.4   Creek   Dinwoody
Peak
11,610'

Downs
Fork
Meadows   Scenic
Pass

Bears Tooth
12,284'   Downs   Fork   1.1

2.5

Baker   Lake   Grasshopper   Creek   Big
Meadows   3.2   Ink   Wells   WILDERNESS

Pixley   Creek   DIVIDE   Grasshopper   Glacier   Klondike
Lake   2.3   Echo
Lake   Ridge   Grassy
Lake

Philsmith
Peak
12,670'   2.4   Dinwoody   Don
Lake

Mt.
Solitude
12,590'   13,450'   Flagstone
Peak

13,155'   ford   Gannett   Creek   Floyd   Wilson   Meadows   Horse   Cub
Lake   Creek   Dry

Desolation
Peak   West
Sentinel
12,585'   3.0   Knoll
Lake

Wells   Creek   Gannett
Peak
13,804'   Dinwoody   Glacier   11,000   Grassy
Lake

Bear left and begin a long climb on 30 sometimes monotonous, but well-graded switchbacks before you reach an open, rolling ridgetop with abundant wildflow-ers and fine views of the brown summits to the west. Hop over a tiny creek

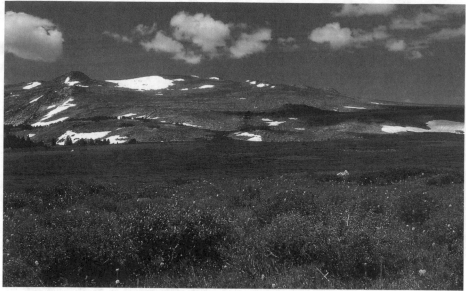

Burro Flat

(possible campsites nearby) then continue gradually climbing in lovely open country to a junction with the old Glacier Trail, which angles in from the left. Keep straight and complete the climb to a 10,895-foot pass. A marvelous, very easy cross-country route leaves the main trail here and goes southwest along the open alpine expanse of Goat Flat, a rolling ridge that offers terrific views of Downs Mountain and countless other high peaks to the west.

The trail now descends over open, alpine terrain to Burro Flat, where there is a small creek and an easy-to-miss junction with the very faint Dinwoody Trail, which starts beside a cairn and goes to the left (east). You stick with the main trail as it descends through a burned forest of whitebark pines to a scenic pond with the rather generous name of Phillips Lake. Larger off-trail lakes are accessible to the west for those looking for a private campsite.

From Phillips Lake the trail descends to irregularly shaped Double Lake. This very scenic lake is backed by several cliff-edged buttes and rock outcroppings and has numerous very good campsites. Since these are the trail's first really good campsites, however, they are usually very crowded. In July the lake plays host to clouds of mosquitoes who find all those tired backpackers a wonderful source of fresh blood.

From Double Lake the trail climbs about 300 feet in a half dozen switchbacks to Star Lake, which also has excellent campsites. Just on the other side of this small lake the trail begins a long downhill, most of it accomplished in tight rocky switchbacks. Along the way you pass rock-rimmed Honeymoon Lake, which is easy to miss since the trail never gets close to the water. At the bottom of the downhill you meet large and roaring Dinwoody Creek, whose waters are full of silt from glacial runoff. An unsigned, easily missed side trail goes downstream here 0.4 mile to a thundering waterfall.

For the next mile the main trail heads upstream, skirting marshy Downs Fork Meadows to a junction. The Downs Fork Trail goes right to some very scenic mountains and lakes. Reaching the best of this country, however, requires cross-country scrambling—great for adventure hikers.

The Glacier Trail goes left at the junction and immediately crosses a bridge over Downs Fork, whose waters are also laden with glacial silt. The trail then climbs through a burned forest away from Downs Fork Meadows, goes around a butte, and comes to very scenic Big Meadows. The often sandy trail now goes around the right side of this large meadow to a possible campsite at the meadow's south end. About 0.5 mile past Big Meadows is a signed junction with the Ink Wells Trail, which goes sharply to the left. There's a good campsite 200 yards down this trail on the other side of a bridge over Dinwoody Creek.

The main trail goes straight at the Ink Wells junction, rounds a corner, and affords you the first good views of distinctive Gannett Peak, straight ahead to the southwest. This tall summit, clearly higher than the many peaks surrounding it, is mantled with large glaciers and is an impressive sight. Over the next few miles you continue to get closer to this mountain, and the views remain outstanding the entire way. Also over these miles are numerous good and exceptionally scenic campsites.

Cross rushing Klondike Creek, where a very rough cross-country route goes right on its way to huge, beautiful Klondike Lake. As the Glacier Trail continues slowly climbing the trees get smaller, the rocks more numerous, and the scenery increasingly grand. The trail goes through mostly flat Floyd Wilson Meadows (more camps here, although they are often crowded with climbers) and comes to a ford of glacial Gannett Creek. Previous hikers have often placed a rope across the creek to help with your balance on this cold, tricky ford.

Above crossing Gannett Creek, the trail's character becomes increasingly alpine as it climbs amid grasses, rocks, and moraine material to the source of Dinwoody Creek where the waters pour out of large Dinwoody Glacier. Unless you brought climbing gear, this is as far as you can go. So take in the scenery for an hour or two, then reluctantly turn around and head back the way you came.

POSSIBLE ITINERARY

	CAMPS & SIDE TRIPS	MILES	ELEVATION GAIN
DAY 1	Double Lake	9.8	3500'
DAY 2	Floyd Wilson Meadows	8.9	1200'
DAY 3	Floyd Wilson Meadows, with dayhike		
	to Dinwoody Glacier	6.8	1300'
DAY 4	Double Lake	8.9	1000'
DAY 5	Out	9.8	1000'

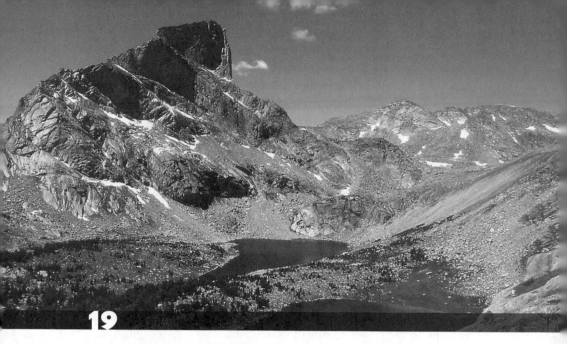

19

DICKINSON PARK
& BEARS EARS TRAIL LOOP

RATINGS: Scenery 10   Solitude 4   Difficulty 7
MILES: 37.1 (38.3)
ELEVATION GAIN: 5500´ (5800´)
DAYS: 3–6
MAP: Earthwalk Press *Southern Wind River Range*
USUALLY OPEN: Mid-July to October
BEST: Mid-July to August
CONTACT: Washakie Ranger District, Shoshone National Forest
SPECIAL ATTRACTIONS: *Awesome* mountain scenery, but hey, this is the Wind Rivers, so what did you expect?
PERMIT: None required for hikers—sign in at the trailhead. Stock users must obtain a permit to stay overnight.

RULES

Fires are prohibited above treeline. Groups are limited to 15 people and 25 stock. Camping is prohibited within 100 feet of streams and 200 feet of lakes or trails. All food and other odorous items must be stored away from bears.

Photo: *Lizard Head Peak and Bear Lakes*

CHALLENGES · · · · · · · · · · · · · · · · · ·

The area has frequent thunderstorms, and this trip has a long section of exposed, above-treeline hiking. Road access is rather poor. Smith Lake Basin has camp-raiding black bears. The first 5 uphill miles are waterless.

HOW TO GET THERE · · · · · · · · · · · · ·

From a junction on U.S. Highway 287 just south of the small town of Fort Washakie, on the Wind River Indian Reservation about 15 miles northwest of Lander, turn west on Trout Creek Road (County Road 294). Drive 5.2 miles to the end of pavement and begin bouncing along on a rutted and bumpy gravel-and-dirt road. After heavy rains this road becomes muddy and quite slick and may be impassable for passenger cars. Drive 0.4 mile to a fork, where you go straight, and begin winding steadily uphill from sagebrush-covered plains to forested hillsides and mountains. At 19.5 miles from Highway 287 turn left at a junction, following signs to Dickinson Park, and soon thereafter enter the Shoshone National Forest. Now on Forest Service Road 329, proceed 1.7 miles and come to the turnoff to the Bears Ears Trailhead near the small Dickinson Park Work Center.

If you have two cars you can save 2.7 miles of walking along the road by leaving the second car at the Dickinson Park Trailhead. To reach it, go straight at the Bears Ears Trailhead turnoff, drive 1.4 miles to a junction just before a campground entrance, turn left, and go another 0.7 mile to the trailhead parking area in a large meadow about 100 yards past the signed trailhead.

To reach the Bears Ears Trailhead, turn right at the junction near the work center and slowly proceed 0.6 mile on a badly rutted, rough, and pothole-filled road to the trailhead.

NOTE: Be sure to begin your hike with plenty of water, since you have plenty of climbing to do before the first reliable source at 5.2 miles.

TAKE THIS TRIP

For a compact three- to four-day loop trip with unparalleled mountain scenery, it would be hard to top this hike in the southeastern Wind River Range. Perhaps the highlight of the trip is the magnificent Bears Ears and Lizard Head trails traverse, unquestionably one of the finest above-treeline rambles in North America. In addition to this scenic treasure, the loop also visits the outstandingly beautiful Smith Lake Basin, with its numerous large lakes set beneath tall granite peaks; explores much of the sparkling North Popo Agie River, one of the best trout fishing streams in the Wind River Range; and comes within an easy side trip of the world-famous Cirque of the Towers, one of the classic beauty spots in the American Rockies. On the down side, the hike is rugged and involves some long ups and downs, but it's hard to complain amid scenery this grand.

Dickinson Park & Bears Ears Trail Loop

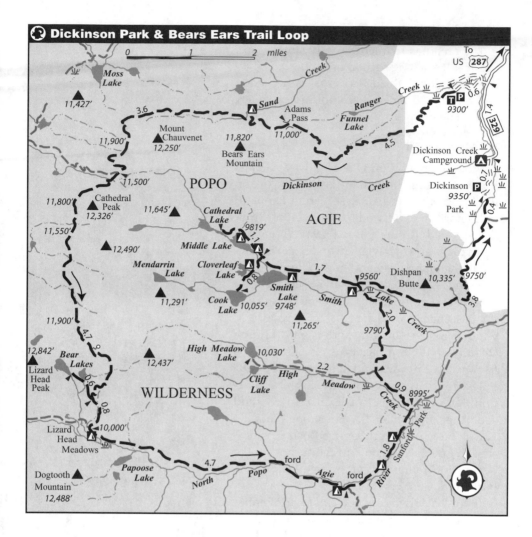

DESCRIPTION

As an enticing preview of what is to come, the trail starts in a beautiful mountain meadow of grasses and low sagebrush with good views to the west of a line of unnamed jagged peaks. The trail soon enters a forest of mostly lodgepole pines and begins gradually climbing in a series of irregularly spaced, lazy switchbacks. At 1.6 miles you enter the Popo Agie Wilderness after which the trail continues its pattern of gently ascending switchbacks in open forest. As you gain elevation the forest changes from mostly lodgepole pines to a mix of Engelmann spruces, subalpine firs, and whitebark pines. The first views come at around 3.5 miles when you reach a sloping, willow-choked meadow beneath a row of rocky pinnacles. The trail loops around the top of this meadow, then curves back to the west and traverses a rocky slope to indistinct Adams Pass. You are now above treeline, so the views are unobstructed and superb. Most striking are the looks down to teardrop-shaped Funnel Lake to the east-northeast and west to Mt. Chauvenet and distinctively shaped Bears Ears Mountain. The summit of the latter peak features a tall pinnacle topped by two lobes that might, with a little imagination, be said to resemble ursine ears.

> **NOTE:** The trail remains above treeline for the next several miles, providing great vistas along one of the best high country walks in Wyoming or, for that matter, anywhere else. On the other hand, this is no place to be if thunderstorms or other inclement weather is expected, so plan accordingly.

After traversing rocks and tundra for 0.5 mile, the trail loses about 150 feet to a lovely meadow near the head of Sand Creek, the first reliable water source of the trip. Good but rather exposed campsites are available here if the weather cooperates. The trail crosses what is left of Sand Creek a little above the meadow and then slowly climbs through an enchanting alpine landscape beneath the pyramid of Mt. Chauvenet. The climax comes at about 7 miles when you finally top the watershed divide above Sand Creek and are treated to a . . . well . . . adjectives fail me, but suffice it to say that it's one heck of a view. Spread out to the west is almost the entire southern Wind River Range with its sheer cliffs, hundreds of rugged peaks, and dozens of sparkling lakes. The most prominent body of water is huge, curving Grave Lake. Sit back and enjoy, although you will probably need a windbreaker since a stiff breeze almost always blows at this elevation.

The trail now turns south, climbs some more to go around the back (west) side of Mt. Chauvenet, contours past several large rock formations, and then switchbacks down to a junction at 8.1 miles. The Bears Ears Trail goes right descending to the lakes country at the headwaters of Little Wind River and providing access to magnificent backcountry adventures of a week or more. If you need a campsite, the closest alternative is about 2.6 miles and 1100 feet down this trail at popular Valentine Lake.

The main loop trail goes left at the junction onto Lizard Head Trail, which ascends around the west side of Cathedral Peak. From here the trail descends 300 feet before beginning an extended, gradual uphill through a view-packed alpine wonderland. The tread is frequently faint amid the rocks and grasses, but numerous small cairns keep you on course. The prominent, bulky mountain to the southwest with a glacier on its north flank is Lizard Head Peak. It will dominate the view for the next few miles and change dramatically in appearance as you make your way around its east side.

You eventually reach a high point right across from looming Lizard Head Peak then begin a long downhill. The trail soon passes a cluster of small springs and then goes steeply down past countless outstanding viewpoints. Nearby Lizard Head Peak dominates the scene, but you can also look west to Lonesome Lake and Cirque of the Towers.

The trail eventually returns to the forest and comes to a signed junction with the good but unmaintained Bear Lakes Trail. This short trail provides a worthwhile side trip to a pair of dramatic lakes, if you have the time. The main trail goes straight and continues downhill to a junction with the North Fork Trail in the trees near Lizard Head Meadows. Extremely scenic campsites are scattered all around this area.

An excellent side trip from Lizard Head Meadows is the short hike up to the world-famous scenery in Cirque of the Towers. It's an easy 1.7-mile one-way stroll up to Lonesome Lake, and from there the exploring, climbing, and photography options are virtually unlimited. Trip 17 (p. 153) in this book describes that area more thoroughly.

To continue the loop, head downstream (east) on North Fork Trail and after just 0.3 mile pass a marshy pond in the lower part of Lizard Head Meadows. This pond provides tremendous early-morning reflections of the massive granite cliffs and pinnacles of Dogtooth Mountain. The trail keeps going mostly downhill, staying in forest well away from the North Popo Agie River but with frequent glimpses of a series of sheer granite walls to the south. At 3.6 miles from Lizard Head Meadows you make a calf- to knee-deep ford of the river and then travel along its south side for 1.1 miles to a fair campsite just before a junction with Pinto Park Trail. Bear left and descend for 0.4 mile to a second ford of North Popo Agie River, also about calf deep.

Soon after the ford you hike beside the long and narrow meadow at Sanford Park, where there are a couple of very pleasant campsites. Sanford Park is a good place to look for moose. About 1.4 miles below the last ford is a junction. Turn left on High Meadow Trail and begin a fairly steep climb on an often rocky trail. After gaining 700 feet in just 0.9 mile top a low rise and reach an unsigned, easy-to-miss junction. The trail to the left goes up to a group of small lakes at the headwaters of High Meadow Creek. Although not as spectacular as many other lakes in these mountains, they are still very attractive and worth a couple of hours of your time.

The main trail goes straight and gently climbs to the top of a forested ridge. You then make a short but steep descent before climbing over a second minor

Cathedral Lake

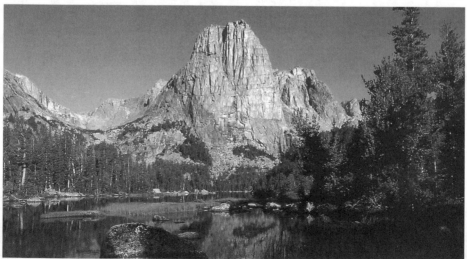

ridge and dropping to a gorgeous little meadow. Here you make an easy ford of Smith Lake Creek just before reaching a good campsite and a junction.

The return route to Dickinson Park goes right here, but if you do that now you will miss the trip's next great scenic highlight. Turn left and walk up a very gentle forested valley for 1.3 miles to some good campsites at the east end of large Smith Lake. Several rugged granite peaks (mostly unnamed) ring the basin holding this and a cluster of other nearby lakes. The area is popular, however, with both people and black bears. In fact, camp-raiding bears have become a problem here—take all necessary precautions to protect your food.

The trail soon leaves Smith Lake and climbs for 0.4 mile to an unsigned but obvious junction. Your only decision here is which way to go first. The path to the left (south) goes 150 yards to a creek crossing and then climbs a bit to Cloverleaf Lake, backed on its west side by a tall granite pinnacle and with a fine campsite above its southeast shore. Beyond Cloverleaf Lake the trail goes steeply uphill for 0.3 mile to trail's end at impressive Cook Lake. This dramatic gem is backed by a 1000-foot cliff and demands plenty of time for awed appreciation.

Back at the junction above Smith Lake the trail that goes northwest almost immediately reaches Middle Lake, yet another spectacular lake in this outstanding basin. Excellent campsites here allow you plenty of time to fish or simply enjoy the views of several nearby granite domes, peaks, and cliffs. The trail then goes around the north side of Middle Lake to another good campsite. From here a rugged, unmaintained path climbs 0.2 mile to Cathedral Lake, which sits in a narrow basin almost directly beneath a huge, towering granite monolith. In a word: *wow!* Once you've had your fill of all these lovely lakes, return to Smith Lake and backtrack 1.3 miles to the junction with High Meadow Trail.

To complete the loop, go straight (east) at the junction and hike down, up, then down again as you work around the south side of Dishpan Butte. The trail then turns north, switchbacks uphill nearly 400 feet to the wilderness boundary, and then gradually descends to a junction with the North Fork Trail. Go straight and cross the marshy meadow at Dickinson Park on a boardwalk to the Dickinson Park Trailhead. If your car is at the Bears Ears Trailhead, you face an easy 2.7-mile roadwalk to finish your trip.

POSSIBLE ITINERARY

	CAMPS & SIDE TRIPS	MILES	ELEVATION GAIN
DAY 1	Sand Creek	5.2	1800'
DAY 2	Lizard Head Meadows, including a side trip to Bear Lakes	9.6	2200'
DAY 3	Smith Lake	10.7	1300'
DAY 4	Out, with a side trip up to Cook and Cathedral lakes and including a 2.7-mile roadwalk back to your car	12.8	500'

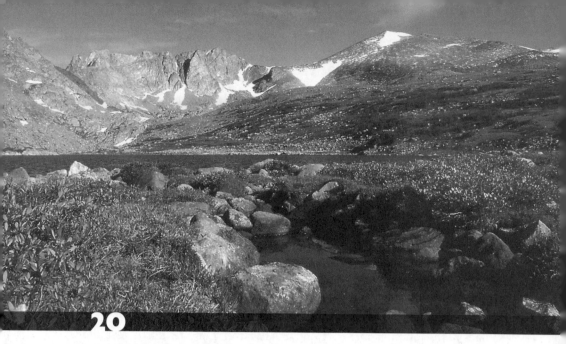

STOUGH LAKES & MIDDLE POPO AGIE RIVER LOOP

RATINGS: Scenery 9 Solitude 6 Difficulty 5
MILES: 31.4 (53.2)
ELEVATION GAIN: 5000´ (8000´)
DAYS: 4–6
MAPS: USGS *Cony Mountain;* Earthwalk Press *Southern Wind River Range*
USUALLY OPEN: July to October
BEST: Mid-July to September
CONTACT: Washakie Ranger District, Shoshone National Forest
SPECIAL ATTRACTIONS: The usual incredibly dramatic sparkling lakes, granite peaks, and alpine meadows that characterize the Wind River Range

PERMIT

None required for hikers—sign in at the trailhead. Stock users must obtain a permit to stay overnight.

RULES

Fires are prohibited above treeline. Groups are limited to 15 people and 25 stock. Camping is prohibited within 100 feet of streams and 200 feet of lakes or trails. All food and other odorous items must be stored away from bears.

Photo: Wind River Peak over Tayo Lake

CHALLENGES · · · · · · · · · · · · · · · · · · ·

Nothing significant. Besides, with this kind of scenery who can nitpick about little problems like mosquitoes or thunderstorms?

HOW TO GET THERE · · · · · · · · · · · · · ·

From U.S. Highway 287 in downtown Lander go southwest on Wyoming Highway 131, which eventually becomes Forest Service Road 300 and climbs into the mountains. At 18 miles from Lander turn right on Forest Service Road 302, following signs to Worthen Meadow Reservoir, and proceed 2.4 miles on this sometimes bumpy gravel road to a fork with a campground access road. Go straight and continue 0.3 mile to the large trailhead parking lot on the right.

DESCRIPTION · · · · · · · · · · · · · · · · · · ·

From the parking lot, walk back along the entrance road for 20 yards to the Stough Creek Lakes Trail and turn west-southwest onto that path. This wide, rather rocky trail slowly climbs through a forest composed mostly of lodgepole pines and, at least initially, without any good views. At 0.8 mile you enter the Popo Agie Wilderness and come to some possible campsites at shallow Roaring Fork Lake. The trail now crosses Roaring Fork Creek just as that stream flows out of the lake of the same name. By late summer it is usually possible to keep your feet dry by rock-hopping the creek a little downstream from the official crossing.

The trail goes around the right (north) side of Roaring Fork Lake, makes four gentle uphill switchbacks, then begins a long, gradual climb through forest and past a couple of pretty meadows. The ascent continues with several gently graded switchbacks through a thinning whitebark-pine forest before finally topping out at a 10,535-foot pass. The view to the west from here of massive Wind River Peak is outstanding.

TAKE THIS TRIP

The Wind River Range is so full of wonderfully scenic hiking opportunities that a guidebook author is sorely tested to come up with original superlatives to describe each hike. All the hikes here are great, with spectacular lakes, tall granite peaks, lovely meadows, view-filled passes, and a host of other mountain joys. Suffice it to say that this fun loop trip is more of the same, and thus well worth every step. It isn't for lack of scenery, but for some reason this part of the range is somewhat less popular than other areas, so solitude seekers may prefer this area to, for example, the overcrowded Cirque of the Towers, Glacier Trail, or Titcomb Basin.

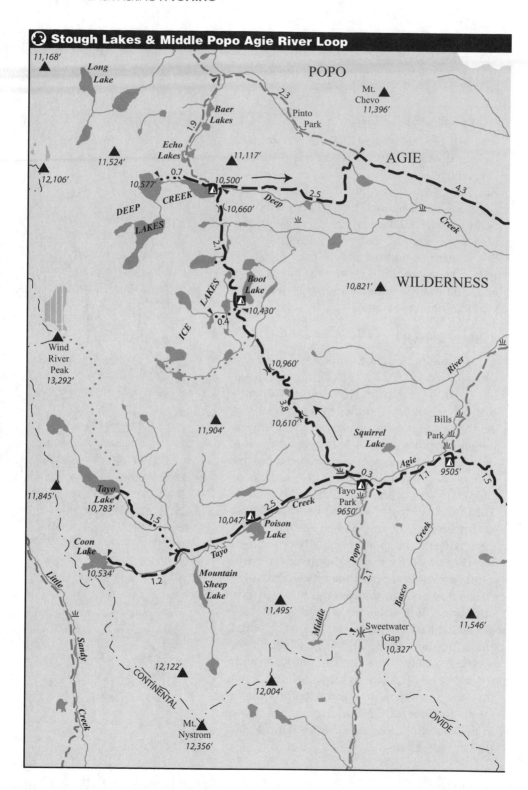

Stough Lakes & Middle Popo Agie River Loop

11,168'

Long
Lake

POPO

Baer
Lakes

2.3

Mt.
Chevo
11,396'

Pinto
Park

1.9

Echo
Lakes

11,524'

11,117'

AGIE

4.3

12,106'

0.7

10,577'

10,500'

2.5

DEEP   CREEK

10,660'

Deep

Creek

LAKES

2.1

Boot
Lake

10,821'   **WILDERNESS**

ICE   LAKES

10,430'

0.4

10,960'

River

Wind
River
Peak
13,292'

3.8

Bills

11,904'

10,610'

Squirrel
Lake

Park

9505'

1.5

Agie

1.1

11,845'

Tayo
Lake
10,783'

0.3

Tayo
Park
9650'

1.5

Creek

Tayo

2.5

10,047'

Poison
Lake

Coon
Lake

Little

10,534'

1.2

Tayo

Mountain
Sheep
Lake

Popo

2.1

Basco

Creek

11,495'

11,546'

Middle

Sandy

Sweetwater
Gap
10,327'

12,122'

CONTINENTAL

12,004'

Creek

Mt.
Nystrom
12,356'

DIVIDE

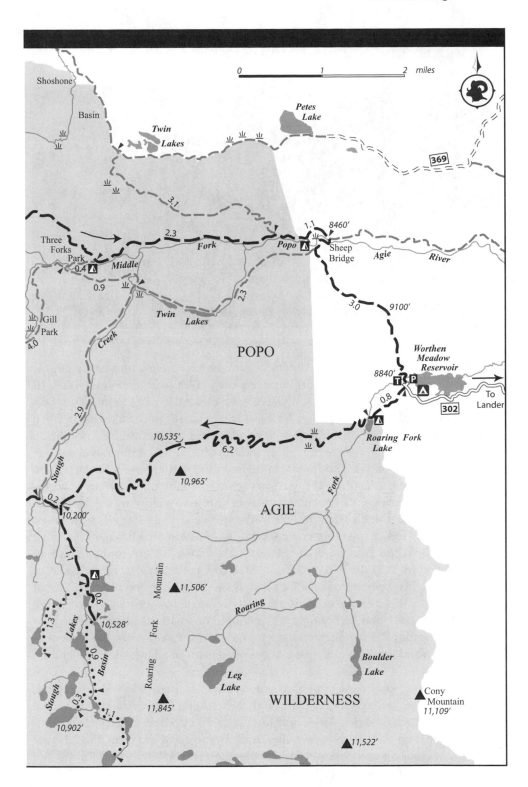

Shoshone

Basin

Twin Lakes

Petes Lake

369

0   1   2   *miles*

3.1

2.3

Three Forks Park

0.4

Middle

0.9

Fork

1.1

Popo

8460'

Sheep Bridge

Agie   *River*

Twin   Lakes

2.3

3.0   9100'

POPO

Gill Park

4.0

Creek

Worthen Meadow Reservoir

8840'

T   P

2.9

Stough

0.8

302

To Lander

10,535'

6.2

Roaring Fork Lake

0.2

10,200'

▲ 10,965'

AGIE

Fork

1.1

Mountain

▲ 11,506'

Roaring

10,528'

0.6

1.3

Lakes

0.6

Basin

Roaring   Fork

Boulder Lake

Leg Lake

▲ Cony Mountain 11,109'

Stough

0.3

1.1

WILDERNESS

10,902'

▲ 11,845'

▲ 11,522'

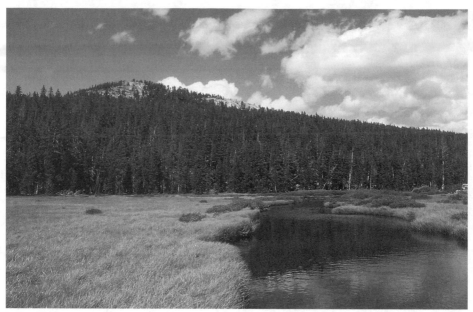

Tayo Park

The trail now goes generally downhill, slowly losing elevation past a couple of meadows and ponds to a poorly marked, easy-to-miss junction at 7 miles. (If you descend to a creek crossing, you have gone about 0.2 mile too far.) The main loop goes straight here, but first make the side trip into Stough Lakes Basin. Turn left and climb through open forest on a winding but gentle trail for 1.1 miles to the first lake, where there are campsites and the official trail ends. Lovely as this lake is, more than a dozen additional lakes lie in the basin above you, each more spectacular than the last. The entire basin is cradled in the rugged arms of horseshoe-shaped Roaring Fork Mountain, with its impressive cliffs and rocky ridges. Relatively easy scramble trails and off-trail routes lead to almost all of the lakes, and you could easily spend several happy days exploring the basin.

Once you've had your fill of the Stough Lakes Basin, return to the main trail and descend for 0.2 mile to a crossing of Stough Creek. You can either make an easy ford of this creek or look for logs across the flow a bit downstream. About 50 yards after the creek crossing is a junction. Veer left, following signs to the Middle Fork Trail, and contour around a couple of small meadows for 0.4 mile before descending at a moderately steep grade. At the bottom of this downhill is a junction and a possible campsite at the upper end of a large meadow known as Bills Park.

Go left here, soon pass through a wooden fence, then follow the tumbling Middle Popo Agie River upstream through fairly dense forest. After 0.5 mile take a bridge over small Basco Creek and then continue up and down before coming to a junction with Sweetwater Gap Trail. If you have the time, the 2.1-mile one-way detour up to the pass at Sweetwater Gap is worth the effort for the fine views it offers of the southern Wind River Range.

The Middle Fork Trail goes right at the Sweetwater Gap junction and quickly leads to a ford of Middle Popo Agie River at a pretty meadow called Tayo Park. The crossing is very cold, but the water is slow moving and rarely more than knee deep. On the other side of the ford are several very attractive campsites that make a good base camp for a dayhike into Coon and Tayo lakes.

The trail now climbs away from Tayo Park for 0.3 mile gaining about 200 feet up a forested hillside to a junction marked by a post at the base of a small meadow. The main loop trail goes straight here on its way to the Ice and Deep Creek lakes. Before heading that way, however, another fun side trip is in order. So turn left on Tayo Creek Trail and follow this route as it intermittently gains elevation. After initially taking you through forest, the path enters a large meadow along Tayo Creek where you gain good views of the nearby rounded peaks. At 1.3 miles from the main trail you reach Poison Lake. Although its name is unfortunate, this lake offers gorgeous scenery and a couple of very nice campsites. Just after you rock-hop a creek at 2.5 miles from the junction above Tayo Park is a signed junction. Both trails lead to lakes and both lakes are worth seeing. The easier trail goes straight and ascends for 1.2 miles to Coon Lake, which sits in a low saddle just below the Continental Divide.

The much more scenic lake, however, lies to the right (north) from the junction at the end of an often faint trail. You will frequently lose the tread, but the general route is usually obvious and the reward at the end is well worth it. This trail goes uphill over meadows and through brush for about 0.5 mile, crosses a creek, and then follows a grassy, sloping bench a little west of the creek. After 1.5 sometimes difficult miles you reach your goal: incredibly dramatic Tayo Lake, which sits in as impressive a setting as almost any other lake in the Wind River Range. The views of tall Wind River Peak to the north and other jagged granite ridges all around are truly outstanding. Unfortunately, the lake is located right at treeline and offers no reasonable camping. From Tayo Lake it is possible to make a long, tiring, but not technically difficult, scramble to the top of Wind River Peak. As you might expect, the view from the top of this, the highest summit in the southern Wind River Range, is absolutely amazing.

After returning to the junction at the meadow above Tayo Park, turn left (north) walk around the little meadow, then begin climbing once again. A little more than halfway up this 900-foot climb, you pass a cluster of tiny ponds with fine views of the peaks to the northwest. Top out at a rocky 10,590-foot pass and then descend almost 200 feet to a lovely basin holding a beautiful but unnamed little lake. From here you climb steeply once again, gaining another 500 feet to a second pass, this one just shy of 11,000 feet and a little above treeline.

From this high point you are treated to a wonderful view of Wind River Peak and the glacier-scoured cliffs backing the numerous rocky cirques of the Ice Lakes basin. You gradually descend into this rather stark basin where you can explore off-trail to a dozen or more dramatically scenic lakes of various shapes and sizes. As their name suggests, several of the Ice Lakes remain at least partially frozen until late July.

The trail misses most of the Ice Lakes as it goes down through pretty alpine meadows, past rocks, and through stunted forests of whitebark pines. You briefly visit Boot Lake with its mediocre campsites and then climb over a minor ridge to visit two smaller lakes. After yet another little pass, the trail descends to the east end of a large lake at the lower end of the Deep Creek Lakes chain. There are good campsites on the north side of this very scenic lake. The next lake up in the Deep Creek Lakes cluster is just above the west end of the lake that you are now enjoying and is easy to reach by angler's paths and a short, very simple off-trail hike. The effort is rewarded with a dramatic rock-lined lake backed by tall granite cliffs and several unnamed peaks.

To continue the recommended loop, go east (downstream) from a junction marked with a post near the outlet of the lowest Deep Creek Lake. Follow this rocky trail as it parallels tumbling Deep Creek, passes a meadow and a small scenic lake, then turns north and climbs around the base of a prominent granite knoll. At 2.5 miles from Deep Creek Lake is a junction. Turn right on the Pin-to Park Trail, and for the next few miles contour gently through an uneventful lodgepole pine forest. Eventually the trail becomes rocky and steeply loses elevation to a junction beside the lazy Middle Popo Agie River at Three Forks Park. There are good campsites in this area.

Keep left and follow the river downstream as the surrounding terrain slowly becomes drier and sagebrush begins to appear amid the thinning forest of pines and aspens. Keep straight where the Shoshone Lake Trail goes sharply left, then pass the wilderness boundary and almost immediately thereafter reach an

Lowest Deep Creek Lake

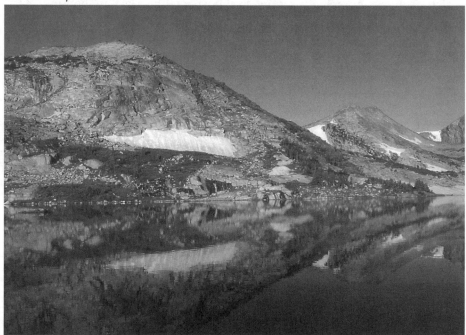

unsigned junction with a side trail that goes right to a small log cabin and some good riverside campsites.

The main trail continues straight and for the next 0.3 mile goes around a meadow with considerable beaver activity. A little past the east end of this meadow you come to a fork in the trail. Bear right on Sheep Bridge Trail and soon cross that path's namesake bridge over the Middle Popo Agie River. The trail then follows the lazy river upstream for 0.2 mile to a junction with Twin Lakes Trail. You go left and begin a moderately steep climb. After 1.4 miles the uphill grade eases and you wander through rolling forested terrain all the way back to the trailhead at Worthen Meadow Reservoir.

POSSIBLE ITINERARY

	CAMPS & SIDE TRIPS	MILES	ELEVATION GAIN
DAY 1	Stough Lakes Basin	8.1	2100'
DAY 2	Tayo Park, including a dayhike in Stough Lakes Basin	12.3	1200'
DAY 3	Tayo Park, dayhike to Tayo and Coon lakes	11.0	1600'
DAY 4	Deep Creek Lakes, including explorations to two of the closer Ice Lakes and the second Deep Creek Lake	8.6	2200'
DAY 5	Out	13.2	900'

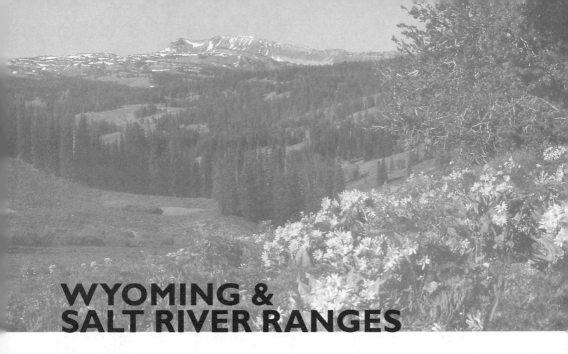

WYOMING &
SALT RIVER RANGES

L ocated in west-central Wyoming, and far from any of the state's main tourist attractions, the Wyoming and Salt River ranges are rarely traveled and
little known except to a handful of locals. But the secret those locals are
keeping is a spectacular one. These ranges contain all of the attributes you could
reasonably want from high mountains, including plenty of sky-scraping peaks,
huge meadows filled with wildflowers, cirque lakes tucked beneath awesome
cliffs, tumbling waterfalls, and plenty of wildlife. But isolation and easier access
to other more famous ranges has kept the trail population here so low that you
may not see another human being in several days of hiking. (In my own almost
three weeks of hiking here at the height of the season, I saw a grand total of two
other people.)

If you come here, however, be prepared for the rigors of hiking in such an
isolated area. Specifically, you can expect the trails (even the main ones) to disappear with frustrating regularity, which forces you to bushwhack, sometimes
for miles at a time, and to have well-developed map-reading and navigation
skills. Your gear, and especially your clothes, will take a beating from all the off-
trail travel and your boots should be both sturdy and well broken in. If all that
doesn't scare you, however, the rewards of hiking here are tremendous. There
may be no better place in the Lower 48 to enjoy pristine mountain scenery while
knowing that you are probably the only person for several miles in any direction.
So if you love both solitude and wild mountain scenery, explore the Wyoming
and Salt River ranges.

Photo: *Deadman Mountain from Cliff Creek Pass (Trip 21)*

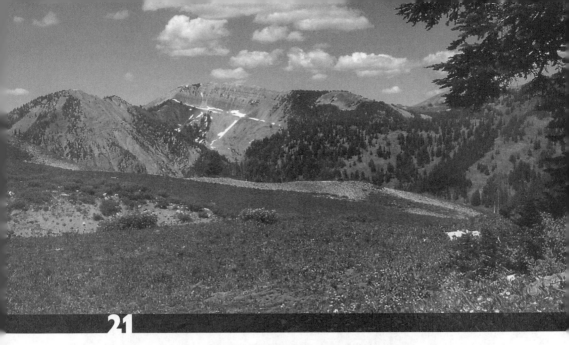

21

LITTLE GREYS RIVER LOOP

RATINGS: Scenery 7   Solitude 9   Difficulty 8
MILES: 30.7 (32.9)
ELEVATION GAIN: 7200´ (8100´)
DAYS: 3–5
MAPS: USGS *Hoback Mountain* and *Pickle Pass*
USUALLY OPEN: July to mid-October
BEST: Mid-July to early August
CONTACT: Greys River Ranger District, Bridger-Teton National Forest
SPECIAL ATTRACTIONS: Lots of solitude; fine mountain scenery; plenty of wildlife; acres of wildflowers in early to midsummer
PERMIT: None required

RULES

The usual no-trace rules apply.

CHALLENGES

The trail is often very sketchy and even disappears for long stretches. Most junctions are unsigned, so patience and good navigation skills are required.

Photo: Clause Peak from camp near head of Hunter Creek

TAKE THIS TRIP

This outstanding loop trip is a typical example of what hiking is like in the Wyoming Range. The mountain scenery, especially in early to midsummer when the wildflowers are blooming, is exceptional. The visitor is also treated to abundant wildlife and countless grand viewpoints. Despite these attractions, however, almost no one hikes here outside hunting season, so solitude is virtually assured. With virtually no one hiking the trails, the proper course is often faint at best and route-finding becomes tricky. Since most of the country is open, experienced hikers who are confident in their map-reading skills and who don't mind spending time wandering around in search of the correct path should not have any problems. If you are the type of person who panics if the tread disappears or who gets frustrated when you have to spend extra time looking for a trail that " . . . the *?#!&* map says has to be around here someplace!", then this trip is probably not for you.

HOW TO GET THERE

From the intersection of U.S. Highways 89 and 26 just across the border from Idaho at the community of Alpine Junction, go 0.6 mile south on U.S. Highway 89 over a bridge spanning the Snake River and into the town of Alpine. Turn left (southeast) on paved Greys River Road, which after 1 mile enters national forest land, turns to good gravel, and becomes Forest Service Road 10138. Follow this road for 7.9 miles to a major junction, turn left on Road 10124 (Little Greys River Road), and proceed 2.2 miles to a fork. Go right on Road 10047 and drive 2.3 miles to the road-end trailhead.

NOTE: When reviewing this trip information, the Forest Service informed me that they were currently putting up white (for nonmotorized trails) or green (for trails open to motor vehicles) diamond-shaped trail markings to assist in navigation. Hopefully, this will make life easier for confused hikers.

DESCRIPTION

The trail starts in an open forest of quaking aspens and lodgepole pines interspersed with small, lush meadows filled with rose and sagebrush bushes and lots of pink geranium, red gilia, yellow balsamroot, blue lupine, greenish horsemint, and other wildflowers.

Remaining on the hillside well above the clear Little Greys River, the trail climbs at an irregular but sometimes fairly steep grade for 1.4 miles to a fork. The main trail goes right, but you turn left (uphill) on the trail to Pickle Pass. Still traveling through lovely forest and meadows, this rather steep trail ascends past fields of early-July wildflowers that include many of the same species as before, but with the colorful addition of white columbine, tall blue larkspur, red paintbrush, green false hellebore, white valerian and coltsfoot, bluebells, and pink vetch, among many others. Views continuously improve as you climb, especially to the south of Deadman Mountain and

Little Greys River Loop

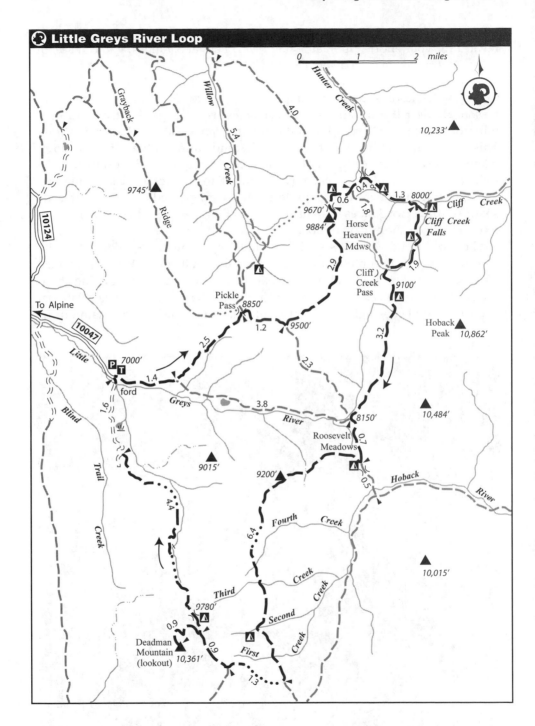

southwest to the rugged Salt River Range. At one point, a little more than half-way up the 1300-foot climb, the trail steeply loses about 100 feet, but for the most part it is a consistent, often tiring uphill. Game trails frequently cross your route, but if you stick with the main path going northeast you should be fine. As a nice reward for your efforts, upon attaining Pickle Pass at 3.9 miles, you can see all the way north to the jagged Teton Range.

Several trails, mostly faint and all unsigned, converge at Pickle Pass. The one to the left that leads to Grayback Ridge is very hard to discern, but the others are reasonably clear. If you want a somewhat longer trip, then go slightly left (downhill) from the pass on the northbound Wyoming Range National Recreation Trail. This very scenic but often sketchy route descends through beautiful meadows where you can often see herds of elk, to a creek crossing and a campsite. The trail then follows Willow Creek, mostly in forest, for 4 miles to a poorly marked junction. Turn right here and climb steeply to a view-packed ridgeline that leads south-southeast for 3 miles to an unsigned junction in a pass where you meet the recommended shorter loop option.

The recommended loop is slightly shorter and requires less elevation gain. To take it, turn right (uphill) at Pickle Pass on the southbound Wyoming Range National Recreation Trail and ascend a partly forested ridge. After gaining about 800 feet in 1 mile you come to a ridgetop junction. The Wyoming Range National Recreation Trail goes right (downhill), but your trail, which is often faint, turns

Cliff Creek Falls

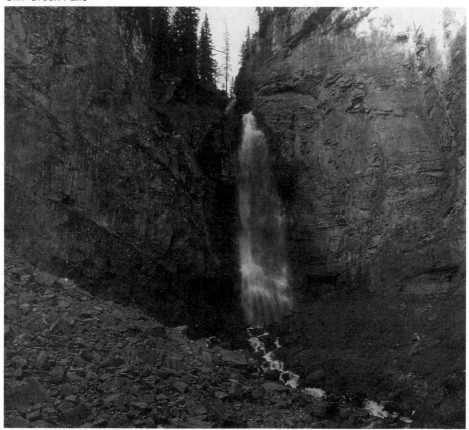

left and goes up and down for the next couple of miles as it curves north. Views are frequent along this trail, with particularly good looks at Hoback Peak to the east and down into the impressive canyons on either side of the ridge. Eventually the trail hugs the east side of a steep ridge well above the sloping grassy expanse of Horse Heaven Meadows. The path then goes around the right (east) side of a high point on the ridge and comes to the unsigned junction in the pass where you meet the longer route described above.

From this pass you take the trail that goes north-northeast and make a downhill traverse of a steep hillside, savoring superb views to the northeast of red-tinged Clause Peak and to the east of the distant Wind River Range. Below the trail is a huge rolling meadowland. Where the trail levels out in the upper reaches of this meadowland are some very scenic camping areas, although the tiny snowmelt creeks here tend to dry up after midsummer. One advantage of camping here is that the almost constant breezes at this elevation help to keep the mosquitoes at bay.

From the meadowland follow the now-faint trail as it goes along the top of a low, rounded ridge that heads generally east-southeast. Ignore an easy-to-miss and (as usual) unsigned trail going sharply right (downhill) and make your way down to a saddle and an unsigned junction with the trail coming up from Hunter Creek.

Turn right and follow this much-more-distinct path as it descends through view-packed meadows and past a large spring to a nice campsite. From here the very rocky trail steeply descends for almost 1 mile to a hop-over crossing of a branch of Cliff Creek, and, 0.1 mile later, an unsigned (but this time obvious) junction.

A short side trip is in order: Drop your heavy pack and take the left fork 0.2 mile steeply downhill to a viewpoint and fine campsite just below the base of Cliff Creek Falls. This tall and very impressive two-tiered falls drops over a colorful cliff face and provides a continuous cool (often downright *cold*) breeze to anyone camped below. Unfortunately, the falls is almost always in the shade, making it difficult to photograph, but it is well worth a visit nonetheless.

Back at the junction above Cliff Creek Falls, turn south (uphill) and immediately set about the task of regaining most of the elevation you so recently lost. Typical of the Wyoming Range, the fairly steep ascent starts off in a forest of pines and spruces and then breaks out into a series of lovely meadows. About 0.5 mile into the climb you pass a spacious campsite and, immediately thereafter, splash across the main stem of Cliff Creek and then a tributary creek. Another stretch of steady climbing in meadows and open forest takes you to a second crossing of Cliff Creek (this one not shown on the USGS map), followed by a gentle ascent in open country to a junction. Go left, immediately cross what's left of Cliff Creek a final time, and soon reach wide Cliff Creek Pass with its inspiring views to the south-southwest of Deadman Mountain.

The trail turns left and briefly ascends a small ridge before turning to the right (south). It then passes a willow-lined pond with a mediocre campsite above it and goes gradually up and down across a rolling, meadow-covered bench. In

July the wildflowers here put on a tremendous show, especially the yellow sun-flowers. A long, mostly gentle downhill takes you to the Little Greys River and a junction with the Wyoming Range National Recreation Trail. Although it is possible to go straight here on an initially faint trail back to the trailhead in just 5.2 miles, I strongly recommend that you take an extra day or two and explore a very scenic loop to the south. Turn left and walk 0.4 mile through forest to where you break out of the trees at lovely Roosevelt Meadows. The trail then takes you around the left (north) side of this meadow to a campsite and junction near a low pass.

Turn right and climb very steeply for the next mile to a beautiful rolling mead-owland. If looking for the often-faint trail doesn't take all your attention, you might watch for herds of elk, common in these meadows throughout the sum-mer. After crossing an intermittent creek, the trail makes one more ascent before topping out on a 9200-foot knoll.

Ups and downs in open country are the rule for the next several miles with nearly constant views and several seasonal and permanent creeks to provide wa-ter. Near the start of this section you pass through one small burn area where you must go straight when a couple of very official-looking fire and game trails cross your route. Even without these distractions, the correct trail is often obscure (at best); keep your contour map handy and check your position frequently to stay on course. The trail makes a series of ups and downs as it takes you to cross-ings of Fourth, Third, Second, and, you guessed it, First creeks, each separated by small ridges you must climb over. All these ups and downs add up to a fair amount of elevation gain, but the meadows and views keep you happily plug-ging along. From the high points between the creeks you'll enjoy good views to the south of the rugged north faces of distant Mt. Fitzpatrick and Rock Lake Peak. On the bench just south of the crossing of Second Creek are some possible places to camp, although there are no established sites. The impressive two-foot-tall spiky plants you see in this area are monument plants, which grow abun-dantly in these high meadows.

Just beyond the high point south of First Creek is an unsigned and almost impossible to find junction. (If you end up hiking along a low ridge that parallels a long drainage going south-southeast, then you have gone about 0.2 mile too far.) Since finding the trail that goes right here is probably beyond the skills of the best tracker, just head uphill to the west-northwest over alpine terrain. For-tunately no trail is needed, as the country is open, the vegetation is low, and the navigation, at least in clear weather, is easy. By the same token, do not attempt this section in bad weather with poor visibility—it is too easy to get lost.

After about 0.5 mile you'll see the top of Deadman Mountain, a good land-mark. In less than 1 mile you should locate the intermittent tread of the official trail as it angles northwest toward that peak. This wildly scenic route leads to a ridgeline just east of Deadman Mountain and provides terrific views of that hulking summit with its short lookout building on top.

When the trail reaches a little basin, which is just below you on the left, there is a fork. Typically for these mountains, the junction is unsigned. The left branch goes 0.9 mile to the top of Deadman Mountain. If the large snowfield you can see on the steep east face of the peak has melted and is not blocking the trail (usually by about mid-July), then by all means make this side trip, because the views are outstanding. If the snowfield is still there, however, the crossing is too treacherous to recommend.

The main trail goes straight, soon tops a minor saddle, and drops to another basin, this one filled with white marsh marigolds and alpine buttercups early in the summer and featuring great views up to the steep-sided north ridge of Deadman Mountain reflected in tiny ponds. Very scenic camping is possible here, although the place is rather exposed so be careful of the weather. The trail now parallels the cliff-edged ridge, staying below its east face as both trail and ridge descend to the north. The path is often hard to find, but with experience and a careful eye you can usually relocate it as it hugs the side of the ridge. If you lose the trail and need a landmark, aim to be a few feet above the west side of the creek when that stream plunges over a tall, cascading waterfall.

Past the waterfall, the trail is somewhat easier to follow for the next 0.5 mile as it descends the heavily vegetated slopes on the east side of the steep ridge. This is only a temporary reprieve, however, as the tread disappears again amid tall grasses and the frustrating blowdown of a burn area. Consoling yourself that scrambling around in search of the tread is all part of the experience on Wyoming Range trails, you eventually make your way down through the burn zone and come to a flatter area near the creek. Here the trail reappears and contours to the northwest, eventually making its way out to the end of a ridge. It then descends once again to a junction with an abandoned jeep track.

Still in the shadeless burn area, go right (north) on the winding jeep road and follow it past a marshy little lake. The track then goes through a fence, reenters unburned forest, and soon reaches the Little Greys River. The ford here is calf deep by mid-July and, while chilly, is not particularly difficult. After the crossing it's an easy 0.1-mile walk back to the trailhead.

POSSIBLE ITINERARY

NOTE: Days 3 and 4 involve some bushwhacking and searching-for-the-trail miles not included in these figures.

	CAMPS & SIDE TRIPS	MILES	ELEVATION GAIN
DAY 1	High meadow at the head of Hunter Creek	8.3	3000'
DAY 2	Roosevelt Meadows, including a side trip to Cliff Creek Falls	8.2	1700'
DAY 3	Alpine meadow below (and including a side trip up) Deadman Mountain	10.6	3100'
DAY 4	Out	5.8	300'

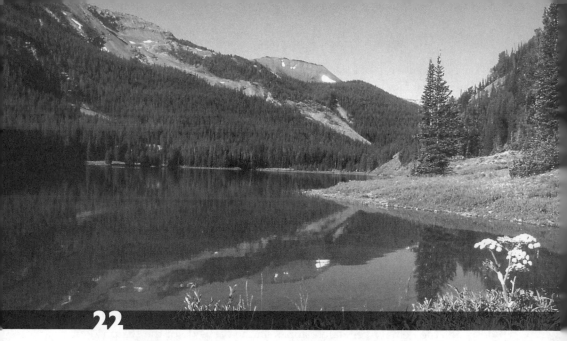

NORTH PINEY CREEK LOOP

RATINGS: Scenery 7   Solitude 9   Difficulty 5
MILES: 33.4
ELEVATION GAIN: 6700′
DAYS: 3–5
MAPS: USGS *Box Canyon Creek, Mount Schidler,* and *Wyoming Peak*
USUALLY OPEN: July to mid-October
BEST: Early July
CONTACT: Big Piney Ranger District, Bridger-Teton National Forest
SPECIAL ATTRACTIONS: Lots of solitude; fine mountain scenery
PERMIT: None required

RULES

The usual no-trace rules apply.

CHALLENGES

This area has several miles of ATV (all-terrain vehicle) trails. The route involves numerous relatively easy but annoying creek fords. A (very) few grizzly bears have recently migrated into this area—camp and act accordingly.

Photo: North Piney Lake

HOW TO GET THERE • • • • • • • • • • • •

From U.S. Highway 189 in downtown Big Piney, turn west on Budd Avenue (a.k.a. Wyoming Highway 350), following signs to North and Middle Piney Creeks. Stay on the main paved road for 10.7 miles to a fork, where you go straight on good gravel County Road 111. After 10.2 miles this road enters national forest land and becomes Forest Service Road 10046. Drive 1.8 miles to another fork, where you keep right, still on Road 10046, go 6.1 miles, and then turn left on Road 10370, following signs to North Piney Cutoff Trail. Slowly drive this bumpy road for 0.6 mile to the road-end trailhead.

DESCRIPTION • • • • • • • • • • • • • • • • • • •

The trail starts as a wide, dusty ATV route through a fairly dense evergreen forest of lodgepole pines, firs, and Engelmann spruces. After 0.5 mile of downhill the trail reaches a junction at the edge of the wide valley of North Piney Creek. Turn right (upstream), staying on the ATV trail, and follow the clear creek past beaver dams and excellent viewpoints of the cliffs on towering Mt. Schideler to the southwest. From this angle this sloping mountain resembles a huge tilted haystack. A worthwhile way to kill some time while enjoying this view is to break out the fishing pole and try to catch some of the creek's abundant trout.

At 1.6 miles, just after you splash across a seasonal tributary creek, a nonmotorized trail goes to the right (north). You stay straight and at 2.2 miles go through a gate in an impressive fence built from large logs. At 2.6 miles is a major junction and the start of the recommended loop.

Turn left (south) and almost immediately come to a campsite just before crossing North Piney Creek. There may be an unstable log across the creek upstream from the official trail crossing, but it is usually safer to brave

TAKE THIS TRIP

Here is yet another wonderfully scenic but largely overlooked hike in the impressive Wyoming Range of west-central Wyoming. Although many of the trails here are wide and dusty due to ATV use, if you hike on weekdays you are unlikely to see any machines (or any people at all, for that matter). If you're a wilderness purist and want to avoid encounters with noisy machines, visit before July 15 or after October 15, because the trail is only open to the two- and four-wheeled terrors between those dates. If the winter's snows haven't been too heavy, early July is a particularly nice time to visit, since the wildflowers will be blooming and the snow streaking the rugged, colorful peaks is extremely photogenic.

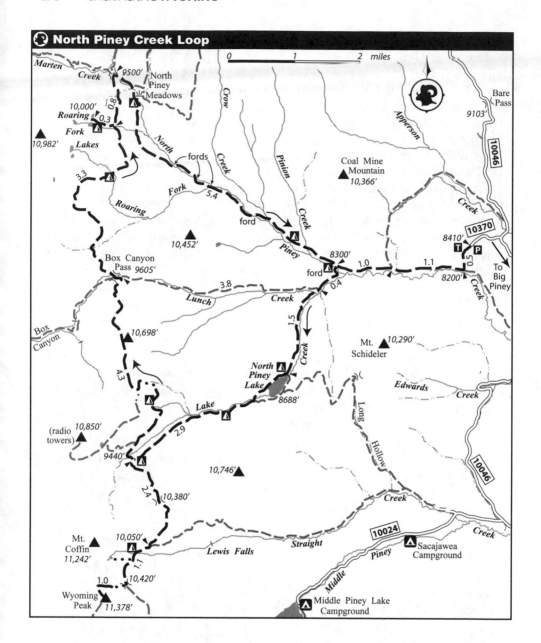

North Piney Creek Loop

Marten Creek 9500' North Piney Meadows

10,000' Roaring 0.8 0.3

Fork Lakes

10,982'

North Fork fords

Roaring Fork 3.3 5.4

Crow Creek

Pinion Creek

Piney Creek

ford

Coal Mine Mountain 10,366'

Bare Pass 9103'

10046

10,452'

Box Canyon Pass 9605'

3.8

Lunch Creek

ford 8300'

1.0 0.4 8200' 1.1

8410' 10370 T P 0.5

To Big Piney

Box Canyon

10,698'

1.5

Creek

Mt. Schideler 10,290'

Edwards Creek

North Piney Lake 8688'

4.3

Lake

2.9

(radio towers) 10,850'

9440'

10,746'

2.4 (10,380')

Long Hollow

Creek

10046

Creek

10024

Straight

Piney

Sacajawea Campground

Mt. Coffin 11,242'

10,050'

Lewis Falls

1.1

1.0 10,420'

Wyoming Peak 11,378'

Middle

Middle Piney Lake Campground

the cold calf-deep ford. Now back in forest, you hike 0.4 mile to another junction, this time with the Lunch Creek Trail, which goes to the right.

Continue straight on the Lake Creek Trail and soon cross Lunch Creek, which may get your feet and ankles wet if you cannot find a convenient log. From here the trail travels through a mix of forest and small meadows as it ascends along rollicking Lake Creek. In the forest openings, and especially the wet meadows near the creek, there are a host of wildflowers. A partial list of species includes cow parsnips, bluebells, larkspurs, paintbrushes, arnicas, and geraniums. At 4.5

miles is a junction near several good campsites at the northeast end of North Piney Lake. This large, scenic, and green-tinged lake offers fine views of a group of reddish peaks on a ridge to the south. ATVs are not allowed beyond this lake, so you will be free of the machines for the next day or two.

Trails go around both sides of North Piney Lake, but the one to the right along the northwest shore is a bit more scenic. Follow it as it closely hugs the lakeshore where the sunny and relatively dry slopes support a different array of wildflowers than in the lush meadows below the lake. Blazing star, yarrow, horsemint, flax, buckwheat, and sunflower all thrive here. At the head of the meadow at the lake's southwest end, ford Lake Creek and rejoin the trail that went around the other side of North Piney Lake.

Gradually ascend mostly in shady forest for about 0.5 mile to a campsite at the base of a very scenic meadow with views of unnamed peaks. Cairns lead you across a small rockslide before the tread picks up again in the forest on the other side.

In the middle of another scenic little meadow at 7.4 miles is a junction with the Wyoming Range National Recreation Trail. You could camp at this meadow and dayhike south to Wyoming Peak, but mosquitoes are a real problem here through most of July. The main loop goes right (north) from this junction, but to do that now would miss some of this trip's best scenery. So turn left and climb steeply, gaining 800 feet through a high-elevation forest of stunted trees to a windswept 10,380-foot pass. The views here are grand, especially east toward the broad Green River plains.

After rapidly losing almost 200 feet, the sometimes sketchy trail contours through lovely subalpine terrain featuring whitebark pines, meadows, and rocky areas. Good camps are possible almost anywhere in this area, with the rocky pyramid of Wyoming Peak and the strikingly red cliffs of Mt. Coffin providing very scenic backdrops. Pass an unsigned junction with a trail that comes up Straight Creek and then wander across the open terrain where cairns keep you on track when the tread disappears. For an excellent side trip wander west about 0.3 mile to a pair of sparkling tarns located directly beneath the rugged cliffs of Mt. Coffin.

The trail ascends to a rocky pass on the northeast shoulder of Wyoming Peak. According to the Forest Service map, a trail leaves from this pass and goes to the summit. Finding this trail is close to impossible, but it is not too difficult to scramble cross-country up a talus slope to the west until you find the tread on the less steep, more stable terrain on the northeast shoulder of the peak. Once you locate this trail, simply follow it to the squat lookout building at the summit. The views from here, as you might expect, are beyond superb. On clear days they extend from the Wind River Range to the east, to the Salt River Range to the west, and for seemingly endless miles in all directions.

Once you've had your fill of the view from Wyoming Peak, return to the Wyoming Range National Recreation Trail and hike back to its junction with the Lake Creek Trail. Go north and briefly descend to a sometimes wet but never difficult crossing of Lake Creek. From here the often faint but discernible trail goes

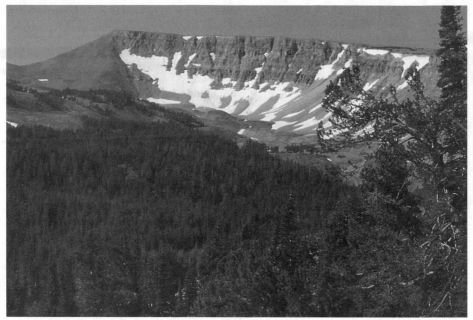

Mt. Coffin from the north, over Lake Creek Valley

northeast, generally staying at or near the same elevation for the next mile or so. Continue straight where an unsigned trail goes sharply back to the left, and then skirt the base of a large talus slope before beginning a long and strenuous ascent. Look back south during this climb for fine views of Mt. Coffin and the top of Wyoming Peak.

After a brief respite beside a tiny but very scenic pond (possible campsites here), the steep climb resumes as you make your way up to a high basin where the tread disappears. Guided by your contour map, wander up to the head of the basin and then make a looping climb back to the south to an easily missed junction with a faint, unsigned trail. You loop back to the right (northwest), still going steeply uphill, all the way to the top of the range. From here you can look west to the strikingly orange cliffs of aptly named Box Canyon and on to the Salt River Range.

WARNING: The winds often howl along this ridgetop, so be prepared to be buffeted around.

The intermittent tread now leads north along the open, alpine crest of the Wyoming Range. For the next 1.5 miles you will be high on this view-packed crest, most of the way above treeline. The scenery is outstanding, but this is no place to be if thunderstorms are in the area. Watch the weather carefully and plan to be off this section before about 1 or 2 P.M.

Following bits of tread and occasional posts, make your way down from the crest losing 1100 feet to a junction near a small, shallow, meadow-rimmed lake at Box Canyon Pass. Turn left and walk 150 yards to the west end of the lake and another signed junction where you turn right (north). Now on a better-defined trail, you gain 300 feet and then begin a long section of gentle ups and downs across wildflower-covered slopes, through open forest, and over tiny snowmelt creeks. At 2.4 miles from Box Canyon Pass you enter a large meadow and pass a campsite just before you hop over small Roaring Fork Creek. From here you round another ridge, hop over a small creek, and come to a junction with an ATV trail. The not-to-be-missed trail to the left goes gradually uphill for 0.3 mile to good campsites at the small and shallow but very scenic Roaring Fork Lakes. This gorgeous group of lakes sits beneath a rugged, rocky line of cliffs and demands some extra time for sitting back and admiring.

To continue the loop, return to the junction below the Roaring Fork Lakes and follow the ATV trail as it curves north and begins going gradually downhill. At 0.8 mile from the Roaring Fork Lakes turnoff, turn right at a four-way junction at a forested pass, still on the main ATV trail, and almost immediately pass a shallow little lake before reaching a junction at the northwest end of North Piney Meadows. A very faint trail goes left here but you keep right and go around the west side of this large green meadow, a good place to see elk, if the ATVs have not scared them away. At the south end of the meadow is a good campsite.

The trail continues downhill through sloping meadows and forest to a flat creekside meadow and an easy calf-deep ford of North Piney Creek. If they are comfortable enough for hiking, it is a good idea to leave your wading shoes on, because in the next 1.4 miles you face a second ford of North Piney Creek, a ford of Roaring Fork Creek, a third ford of North Piney Creek, and a shallower crossing of Crow Creek. The crossings are all easy and no doubt splashing fun for the ATV crowd, but they are very inconvenient for hikers who are constantly changing between boots and wading shoes.

Apart from all the annoying fords, the hiking is easy and nearly flat as you wander very gradually downhill in the sagebrush- and willow-lined meadows along North Piney Creek. Shortly after passing a well-developed hunter's camp, you cross Pinion Creek (no need to get your feet wet this time) and continue to the junction with Lake Creek Trail and the close of the loop. Go straight and return the 2.6 miles to the trailhead.

POSSIBLE ITINERARY

	CAMPS & SIDE TRIPS	MILES	ELEVATION GAIN
DAY 1	Meadow below Mt. Coffin	10.0	2400'
DAY 2	Pond along Wyoming Range Trail, including a side trip up Wyoming Peak	8.0	1950'
DAY 3	Roaring Fork Lakes	6.3	2000'
DAY 4	Out	9.1	350'

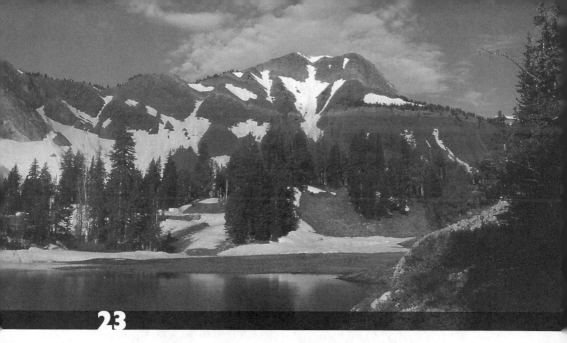

MOUNT FITZPATRICK LOOP

RATINGS: Scenery 8   Solitude 9   Difficulty 9

MILES: 39.3 (plus plenty of extra bushwhacking miles)

ELEVATION GAIN: 12,000´

DAYS: 4–7

MAPS: USGS *Box Canyon Creek, Park Creek, Red Top Mountain,* and *Rock Lake Peak*

USUALLY OPEN: July to mid-October

BEST: Mid-July to early August

CONTACT: Greys River Ranger District, Bridger-Teton National Forest

SPECIAL ATTRACTIONS: Lots of solitude; gorgeous mountain lakes amid generally fine mountain scenery; plenty of wildlife

PERMIT: None required

RULES ·

The usual no-trace rules apply.

CHALLENGES ·

In places the trail ranges from sketchy to nonexistent, and most junctions are unsigned, so plenty of patience, some bushwhacking, and good navigation skills are required. ATVs (all-terrain vehicles) are allowed on a few trails.

Photo: Tarn below Rock Lake Peak

HOW TO GET THERE ·····································

From U.S. Highway 89 in downtown Ashton, on the west-central border of Wyoming, turn east on Second Avenue. Drive 1.2 miles to the end of pavement where the road enters national forest land and becomes Forest Service Road 10211. From here follow a good gravel road through a narrow but extremely scenic canyon past dramatic rock formations along aptly named Swift Creek. This spectacular but short drive ends after 4.4 miles at the road-end trailhead.

> **NOTE:** When reviewing this trip information, the Forest Service informed me that they were currently putting up white (for nonmotorized trails) or green (for trails open to motor vehicles) diamond-shaped trail markings to assist in navigation. Hopefully, this will make life easier for confused hikers.

DESCRIPTION ·····································

Most people visiting this trailhead take the easy trail that leaves from the east end of the large parking lot and travels upstream beside the clear waters of Swift Creek. This wide, very gentle route goes 0.7 mile to a picnic table and interpretive sign beside Periodic Spring.

For this trip, however, you take the signed Swift Creek Trail, which departs from the north side of the parking lot near the restroom building. This narrow and rocky but well-maintained path follows a scenic route across the steep slopes above Swift Creek as that stream rushes through a deep, impressive canyon. The terrain is a mix of rocky and/or brushy areas and evergreen forest mostly composed of Engelmann spruces, Douglas firs, and Rocky Mountain junipers. For

TAKE THIS TRIP

Like the neighboring Wyoming Range just a few miles to the east, the Salt River Range lies hidden along the western border of Wyoming and, despite offering plenty of outstanding scenery, is virtually ignored by the hiking public. These mountains offer numerous worthwhile destinations and many miles of beautiful hiking, and lake lovers can revel in the scenery without the crowds often associated with mountain lakes. Unfortunately, the trails here are, if anything, even more rugged than those in the Wyoming Range, with somewhat more brush and, therefore, more difficult bushwhacking when (and that is definitely a "when" not an "if") you lose the trail.

So, if you want to get away from the crowds and don't mind paying a price for that solitude, the Salt River Range is a terrific place to go. This loop offers only a sampling of the many wonders found in these mountains, but it's a glorious sampling with several spectacular lakes, wildflower-covered meadows, small waterfalls, excellent mountain scenery, and even a geologically unique fluctuating spring.

Mount Fitzpatrick Loop

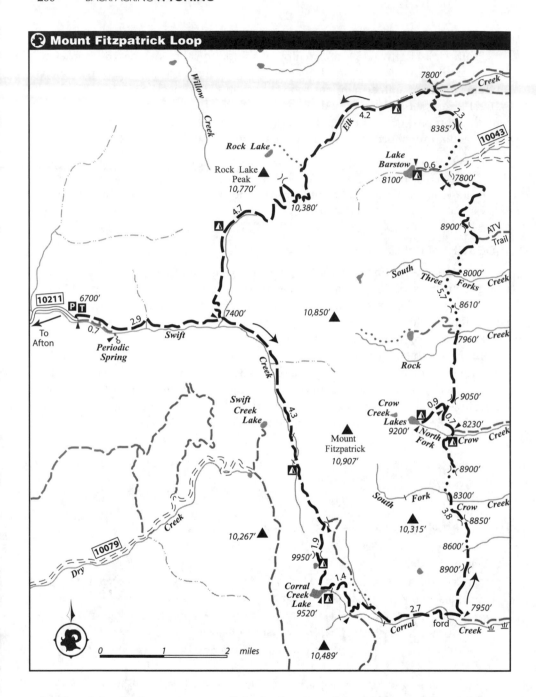

the first 0.6 mile your route parallels the lower trail beside the creek, until you come to a junction with a short but very steep path down to a junction with that lower path just downstream from the bridge over the creek at Periodic Spring. It is worth making this side trip to visit this geologic oddity, which is sometimes referred to as a cold water geyser and is the largest of only three known intermittent or fluctuating springs in the world. Geologists aren't sure how it works, but in the latter part of the year the spring flows only at regular intervals every 12 to 20 minutes. In spring and early summer it may flow almost continuously, depending on how wet the winter has been. The huge quantities of water it pours out of a fissure in the south canyon wall contributes a large percentage of Swift Creek's considerable volume.

Shortly after the junction with the side trail, the Swift Creek Trail passes a fine viewpoint of Periodic Spring before continuing up the main canyon of Swift Creek. About 0.5 mile later the trail briefly detours into a meadow- and wildflower-filled side canyon before returning to the hillside above Swift Creek. The trail here has many ups and downs, which adds significantly to the total elevation gain.

At 2.9 miles the trail splits at the start of the recommended loop. The Rock Lake Peak Trail goes left, but you bear right (initially downhill) and soon either find a log or make a calf-deep ford of an unnamed tributary creek. For the next 1.5 miles the trail travels close to Swift Creek often in lush, overgrown meadows or willow flats, excellent moose habitat—keep an eye out for these gangly but impressive animals. During this section the trail and canyon gradually curve until you are hiking south. Another noticeable change results from the relentless gain in elevation: The landscape changes from forest to meadows that are carpeted with July-blooming wildflowers. Look for geranium (both white and pink varieties), bluebell, forget-me-not, fernleaf, wild carrot, columbine, ballhead waterleaf, paintbrush, lupine, and valerian, among a host of others. Views also improve, especially of the surrounding ridges and of several small waterfalls that tumble down the canyon walls on both sides of Swift Creek. It all adds up to some fine mountain scenery.

At 5.6 miles you cross now-fairly-small Swift Creek just below a cascading waterfall, then cross the creek again 0.5 mile later near an even larger sliding falls. There is a fair campsite just above the second crossing. If you turn around at this point and look north, you will enjoy your first views of (from this angle) pyramid-shaped Rock Lake Peak and see the less distinctive hump of Mt. Fitzpatrick along the top of the canyon wall. At 7.2 miles you reach a trail junction at a pass. The views from here up and down the canyons, ridges, and peaks of the Salt River Range are awe inspiring.

From the pass an old trail goes sharply left and downhill. You, however, turn right (south-southwest) on Corral Creek Trail and gradually gain elevation as you cross mostly open slopes usually covered by snowfields until mid-July. After 0.7 mile you reach a second pass, this one almost directly beneath a line of striated cliffs. The trail now makes a short but very steep descent to a cliff-backed little lake with no name but a fair campsite above its outlet creek. Climb over another minor ridge and then steeply drop to teardrop-shaped Corral Creek Lake at 9.1 miles. Backed by 1000-foot cliffs on three sides and with icebergs floating in its waters until at least early to mid-July, this lake is quite a spot. To allow for more leisurely appreciation of its scenic beauty, the lake has good campsites above its north and southeast shores.

Sadly leaving Corral Creek Lake behind, take the trail that follows the north side of Corral Creek Lake's outlet creek (not surprisingly, named Corral Creek) and descend a series of irregularly spaced switchbacks. You soon pass a waterfall dropping out of the lake's cirque and then descend through some sloping meadows to a confusing and unsigned junction in a small basin beneath a line of cliffs. Go left and make several rounded, downhill switchbacks to a hop-over crossing of a small creek. From here you pass above a nice waterfall on Corral Creek and then parallel that stream to a bridgeless but easy crossing. After another set of downhill switchbacks, from which you can see a large willow-choked meadow to the east, you come to another crossing of Corral Creek. Through most of July this crossing requires a chilly knee-deep ford of swift water. In a meadow just 0.15 mile below this ford is a junction.

Turn left at a small sign for Way Trail #079 and immediately face the pattern this trail will offer for the next dozen or so miles: usually steep, and always tiring, ups and downs as it tackles the numerous ridges and creek canyons on the east side of the Salt River Range. It begins on a trail sometimes used by ATVs that makes a 950-foot ascent to a forested, viewless ridgetop. After a rapid descent of 300 feet to a tiny creek in a meadow, the trail pulls the first of its many disappearing acts. When you lose the trail along this route (and you *will* lose it from time to time) it can be both frustrating and difficult to find it again. Expect to do a fair amount of head scratching, map reading, and bushwhacking as you search on steep slopes for the correct route. Most of the time this cross-country travel is in open forest that is fairly easy to travel through, but it can still become frustrating, especially if you are accustomed to hiking on smooth, well-maintained trails. That is why I recommend this trip only for experienced hikers with good navigation skills.

To find the trail this time, stay near the top (west side) of the meadow, carefully ignoring several game paths that tend to erroneously lead you downstream, and look for the tread reentering the forest near the northwest corner of the meadow. From here it is a 250-foot climb to the top of another ridge, which is followed by an elevation loss of almost 600 feet to South Fork Crow Creek, the crossing of which is an easy ankle-deep affair. Expect to lose the trail amid the lots of very confusing game trails on the north side of this crossing and to have to use your instincts to find it again. The very faint trail closely follows the north bank of South Fork Crow Creek for almost 0.3 mile, then charges up the ridge to the north. You will probably lose the trail here, but if you climb cross-country through the open forest toward the low point in the ridge you should find it again. From the ridgetop the trail is obvious once again as it descends over 650 feet to a scenic meadow and a possible campsite just before the step-over crossing of North Fork Crow Creek.

About 160 yards after the crossing of North Fork Crow Creek turn left at a junction. Turn left and gear down once again because, you guessed it, there is another steep uphill coming. This one takes you up 830 feet. On the plus side, the trail is obvious for a change and the views toward the cliffs of Mt. Fitzpatrick are very impressive.

A little before you reach the next pass is a junction with an unsigned side trail easily confused with the faint main trail—you may end up on the side trail without even realizing it. But that's okay because you won't want to miss this superb side trip, which goes up and down across an open hillside for 0.9 mile to the lower and larger of the two Crow Creek Lakes. Sitting at the base of a hulking side peak of Mt. Fitzpatrick, and with a glimpse of the main summit to the west, this lake is a real showstopper. There are possible campsites near the outlet if you want to savor a night here, a decision that I highly recommended. Reaching smaller Upper Crow Creek Lake requires some steep scrambling and so is recommended only for determined hikers.

Back on the main trail, go through a little pass and then resume your now-familiar up-and-down pattern. First up is a long 1100-foot descent on well-defined trail to the easy calf-deep ford of Rock Creek. Immediately on the other side of this crossing you have another excellent side trip option. At the top of the small meadow near the ford and a little to the left (west) a small cairn marks the start of a steep and reasonably well-defined trail, not shown on either the USGS or Forest Service maps, that leads to a scenic but unnamed lake. From here you could spend hours or days exploring cross-country into the very scenic, but very rough, upper basin of Rock Creek.

The harder-to-find official trail goes uphill and to the north from the ford of Rock Creek, often disappearing as it ascends 900 feet to a ridgetop. From there the trail supposedly goes down a long gully to South Three Forks Creek. Since this section receives almost no use or maintenance, however, it is really more of a cross-country hike. Fortunately, the descent is not particularly difficult as it travels through open forest and small meadows with only a little brush. Finding the occasional cut log or red plastic flag marker along the way is a rare but welcome treat. Once at the bottom, locating the trail to the top of the next ridge is yet another challenge. The easiest thing to do is to go downstream on a good game trail for about 0.2 mile, then make a steep cross-country climb up a long grassy gully. After gaining 450 feet you should find the official trail near the top of the grassy swale. This trail travels through meadows for 0.4 mile then intersects a lightly-used ATV track. Turn left and follow this track over the ridge and down the other side as it very gradually winds downhill to a junction at the end of a rough dirt road and a signed trailhead for Lake Barstow.

Turn left and follow this dusty ATV trail for 0.2 mile to a small wooden bridge over North Three Forks Creek. You can continue on the ATV trail another 0.4 mile to the campsites at attractive Lake Barstow, but theses sites are typically trashed by the machine-riding crowd.

To continue with the recommended loop turn right about 100 yards past the bridge on another very sketchy, unsigned trail. Expect this trail to disappear once again rather quickly leaving you to bushwhack through a tangle of blowdown and some brush. The proper course angles uphill to the northeast. You will probably run across the intermittent tread of this rarely maintained trail as it climbs steeply up to a pass on the ridge. If you do not find the trail, make your way up through open forest traveling cross-country to the pass.

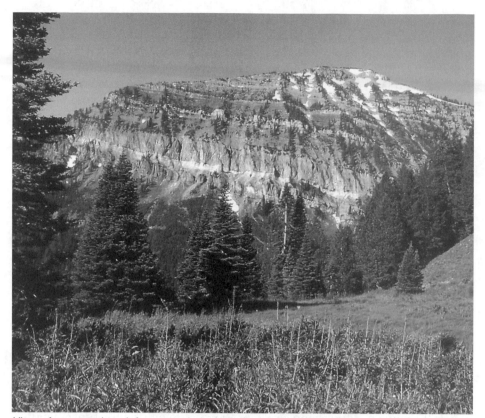

View of unnamed peak from meadow above South Three Forks Creek

Once at the pass the major route-finding problems of the trip are finally over, as you follow a fairly good trail that cuts around the left (west) side of an old logging scar and then contours for a bit before descending to a junction with an ATV trail near Elk Creek. The creek here flows underground for most of the summer, so there is no nearby water. Turn left on the ATV trail as it curves north and east to an unsigned but obvious junction on the other side of Elk Creek's drainage. Turn left on what is initially an ATV trail, but which soon devolves into a narrow footpath that ascends the slope just south of Elk Creek to a long, gently sloping meadow. Once again the creek comes and goes here, sometimes flowing beneath rocks and sometimes on the surface. There are nice views up the meadow to Rock Lake Peak to the southwest. Although there are no established sites, there are plenty of nice spots to camp in the upper part of this meadow and for the next mile or so above that.

After crossing small Elk Creek, the trail climbs steadily into the rocks, snowfields, and increasingly alpine country below Rock Lake Peak. The views and mountain scenery improve with every step. At about 3 miles from where you started on the trail up Elk Creek there is a small snowmelt pond that often floods the tread in early summer, but which provides fine reflections of the surrounding peaks. From here you can make a worthwhile cross-country side trip to the northwest gaining about 500 feet over rocky terrain to dramatic Rock Lake, high on the north side of its namesake peak.

The main trail goes south from the pond into a deep gully of rocks and snow. At the top of the gully a series of fairly long switchbacks take you to treeline and the top of the ridge at 10,380 feet. Not surprisingly, the views in all directions are excellent.

The trail now goes north-northwest, descending near the top of the ridge to a point just below the actual pass, fully 300 feet lower than where the trail went over the ridge. Descend four long switchbacks across steep slopes and then cross the small creek that flows from this high basin. Another mile of easy hiking through gorgeous sloping meadows takes you to a well-developed hunter's camp complete with a small corral. The trail now remains on the forested hillside above a growing but unnamed creek, descending for the next 1.9 miles back to the junction with the Swift Creek Trail and the end of your loop. Turn right and retrace your steps 2.9 miles back to the trailhead.

POSSIBLE ITINERARY

NOTE: Days 2 and 3 involve a lot of bushwhacking and searching-for-the-trail miles not included in these figures.

	CAMPS & SIDE TRIPS	MILES	ELEVATION GAIN
DAY 1	Corral Creek Lake	9.1	3700'
DAY 2	Crow Creek Lake	9.5	3000'
DAY 3	Lower Elk Creek	9.7	2700'
DAY 4	Out	11.0	2600'

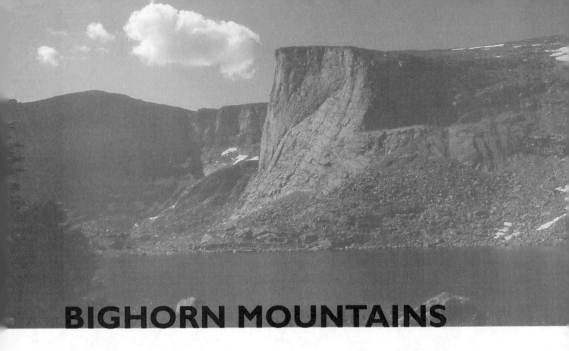

BIGHORN MOUNTAINS

For those driving west across the seemingly endless Great Plains of the Dakotas and northern Wyoming, the high, snow-covered peaks of the Bighorn Mountains are the first "real" mountains that you encounter. (No offense to South Dakota's Black Hills—they're pleasant, attractive, and all that—but they aren't what you would call "real" mountains.) And they represent a truly spectacular introduction to the genre. With outstandingly beautiful canyons, towering cliffs, high cirque basins with lakes, tall granite peaks, wildflower-covered alpine meadows, and even a tiny remnant glacier, these mountains contain all the same wonders commonly associated with the other more famous mountains of the American West. The trailhead parking lots here are often filled with vehicles sporting license plates from Iowa, Illinois, Wisconsin, and other flat states in the upper Midwest whose owners are looking to salivate over scenery taller than a grain silo and infinitely more spectacular (and better smelling) than a dairy farm. Few, if any, leave without a host of great memories, hundreds of fine pictures, and a renewed sense of wonder at the splendors of the western mountains. On the down side, it is also the rare visitor who doesn't initially suffer from at least some altitude sickness, since many trails here are higher than 10,000 feet, an altitude with which most Midwesterners have little experience.

By Wyoming standards, many of the trails here are heavily used. In addition, studies have shown that the lakes in these mountains are more susceptible to acid deposition than anywhere else in the Rocky Mountains. As a result, the no-trace rules you should follow everywhere you hike, as well as the U.S. Forest Service restrictions on this area, are especially important to protect the health of these mountains. See the rules and regulations section of the individual trips for details.

Photo: *Lower Lost Twin Lake (Trip 25)*

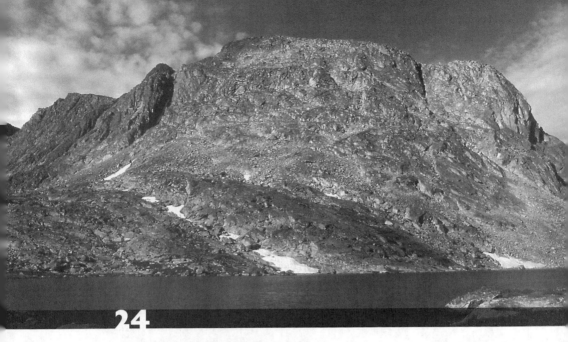

24
NORTH BIGHORN MOUNTAINS LOOP

RATINGS: Scenery 8   Solitude 5   Difficulty 5
MILES: 32.8 (39.8)
ELEVATION GAIN: 4000′ (5100′)
DAYS: 4–6
MAP: Trails Illustrated *Cloud Peak Wilderness*
USUALLY OPEN: Mid-July to October
BEST: Late July to early August
CONTACT: Powder River Ranger District, Bighorn National Forest (Although most of this hike is actually in the Medicine Wheel/Paintrock Ranger District, the Powder River District manages the entire Cloud Peak Wilderness as a single unit and has the latest information.)
SPECIAL ATTRACTIONS: Fine mountain scenery; good fishing
PERMIT: Required—free at the trailhead

RULES •

Fires are prohibited above 9200 feet, which includes virtually all of this trip. Groups are limited to 10 people. Camping is prohibited within 100 feet of water.

Photo: Lake in basin above Lake Elsa

TAKE THIS TRIP

Anywhere you hike in the Bighorn Mountains will treat you to outstanding mountain scenery, plenty of lakes, and miles of beautiful meadows. This loop through the northern part of the Cloud Peak Wilderness boasts some of the best of all three of those features, making it a real winner. And although you won't have the trails all to yourself, somewhat longer and rougher road access ensures that the human trail population is a little less than in the southern part of the range. The animal population is quite large, however, so you should not be surprised to see moose, elk, marmots, and other four-legged residents. Unfortunately, at the start of the trip, the most common four-legged animals are cattle, so be sure to treat your water and expect to be temporarily diverted by confusing livestock trails.

CHALLENGES

The road access is bumpy, and the area has the usual mosquitoes, but otherwise there are no significant problems. (Isn't that a relief? No horror stories to tell upon your return).

HOW TO GET THERE

From Greybull, go 31.6 miles east on U.S. Highway 14 to a prominent junction with Forest Service Road 17 (Paint Rock Road). If you are coming from the east, this junction is about 67 miles west of Sheridan. Turn right (south) on this very scenic gravel road, which wanders up and down in beautiful mountain meadows, over ridges, and through open forest. The road is often rough, but is maintained for passenger cars. After 24.2 miles you reach the well-signed Edelman Trailhead; continue driving another 0.2 mile to reach the trailhead parking lot on the right (west). If you have two cars, leave one at the Lower Paint Rock Trailhead another 1.5 miles along Road 17.

NOTE: Throughout the Cloud Peak Wilderness, trails are signed only with their number. No trail names or destinations are listed. Therefore, to assist in navigation when you reach a junction in the wilderness, I generally refer to trail numbers rather than trail names in the following description.

DESCRIPTION

Walk back down the road 0.2 mile to the start of the Edelman Trail (#025) and head northeast. The trail begins in, and spends its first few miles traveling through, a wide meadow bordered by a lodgepole pine forest. After about 0.8 mile you enter the Cloud Peak Wilderness and continue gradually climbing through the huge meadow going up the drainage of Medicine Lodge Creek. Relatively low, rocky ridges and peaks rise on either side of the meadow, providing good if not terribly dramatic scenery. Cattle graze in these

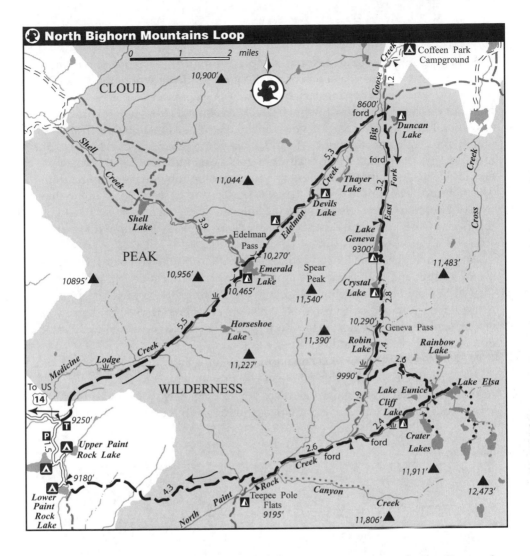

North Bighorn Mountains Loop

0   1   2 miles

CLOUD

10,900'

Coffeen Park
Campground

8600'
ford

Duncan
Lake

PEAK

11,044'

Shell
Creek

Shell
Lake

Edelman
Pass

10,270'

10,956'

Emerald
Lake

10,465'

10895'

Medicine   Lodge   Creek

To US
14

9250'

Upper Paint
Rock Lake

9180'

Lower
Paint
Rock
Lake

North   Paint

Teepee Pole
Flats
9195'

Rock   Creek   ford

Canyon

Creek

11,806'

WILDERNESS

Horseshoe
Lake

11,227'

Spear
Peak
11,540'

Devils
Lake

Thayer
Lake

Lake
Geneva
9300'

Crystal
Lake

11,390'

Robin
Lake

9990'

Cliff
Lake

Lake Eunice

Geneva Pass

Rainbow
Lake

Lake Elsa

Crater
Lakes

11,911'

12,473'

11,483'

Cross   Creek

East   Fork

Big   Creek

Goose   Creek

meadows during the summer; expect to encounter some confusing livestock trails, but keep going northeast and you will be fine.

At about 3 miles step over small Medicine Lodge Creek, then near 3.5 miles the narrowing meadow finally ends and the pace of your climbing noticeably increases. After passing a lovely little meadow with a marshy pond at 4.7 miles climb over a 10,465-foot high point and descend to a junction beside Emerald Lake at 5.5 miles. This beautiful, two-lobed lake is surrounded by rocky buttes and offers exposed but decent campsites.

Go straight at the junction, still on Trail #025, cross Emerald Lake's outlet, and walk through a low saddle named Edelman Pass. From here the often rocky trail descends steeply for 0.3 mile to a couple of gorgeous, wildflower-filled alpine meadows with campsites and great views of the granite buttes and canyon walls above. Moose spend their summers up here, so keep an eye out for these large, awkward-looking animals.

Soon reenter forest and descend steeply through this shady environment. Along the way you pass a series of small, lush meadows where the views improve and your knees get a rest as the trail is less steep in these places. Throughout your descent you follow Edelman Creek, crossing its flow several times with easy rock-hops. At about 8 miles you come to the signed junction with Trail #123, which goes right and in about 0.1 mile takes you to a camp beside scenic, but often buggy, Devils Lake. The main trail goes straight at the Devils Lake junction and leads in another 1.4 miles to an unsigned but obvious junction with the 0.9-mile unofficial trail to Thayer Lake. Keep left and descend to an ankle-deep ford of Edelman Creek followed just 0.2 mile later by a log crossing of East Fork Big Goose Creek. About 150 yards after this crossing is a junction with Solitude Trail #038.

Turn right and begin a long, gradual climb. After 0.5 mile you pass a collapsed miner's cabin and then come to a junction. A worthwhile side trip goes left on Trail #125 from here, traveling 0.4 mile to a nice campsite beside Duncan Lake. Although surrounded by forest, this lake offers excellent views to the southwest of a cluster of snowy peaks. In addition, much of the lake is covered with attractive yellow-blooming pond lilies.

Back on Trail #038, you soon come to another crossing of East Fork Big Goose Creek. Since there is no log this time you will probably have to get your feet wet. Another 1.5 miles of gradual uphill takes you to long, narrow Lake Geneva. This lovely lake has fine views of craggy peaks to the southwest but is heavily used

Emerald Lake

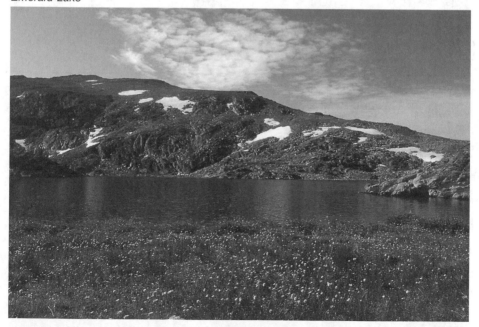

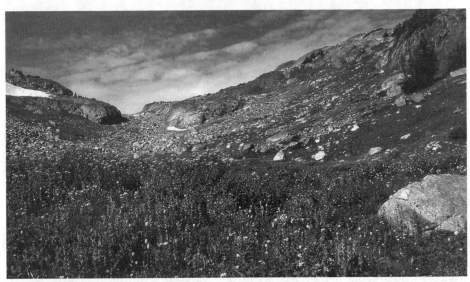

Meadow below Edelman Pass

so be especially careful to follow all the "no trace" rules. The trail hugs the east shore of Lake Geneva to some excellent campsites at the lake's south end and then begins a fairly steep ascent. After gaining 450 feet in a series of switchbacks, you reach an unsigned junction with a side trail that goes right about 150 yards to several good campsites and a pretty meadow beside dramatic Crystal Lake. Beneath the hulking ramparts of an unnamed mountain, this clear gem is high on any hiker's list of great places.

Your climbing is not done yet, so after a good rest stop (or night) at Crystal Lake get back on Trail #038 and keep trudging uphill. After going through a gorgeous alpine meadow, the trail snakes up to and through the narrow defile called Geneva Pass.

A gentle downhill from Geneva Pass takes you across the open slopes above beautiful, teardrop-shaped Robin Lake then past a group of smaller unnamed ponds to a junction. Turn left on Trail #060, which drops briefly to cross the headwaters of North Paint Rock Creek, then slowly winds up to a minor saddle. A little more up-and-down hiking through alpine meadows, over rocky areas, and past small tarns takes you to the campsites and fine scenery around Lake Eunice. The trail then turns to the southwest, descending along a rushing creek to aptly named Cliff Lake, which sits beneath a towering buttress of dark rock. There are numerous excellent but popular campsites near the west end of this very scenic lake.

Cliff Lake is an ideal place for a base camp while you spend a day or two exploring some of the many wildly scenic off-trail lakes in this area. With a contour map you can pick out all kinds of enticing destinations. The easiest to reach is Rainbow Lake. To get there, follow a sketchy use path from the north shore of Lake Eunice that parallels that lake's inlet creek for about 1 mile to meadow-rimmed Rainbow Lake. For more dramatic scenery, don't miss the two Crater

Lakes. To find them, cross the stream leading into Cliff Lake and scramble up a rocky incline to the south for 0.3 mile, staying to the east of a cascading waterfall, to Lower Crater Lake. Upper Crater Lake lies a difficult 0.5 mile to the south. Both lakes are nearly encircled by stupendous cliffs and steep snowfields, especially on their west and south sides. Yet another worthy goal is the string of wonderfully scenic large lakes that lie in a series of rocky cirques southeast of Lake Eunice. The first one in this chain, Lake Elsa, is visible from the trail between Lake Eunice and Cliff Lake and is easily reached by a nearly level meadow walk, partly on a good boot-beaten path. To reach the upper lakes, scramble up a steep rocky gully from the southeast shore of Lake Elsa. The lakes are progressively more dramatic the farther up you go. Some boulder hopping is needed to attain the highest lakes, but the lower ones are not too difficult to reach and are well worthwhile.

After your fill of exploring, get back on Trail #060 and head downstream (west) from Cliff Lake, past a narrow, marshy lake, and then through open forest and pretty meadows to a calf-deep ford of the creek you have been following. From here it's more downhill for 0.3 mile to a reunion with Solitude Trail #038.

Turn left and continue descending mostly in forest for 0.5 mile to an easy ford of North Paint Rock Creek. From here it is 2 miles, mostly in forest near the creek, to a junction just before you enter the large meadow at Teepee Pole Flats, a popular campsite for equestrian groups.

Turn right on Trail #059 and for the next 4.3 up-and-down miles travel through pleasant but unspectacular forested and meadow terrain to the Lower Paint Rock Trailhead. From here it's an easy, mostly uphill, 1.5-mile roadwalk back to the Edelman Trailhead parking lot.

POSSIBLE ITINERARY

	CAMPS & SIDE TRIPS	MILES	ELEVATION GAIN
DAY 1	Meadow below Edelman Pass	6.8	1300'
DAY 2	Crystal Lake	9.0	1200'
DAY 3	Cliff Lake	7.2	1000'
DAY 4	Cliff Lake, with dayhike to the Crater Lakes and lakes above Lake Eunice	7.0	1100'
DAY 5	Out, including the 1.5-mile roadwalk back to the Edelman Trailhead	9.8	500'

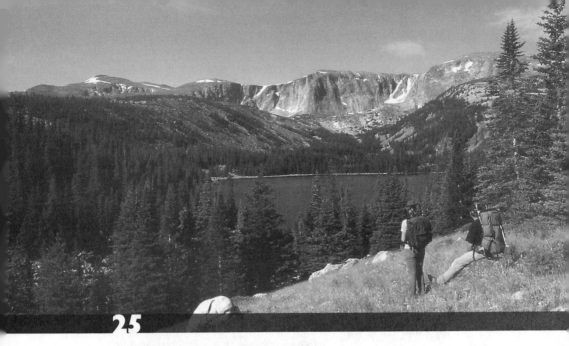

25

SOUTH BIGHORN MOUNTAINS LOOP

RATINGS: Scenery 8   Solitude 3   Difficulty 7
MILES: 31.2
ELEVATION GAIN: 5800´
DAYS: 3–6
MAP: Trails Illustrated *Cloud Peak Wilderness*
USUALLY OPEN: Mid-July to October
BEST: Late July to early August
CONTACT: Powder River Ranger District, Bighorn National Forest
SPECIAL ATTRACTIONS: Fine mountain and canyon scenery; good fishing
PERMIT: Required—free at the trailhead

RULES

Fires are prohibited above 9200 feet, which includes virtually all of this trip. Groups are limited to 10 people. Camping is prohibited within 100 feet of water.

CHALLENGES

A fairly long but not overly difficult cross-country section requires almost 2 miles of boulder hopping. Portions of this hike are quite crowded, especially around Lake Helen, Mistymoon Lake, and the Seven Brothers Lakes.

Photo: Backpackers overlooking Seven Brothers Lakes

TAKE THIS TRIP

Because it has easier road access, the southern half of the Cloud Peak Wilderness is more heavily used than the northern part of this preserve. While solitude is a little harder to find, the scenery includes not only the same sorts of dramatic cliffs and sparkling lakes found to the north but, in Florence Canyon, one of the most impressive high-elevation canyons in the state of Wyoming. Wildflowers and wildlife are also common, so hikers can experience the full range of attractions that the magnificent Bighorn Mountains offer.

The recommended loop involves a fairly long cross-country section, so those who are uncomfortable with off-trail travel might choose a different trip. Experienced backpackers, however, and especially those who are good at boulder hopping, should have little trouble negotiating the relatively straight-forward off-trail crossing of the range.

HOW TO GET THERE

From Exit 299 off Interstate 25 in Buffalo, drive 48.2 miles west on U.S. Highway 16 to a junction near Milepost 44. (Coming from the west, this junction is 43.5 miles east of Worland.) Turn right (west) on Forest Service Road 27 (West Tensleep Road), and follow this good gravel road for 1.1 miles to a fork. Go right, staying on Road 27, and proceed 6.1 miles to another fork. Go right again and drive 0.5 mile to the large trailhead parking lot.

NOTE: Throughout the Cloud Peak Wilderness, trails are signed only with their number. No trail names or destinations are listed. Therefore, to assist in navigation when you reach a junction in the wilderness, I generally refer to trail numbers rather than trail names in the following description.

DESCRIPTION

The very popular trail begins beside the self-issuing registration station at the north end of the trailhead parking lot. After 25 yards the trail splits at the start of your loop.

Go left on Trail #063 and follow this wide and gentle path through a dense forest of Engelmann spruces and lodgepole pines. You soon pass the northeast side of meadow-rimmed West Tensleep Lake, where on a quiet summer morning mule deer may bound away at your arrival and squirrels will angrily chatter at your passing. You may also be fortunate enough to see a moose in the meadow at the north end of the lake.

At 0.8 mile you cross West Tensleep Creek. The bridge here has been removed, so expect to make an easy, but cold, calf-deep ford. Immediately after the crossing a sign points to the Tensleep Cutoff Trail, which supposedly goes to the left toward Bald Ridge, although the trail is so little used it is hard to locate the tread.

Stick with the sometimes-rocky main trail and gradually climb through a mix of dense forest and occasional meadows. The meadows

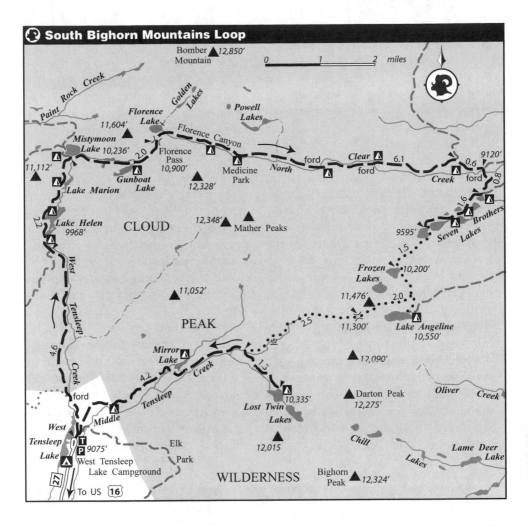

South Bighorn Mountains Loop

provide the potential for wildlife sightings (look for both elk and moose), as well as increasingly tantalizing views of the high peaks ahead. Off to your right, cascading West Tensleep Creek can often be heard but is rarely seen.

At 4.6 miles is a junction with Trail #097, which goes uphill to the left. Keep right, still on Trail #063, and 0.2 mile later reach a possible campsite at the south end of Lake Helen. This mostly rock-lined body of water is the trip's first alpine lake, and it's a nice introduction with the rounded snowy summits of several peaks and ridges reflected in the lake's waters.

Passing more potential campsites, the trail winds along the west side of Lake Helen before pulling away from the water and entering increasingly alpine terrain with fewer trees and more meadows and rocks. You walk past irregularly shaped Lake Marion (more campsites) before climbing in open country to a junction at 6.8 miles beside poetically named Mistymoon Lake. This lovely spot earns its beautiful name with a beautiful setting featuring great views of open slopes and the hulking mass of Cloud Peak to the north. Since the land near the lake is sloping and very fragile, it is better to camp at least 0.2 mile away from the lake on some relatively flat rocky benches.

Mistymoon Lake is a good base camp for hikers who want to climb Cloud Peak, the highest point in the Bighorn Mountains. The ascent, which actually starts from near Lake Solitude about 2 miles west of Mistymoon Lake, is very exposed (do *not* go if the weather is at all questionable) and requires some tricky scrambling and boulder hopping, but the views are beyond description.

To continue the loop, take Solitude Trail #038 going east from Mistymoon Lake, which heads up a narrow rocky canyon. After 0.6 mile, and now above treeline, the climb levels out as you pass narrow Fortress Lake. Just above this lake is an alpine basin, which holds both a narrow unnamed lake immediately on your left and, a short distance to the right (south), dramatic Gunboat Lake. The latter lake sits beneath a tall cliff of very dark rock and has some possible campsites.

The trail now climbs 350 feet over rocks and tundra to 10,900-foot Florence Pass. Less than 0.1 mile down the other side of the pass is stark but very beautiful Florence Lake. The exposure, rocks, and lack of level ground make camping here problematic, but you will still want to admire the views of bulky peaks all around and a small waterfall that tumbles into the lake.

North Clear Creek flows out of Florence Lake and almost immediately drops into steep-walled, impressively deep Florence Canyon. The trail follows suit and you will soon be suffering from neck pain from craning upward. You cross the creek several times, often at places where the water disappears beneath piles of huge boulders that have fallen off the canyon walls. About 1.5 miles below Florence Lake, and once again below treeline, you reach a small meadow where there is a nicely sheltered campsite. Even better, or at least more numerous, campsites are found 0.4 mile farther along at a larger meadow called Medicine Park.

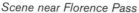

Scene near Florence Pass

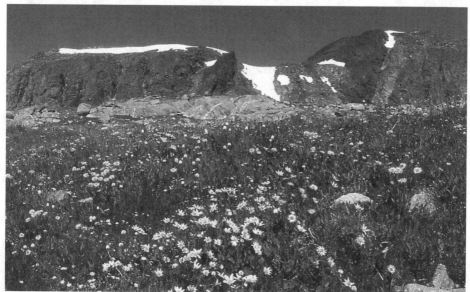

From Medicine Park go downhill some more, steeply at first then more gradually through forest, to an easy calf-deep ford of North Clear Creek at 12 miles. There is a nice campsite right after this crossing. The canyon widens and the steep walls fade as you increasingly find yourself traveling on a gentle trail through a wide, forested valley.

A little less than 1 mile below the first ford you cross North Clear Creek again. As with the first crossing, there is a comfortable campsite just after the ford. About 2 miles of gentle up-and-down forest walking now takes you to a junction. Trail #038 goes sharply left, but you veer right on Trail #024 and walk 0.6 mile through a meadow and past possible campsites to a second junction. Turn right on Trail #044 and immediately ford North Clear Creek for a third and final time.

Back in forest, the trail now follows switchbacks to the top of a minor ridge and immediately on the other side reaches a junction beside the first of the Seven Brothers Lakes. From this first rock-lined lake you have nice views of the cliffs and peaks to the west and these vistas only improve with each new lake in the chain that you reach.

To make that journey, turn right (west) at the junction onto Trail #045 and begin passing above or beside a string of relatively large lakes. All the lakes have campsites (including the ones reachable only by good user paths) and the fishing is very good. To protect from overuse, the Forest Service prohibits all camping and horse use on the west end of the sixth lake and anywhere around the seventh and last lake, where the trail ends.

Continuing the recommended loop beyond the last of the Seven Brothers Lakes requires cross-country travel and quite a bit of boulder hopping. It is long, but not excessively difficult and, in good weather, the navigating is easy. To start your off-trail adventure, cross the lake's outlet creek and walk around the east and south shores, mostly on solid, lichen-covered boulders. About halfway around the south shore climb away from the lake uphill and southwest through a large boulder field. The hiking is tiring, but if you carefully check the stability of each boulder before stepping on it, the going is not especially dangerous. After a little more than an hour of rough walking you reach the cirque containing Lower Frozen Lake. The rockiness of this area makes camping here next to impossible but the staggering views west across this lake to a series of tall cliffs are well worth at least an hour or so of gawking. Upper Frozen Lake, arguably even more dramatic, sits directly beneath the aforementioned cliffs and can be reached by more boulder hopping from the west end of Lower Frozen Lake.

The open, remarkably gentle ridge you will follow back over to the west side of the range is readily apparent starting a little south of the Frozen Lakes. Before heading up, however, check out large Lake Angeline in another scenic cirque on the south side of the ridge. The lake is easy to reach by boulder hopping and tundra walking and has a sketchy trail leading to it from the east. Camping here is very exposed and the ground is fairly rocky, but it is easier to find a level spot here than at the Frozen Lakes.

In good weather the cross-country route up the ridge to the west is obvious and straightforward. (Do *not* try this exposed climb in bad weather in any case, especially if any thunderclouds are around.) Simply follow the wide alpine ridge as it gradually heads uphill toward a rounded knob. The terrain consists of boulders and tundra and is neither technical in nature nor very difficult. In fact, the traveling is much easier than what you encountered crossing the large boulder fields on the way up to Lower Frozen Lake. Life in this alpine world is rather limited. A few low-growing wildflowers such as bistort, cinquefoil, alpine buttercup, moss campion, and aster grow in the small patches of ground, while pikas live in the rocky areas and at least two species of birds—rosy finches and water pipits—spend their summers up here. Not at all limited, however, are the views: down into the basins of Lake Angeline and the Frozen Lakes, up and down the Bighorn Mountains, and across the vast Great Plains to the east. Once you get near the top of the knob, skirt its left (south) side and descend a bit to walk through a broad, tundra-covered pass.

The way down the west side of the pass is even easier than the way up was. Follow a relatively gentle slope, mostly on cushy tundra with a few rocks, staying in the drainage between two rounded ridges. About two-thirds of the way down, just as you get below treeline, work your way around the right (north) side of a large marshy area, and then follow game trails downhill until you hit the popular Lost Twin Lakes Trail #065.

A mandatory side trip from here, either for an overnight stay or just to look, goes left and ascends through meadows and rocky areas for about 1.3 miles to the first Lost Twin Lake. Awe-inspiring cliffs, some higher than 1000 feet, rise above the south and west sides of this alpine jewel as well as its higher twin another 0.5 mile to the southeast. Good to excellent campsites abound at both lakes although they can be busy on weekends.

Lake Angeline

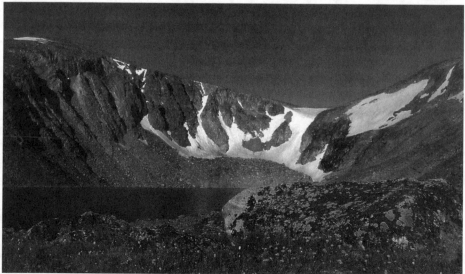

To exit the trip, walk downhill on Trail #065 as it gradually curves to the west then southwest following Middle Tensleep Creek. The way down is an even mix of forest and meadows and continuously pleasant. About 2.6 miles below the Lost Twin Lakes you pass unseen Mirror Lake 0.2 mile north of your trail, which has some nice campsites if you are willing to explore to find them. The main trail soon climbs over a mostly wooded ridge, steeply drops to a campsite near a meadow along Middle Tensleep Creek, and then climbs to the top of a second forested ridge. After following the top of this ridge for about 0.4 mile, pass an unsigned but obvious junction. Go straight and walk another 0.1 mile to reach the junction at the start of the loop only 25 yards from the trailhead.

POSSIBLE ITINERARY

	CAMPS & SIDE TRIPS	MILES	ELEVATION GAIN
DAY 1	Lake Marion	5.8	1200′
DAY 2	Lower Seven Brothers Lakes	10.5	1500′
DAY 3	Lost Twin Lakes, including a short side trip to Lake Angeline	9.4	2600′
DAY 4	Out	5.5	500′

VARIATIONS

Probably the most popular long backpacking trip in the Bighorn Mountains is the 60-mile Solitude Trail Loop, which includes parts of both the shorter north and south loops (this trip and Trip 24, p. 209) described in this book and generally encircles the outer portion of the Cloud Peak Wilderness. Without taking several side trips, however, especially to the lakes in the heart of this range, the loop misses some of the best scenery in these mountains. Even so, it's quite beautiful and well worth it. The usual itinerary is to start at the West Tensleep Trailhead described here, hike 6.8 miles north to the junction with the Solitude Trail at Mistymoon Lake, and then make a long counterclockwise circuit. Numerous other access points provide countless other options.

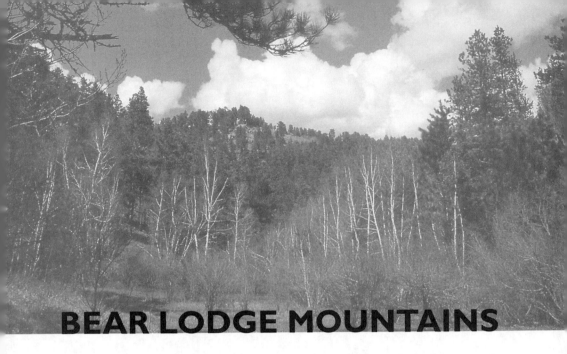

BEAR LODGE MOUNTAINS

The Bear Lodge Mountains in northeast Wyoming are an offshoot of the Black Hills, most of which are in neighboring South Dakota. Like their better-known parent range, the Bear Lodge Mountains consist of attractive hills covered with open meadows and ponderosa pine forests. Although not as ruggedly spectacular as the higher mountains in other parts of Wyoming, this range provides some fine hiking, especially early and late in the season when those taller ranges are buried in snow. This area is also rich in animal and plant life with a unique and interesting mix of species from both the Rocky Mountain region to the west and the grasslands of the Great Plains to the east and south.

The best-known natural feature in this area is Devils Tower, an awe-inspiring 867-foot-tall basalt tower set aside in 1906 as the first national monument in the U.S. Although a distinctive and very impressive landmark that every traveler to the region should visit, the tiny monument that surrounds this monolith offers only dayhiking and, as a result, is not described in detail in this book.

Until fairly recently, longer hiking trails on the Bearlodge Ranger District of the Black Hills National Forest were few and far between. For the most part the scant acreage here not turned over to logging had been the playground of mountain bikers and hunters. In the last couple decades, however, the ranger district has developed a fun, interesting network of hiking and equestrian trails just north of the city of Sundance that cobble together old settler's routes, closed and existing logging roads, and a few newly constructed paths, adding up to more than 50 miles of scenic, interesting hiking. The scenery consists not only of the expected views of rolling, forested mountains surrounded by the seemingly endless prairies, but also some surprisingly rugged and dramatic stream canyons. All and all it is a fun place to explore, and since it is well away from the usual hiking destinations in Wyoming, the area offers plenty of solitude as well.

Photo: *Along Ogden Creek (Trip 26)*

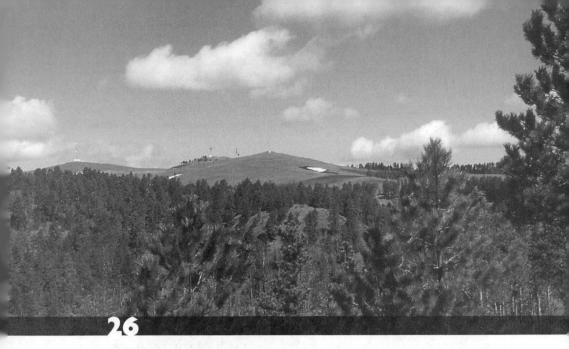

26

SUNDANCE TO OGDEN CREEK LOOP

RATINGS: Scenery 6   Solitude 9   Difficulty 5
MILES: 16.6, with countless other options
ELEVATION GAIN: 2700´
DAYS: 2–5
MAPS: USGS *Sundance East* and *Sundance West*
USUALLY OPEN: May to November
BEST: Mid-May to mid-June and late September
CONTACT: Bearlodge Ranger District, Black Hills National Forest
SPECIAL ATTRACTIONS: Good canyon scenery; interesting mix of flora and fauna from both the Rocky Mountains and the Great Plains; good early or late season hiking; nice fall colors
PERMIT: None required

RULES

The usual no-trace rules apply.

CHALLENGES

The route requires some walking along the road. Some trails are obscure and poorly marked. Water is limited late in the year.

Photo: Warren Peak from the south

HOW TO GET THERE ·

Take Interstate 90 to the town of Sundance, then follow U.S. Highway 14 (the main drag) to the east end of town and a junction exactly 0.1 mile east of the Bearlodge Ranger Station. Turn left (north) on paved Government Valley Road, which soon leaves town and turns to gravel. After 4.2 miles turn left into Sundance Campground and drive about 75 yards to a T-junction and the signed trailhead.

DESCRIPTION ·

The Sundance Campground and trailhead is located in open grassland at the edge of the Wyoming prairie. Just a few yards to the west, however, the forest begins, so this is a good place to appreciate the diversity of the Bear Lodge Mountains and to do some wildlife watching. Here you will see birds from both the Rocky Mountains, such as western tanagers and mountain bluebirds, and those from the Great Plains like bobolinks and lark buntings. The plants are fascinating as well, as they make a rapid transition from prairie grasses to mountain forests. But even those forests are unusual, in particular for their uniformity. Unlike the evergreen forests found elsewhere in Wyoming with the mix of pines, spruces, and firs, the conifers here consist only of a few scraggly junipers and continuous stands of stately ponderosa pines. Deciduous trees are more varied with different species found at different elevations. Look for bur oak at lower elevations along with hackberry and chokecherry. At higher elevations quaking aspens become more common as does water birch. Wildlife is common throughout the mountains. Some of the more interesting species you are likely to see are wild turkeys and white-tailed deer (both abundant) and Rocky Mountain elk.

TAKE THIS TRIP

The Bear Lodge Mountains, an offshoot of South Dakota's Black Hills, offer a relatively gentle but very pleasant landscape of pine-covered hills and impressive canyonlands. And while these mountains lack the dramatic crags and high alpine lakes commonly found in the taller ranges of Wyoming, they contrast sharply with the grassy prairies that extend for countless miles in all directions. Although these mountains are too compact for extended backpacking trips, a fine network of trails not far from the town of Sundance provides hikers with attractive, fun backpacking options, especially in spring and fall when the state's higher ranges are covered with snow.

There are dozens of loop possibilities in this area. The one described here traces the outer perimeter of the trail system and is one of the more scenic alternatives, but you could easily spend a week exploring all the worthwhile paths. For a complete list of the many alternatives, pick up a copy of the free handout entitled *Sundance & Carson Draw Trails*, which is available at the Bearlodge Ranger Station.

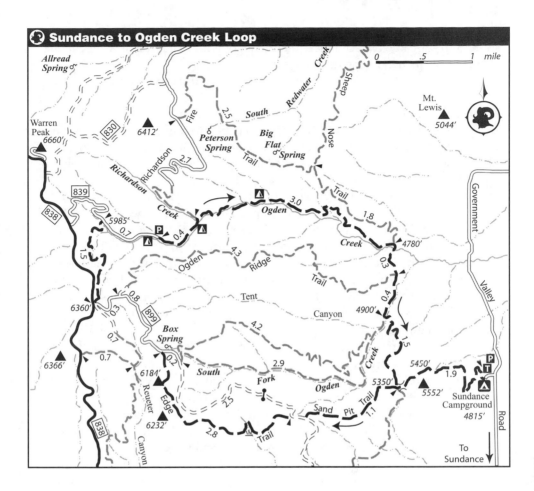

Sundance to Ogden Creek Loop

Fully appreciating this diverse range of flora and fauna, you soon enter a forest of short ponderosa pines and bur oaks, pass through a gate, and begin an extended moderately steep uphill. In late May these slopes are bursting with life. In the air are the constant sounds of songbirds, including chipping sparrows, meadowlarks, and various warblers and vireos. Even more impressive is the show of wildflowers. Some of the more common blossoms are those of phlox, Oregon grape, and balsamroot. For added interest and inspiration as you ascend, the trail offers frequent views of the prairies and ranchlands to the east and the aptly named Black Hills to the southeast.

After two fairly long switchbacks the trail turns west, becomes less steep, and passes through its first groves of quaking aspens. In late September these trees provide excellent fall color as the leaves turn yellow and orange. You top out on a knoll covered with rolling meadows and scattered groves of trees where you gain the first good vistas to the west of the unspectacular but very inviting Bear Lodge Mountains. In late May the meadows here host wildflowers such as larkspur, shooting star, a yellow-blooming pea, and *agoseris* (for the uninitiated, that's a fancy Latin way of saying a type of dandelion). Turkeys are also common in this area, so expect to hear plenty of gobbling. The trail now descends to a four-way junction in a wide grassy saddle.

Numerous attractive loop options start at this saddle, so you can't go wrong. For the recommended outer loop, go straight on Sand Pit Trail and gradually climb a rolling ridgeline. Most of this route is open and offers excellent views of the rugged canyon of South Fork Ogden Creek to the north and the town of Sundance to the south. After 1 mile of this easy, superb walking you come to an abandoned road. Turn right on the road and continue 0.1 mile to a possibly unsigned junction with a foot trail that veers left (uphill).

You could continue walking the road, but for better scenery turn left on Edge Trail. This often faint trail goes steeply uphill in forest and then levels out and passes a fine viewpoint. At about 0.6 mile from the road you reach a lush little meadow with a seasonal trickle of water. At the upper end of the meadow the trail becomes sketchy. The correct route makes a sharp left turn back along the west edge of the little meadow, then angles to the right and enters a relatively open forest that many years ago was selectively logged. The trail is often obscure in this area, so keep a careful eye out for trail markings, including orange flags, blue paint marks on trees, and brown signposts. These signposts, marked with a distinctive bear paw print, direct you across an old jeep road at 4.2 miles and through a fence line at 4.6 miles. Shortly after this fence line you reach and follow an abandoned jeep track for 0.2 mile, then angle to the left back onto a foot trail. The open forest here is alive with birds, including robins, juncos, various woodpeckers, sparrows, ruby-crowned kinglets, yellow-rumped warblers, and nuthatches.

At 5.8 miles the Edge Trail reunites with the road, which here is open to vehicles, so you may have to share your route with machines. Go left, following Road 899 as it gradually ascends for 0.8 mile to the junction with Ogden Ridge Trail, an alternate shorter loop route with good views. For the recommended loop, stick with the road for another 0.3 mile to a multiway junction just before you reach paved Road 838. There are some fine views in this area north to bald-topped Warren Peak, the top of which features a distinctive fire lookout tower and the usual cluster of unattractive electronics towers found on so many peaks these days.

Turn right at this junction onto an abandoned jeep track, signed as UPPER OGDEN TRAIL, which goes downhill for 100 yards to a little grassy flat. Bear left at a sign saying OGDEN CREEK and follow this gently graded mostly downhill route that soon narrows to a trail. For the next 1.5 miles this trail wanders around attractive meadows, travels through groves of quaking aspens and ponderosa pines, crosses a couple of small seasonal creeks, and finally takes you to a wooden bridge over small Ogden Creek just before coming to a junction with gravel Road 839.

Turn right (downstream) on the road and follow it for 0.7 mile as it parallels a telephone wire and Ogden Creek into an increasingly steep-sided, scenic canyon. Along the way you pass numerous lovely creekside meadows and visit a fenced gravesite with a sign commemorating EMIL REUTER, PIONEER MINER, 1845–1926, an exceptionally long life for someone in his era and line of work. The road ends at a trailhead.

Continue downstream, now on a pleasant trail that passes several possible camping spots for 0.4 mile to a bridge over tiny Richardson Creek and a junction with Richardson Fire Trail. This rugged route climbs to several fine viewpoints but requires some walking along the road, and is a longer, more difficult alternate to the recommended Ogden Creek Trail.

Your trail goes right at this junction, remaining close to splashing Ogden Creek for another 0.3 mile before making the first of four crossings of the stream over about 1 mile. Although never difficult, these bridgeless crossings may get your feet wet during spring runoff. Just past the last crossing is a small flat that would make an ideal campsite. A little less than 1 mile past this possible campsite the trail abruptly enters the radically different environment of Ogden Creek's lower canyon. Here the forest mostly disappears and is replaced by open slopes with wildflowers and good views. The canyon is also much steeper with many colorful cliffs and contorted rock formations. In spring and early summer look for flocks of nesting swallows swooping around these cliffs. On the down side, this area can be hot on summer days and you need to keep an eye out for rattlesnakes.

At 12.5 miles you meet the Sheep Nose Trail, where the alternate Richardson Fire Trail rejoins your loop. Go right on Tent Canyon Trail and just 150 yards later ford Ogden Creek a final time.

Avoiding private land just downstream, the trail climbs briefly away from Ogden Creek and goes south through a lovely transition zone between the prairie to the east and the forest to the west. At 0.3 mile from Ogden Creek go straight at a signed junction with the faint Ogden Ridge Trail and then follow South Fork Ogden Creek upstream through a lush grassy meadow rimmed with bur oak.

At 13.2 miles turn left on South Fork Tent Canyon Trail, immediately cross a culvert over South Fork Ogden Creek, and then begin a long, steady, but not overly steep uphill. This ascent crosses a mostly open slope where the forest has never fully recovered from a decades-old fire. As a result, the climb can be quite hot in midsummer, but since it only gains 450 feet in the next 1.5 miles it is not overly steep or difficult. Bur oaks, a few short ponderosa pines, and one grove of quaking aspens provide limited but welcome shade along the way. Also of note are the increasingly good views to the west of rugged Tent Canyon. At the top of the switchbacking ascent is the grassy saddle where you close the loop at the junction with the Sundance and Sand Pit trails. Turn left and return the 1.9 mostly downhill miles to the trailhead.

POSSIBLE ITINERARY

	CAMPS & SIDE TRIPS	MILES	ELEVATION GAIN
DAY 1	Ogden Creek	9.4	1900'
DAY 2	Out	7.2	800'

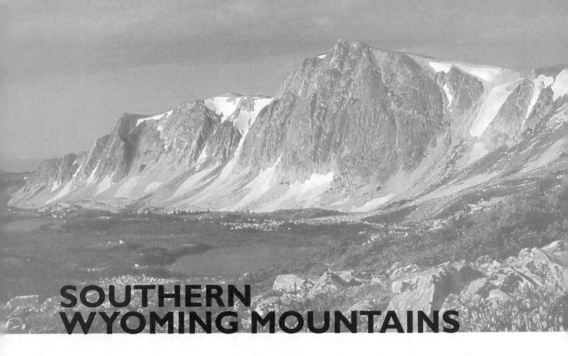

SOUTHERN WYOMING MOUNTAINS

Although not nearly as famous as the state's mountains, the vast deserts of central and southern Wyoming hide a wealth of rarely visited but first-class attractions. Hikes to such remote destinations as Killpecker Dunes, Adobetown, the Sweetwater River Canyon, the Honeycombs, the Jack Morrow Hills, and Boars Tusk (among many others) will reward you with superb desert scenery and plenty of solitude. Unfortunately, road access to these places is generally awful, trails are nonexistent, and water is nothing but a rumor. Dayhikes are the usual choice of the few people who come here since it is considerably easier to carry enough water for a day's journey than an overnight hike. Long-distance hikes of the duration highlighted in this book are possible, but they are logistically difficult and are rarely feasible or advisable for the average backpacker.

The higher mountains of southern Wyoming, in particular the Sierra Madre and Medicine Bow Mountains west of Laramie, offer much better prospects for the backpacker. Here you encounter wonderfully scenic forested mountains with impressive river canyons and even a few eye-popping jagged peaks. The wild areas here are generally small, so really long hikes are not possible, but there is enough roadless terrain to make for some outstanding short to medium-length overnight adventures. Canyon lovers and anglers should not miss, for example, the quite beautiful trail along the Encampment River in the heart of the Sierra Madre. Those who prefer high peaks and sparkling mountain lakes will get more than their fill of both in the compact but spectacular Snowy Range, the highest and most impressive summits in the Medicine Bow Mountains.

Photo: *View south from trail up Medicine Bow Peak (Trip 28)*

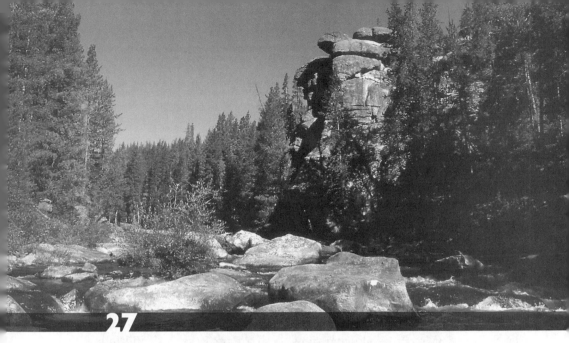

27

ENCAMPMENT RIVER TRAIL

RATINGS: Scenery 7   Solitude 7   Difficulty 6

MILES: 18.2 as an out-and-back hike to Box Canyon Creek
15.4 one-way for the full trail

ELEVATION GAIN: 1300´ as an out-and back hike; 500´ one-way, starting
from the upper (southern) trailhead and going downhill

DAYS: 2–4

MAPS: USGS *Dudley Creek* and *Encampment*

USUALLY OPEN: May to late October (for lower trail); mid-June to
October for the full trail

BEST: Mid-May to mid-June, September, and October

CONTACT: Brush Creek/Hayden Ranger District, Medicine Bow
National Forest; Rawlins District, Bureau of Land Management

SPECIAL ATTRACTIONS: Dramatic canyon scenery; good early or late
season hiking, especially in the lower canyon; excellent fishing

PERMIT

None required—just sign the trail register at Purgatory Gulch.

RULES

Groups are limited to 15 people.

Photo: Encampment River near Hog Park Creek

CHALLENGES •

If the trip is done as a one-way hike, it involves a fairly long car shuttle. Early in the season several fords of tributary streams can be difficult.

HOW TO GET THERE •

From Exit 235 on Interstate 80 east of Rawlins, go 28 miles south on Wyoming Highway 130, then another 10 miles south on Wyoming Highway 70 to a junction in the town of Riverside. Turn right (west), still on Highway 70, and proceed 1.7 miles through the town of Encampment to a junction with County Road 353. Turn left (south) at a sign directing you to the Encampment River Campground, and follow this good gravel road for 2 miles through a ranch property and a pleasant BLM campground to the trailhead parking lot on the left just before the road enters a gated private camp.

To reach the southern trailhead at Commissary Park, return to Wyoming Highway 70 and continue east another 5 miles to a junction with Forest Service Road 550 immediately adjacent to a sign identifying where you enter national forest land. Turn left (south), following signs to Hog Park Reservoir, and follow this good gravel road for 16.2 miles to a junction. Go straight, now on Road 496, drive 4 miles, and then turn left at a sign for Encampment River Trail. Proceed 0.1 mile to the road-end trailhead parking lot in the large meadow at Commissary Park.

DESCRIPTION •

The wide trail goes upstream about 30 yards, past a large trailhead signboard and restroom building, to a metal bridge over the rushing Encampment River. An angler's path goes downstream from here, but the main trail turns right and

TAKE THIS TRIP

The joyful Encampment River tumbles down out of the heavily forested Sierra Madre through a beautiful and diverse wilderness canyon to the semidesert lands near the town of Encampment. An excellent, very scenic trail follows the river throughout its wilderness course, providing an interesting, exciting hike that is often best in the "shoulder seasons" when trails in the higher mountains are still blocked by snow. For anglers, the river provides blue-ribbon trout fishing, and for wildlife enthusiasts the canyon is home to plenty of elk and deer, as well as a wide variety of nesting birds and such interesting smaller mammals as pine martins, porcupines, river otters, and beavers.

If you have two cars and don't mind making a fairly long shuttle, this hike can be done as a one-way, point-to-point trip, starting from the southern trailhead at Commissary Park. Since one of the joys of this area, however, is the excellent early season hiking through the much-more-scenic lower portion of the canyon, the trip is described here as an out-and-back adventure starting from the lower trailhead.

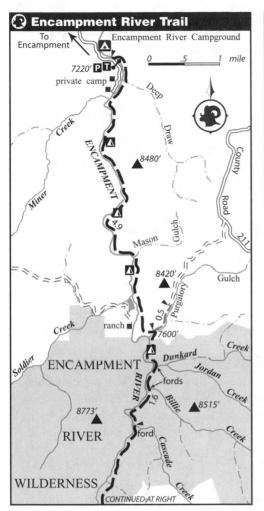

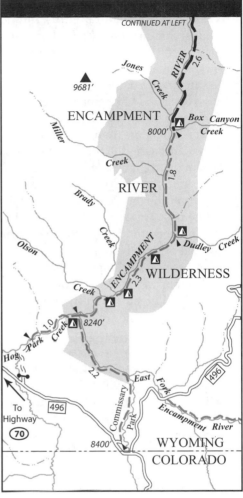

continues upstream. The surroundings here are stark but impressive. The slopes on either side of the canyon, which gradually become steeper and higher as you hike, are covered with sagebrush, grasses, rocks, and wildflowers with a few scattered prickly pear cacti, a reminder that this is a near desert. Considerably more vegetation grows in the riparian zone beside the water, with the most common species being junipers, willows, serviceberry, and cottonwoods. Nesting songbirds are abundant, especially in the riparian shrubbery during May and June. The variety of birds is impressive and includes several species of warblers, vireos, hummingbirds, orioles, sapsuckers, towhees, and countless others. Ticks, a much less welcome form of wildlife, are also abundant in the spring. Check frequently for these nasty little bloodsuckers. It is also wise to keep an eye out for the occasional rattlesnake.

After 0.2 mile you pass through a gate and then hop over a seasonal tributary creek flowing out of Deep Draw. For the next 0.5 mile you pass several buildings and roads that are part of a private camp on the other side of the river. Once beyond these unnatural intrusions, however, you are treated to a wonderfully wild, scenic canyon. The farther you hike the higher and wetter the terrain becomes with gradually increasing numbers of conifers, especially Douglas firs, ponderosa and lodgepole pines, and Engelmann spruces. Quaking aspens also become more common as you climb in the canyon. Through all of these vegetation zones, the trail remains scenic and very pleasant and although consistently uphill it is rarely steep.

At a little more than 1.3 miles the trail goes through a second gate and shortly thereafter passes the first of several good campsites. This one is in a shady grove of conifers right beside the water. You pass the next good campsite at about 2.6 miles, and then follow the river around a couple of sweeping turns before hopping over the tiny seasonal creek draining Mason Gulch.

Just past Mason Gulch the trail crosses a sagebrush-covered hillside above a cottonwood-studded flat that would make a decent campsite, although it is often flooded during the high water of spring and early summer. At a little more than 4 miles you pass a large lake and private ranch on the other side of the river. The trail climbs to a nice viewpoint, ducks into a side canyon, then reaches the junction with Purgatory Gulch Trail at 4.9 miles. Keep right on Encampment River Trail, hop over the small creek in Purgatory Gulch, and then continue upstream, now on Medicine Bow National Forest land.

The increasingly forested terrain here provides different, but no less scenic, surroundings than the drier, more open country downstream. Just beyond Purgatory Gulch you enter the Encampment River Wilderness and then pass an excellent riverside campsite. If you are doing this trip as a three-day out-and-back hike early in the season, this camp is a good place to spend a couple of nights with a dayhike upstream on the second day.

At 5.5 miles wade easily across Dunkard Creek, where a careful examination of the willows along the stream is likely to reveal beaver activity. Just 0.4 mile past this crossing takes you to Billie Creek, which during heavy spring runoff presents quite a challenge with its swift, thigh-deep water. There may be narrow logs across the creek, but it is difficult and dangerous to cross these unstable "bridges," so plan to get wet and possibly even to have to turn around and head back if it is a particularly wet year.

Above Billie Creek the canyon remains wild and extremely scenic with frequent rock formations and views of the high ridges to the west. Just 0.3 mile beyond Billie Creek pass the remains of an ancient, broken-down log cabin, then closely follow the cascading river around a sharp turn and reach swift-flowing Cascade Creek, which also requires wading and may be thigh deep in June.

Above Cascade Creek the canyon and surrounding slopes are heavily forested so views are less frequent. Also less frequent, at least for the next couple of miles, are campsites as the trail stays high on the canyon walls avoiding the narrow, rocky channel below. You go up and down in this fashion enjoying more than a few looks down to the river until 9.1 miles when you reach a large, comfortable campsite just before the hop-over crossing of Box Canyon Creek. For hikers making this an early or late season out-and-back hike, Box Canyon Creek is the logical turnaround point.

If you are continuing south from Box Canyon Creek, the trail alternates between staying close to the river and crossing steep, often rocky slopes above the water for 1.8 miles until you reach another spacious, comfortable campsite just before the easy crossing of Dudley Creek. From here you walk up and down for 2.3 miles, mostly on a forested hillside. For variety, this pleasant section includes a couple of impressive rock formations and passes several grassy river-level flats, all with good campsites. At 13.2 miles is a bridge over the river and a campsite beside the junction with the Hog Park Creek Trail. A significant percentage of the trees in this area are dead, which gives the forest a mottled green and brown appearance—the result of a mountain pine beetle infestation that has killed many of the lodgepole pines throughout the Sierra Madre. Although this is a natural phenomenon, the millions of dead trees are a sad sight.

If you are continuing to Commissary Park, turn left at the junction and keep walking upstream now on a very gentle trail. The only significant impediments to your progress are frequent cow pies on the trail. These smelly land mines are the inevitable result of heavy cattle grazing during the summer months and serve as a useful reminder to always treat your water. After about 1.4 miles of forest hiking you enter Commissary Park, a large open expanse of sagebrush, grasses, wildflowers, and scattered trees. The trail's last 0.8 mile take you through this meadow on a dusty path that parallels the meandering river to the upper trailhead.

POSSIBLE ITINERARY

	CAMPS & SIDE TRIPS	MILES	ELEVATION GAIN
DAY 1	Near Dunkard Creek	5.3	600'
DAY 2	Near Dunkard Creek, dayhike		
	upstream to Box Canyon Creek	7.6	500'
DAY 3	Out	5.3	200'

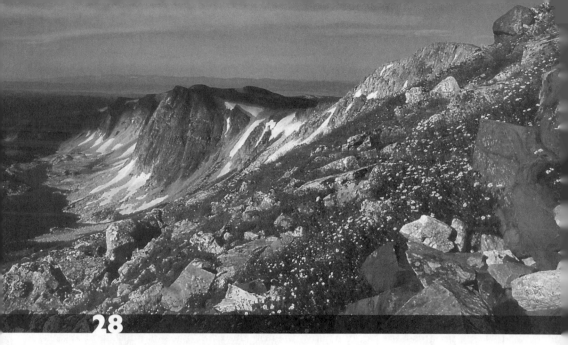

SNOWY RANGE HIGH LAKES LOOP

RATINGS: Scenery 9   Solitude 4   Difficulty 5
MILES: 22.3 (for the full figure-eight)
ELEVATION GAIN: 3400´
DAYS: 2–4
MAPS: USGS *Centennial, Medicine Bow Peak, Morgan,* and *Sand Lake*
USUALLY OPEN: July to October
BEST: Mid-July to early August
CONTACT: Brush Creek/Hayden Ranger District, Medicine Bow National Forest
SPECIAL ATTRACTIONS: Excellent mountain scenery; dozens of beautiful lakes; good fishing; the chance to climb the highest mountain in southern Wyoming
PERMIT: None required

RULES

The usual no-trace rules apply.

CHALLENGES

The trail can be fairly crowded, especially on weekends. Thunderstorms are frequent throughout the summer.

Photo: View south from near summit of Medicine Bow Peak

HOW TO GET THERE • • • • • • • • • • • • •

From Exit 311 off Interstate 80 in Laramie, go 43.5 miles east on Wyoming Highway 130 to the turnoff for the West Lake Marie Trailhead near milepost 42. Turn right and park in the large lot here.

DESCRIPTION • • • • • • • • • • • • • • • • • • •

The majority of hikers who start at the West Lake Marie Trailhead go west and head up the trail on the direct route to the summit of Medicine Bow Peak. Weather permitting, you will come back that way. For now, however, take the paved trail from the north end of the parking lot and parallel the highway as you follow the east shore of gorgeous Lake Marie. Backed by the towering cliffs along the ridge south of Medicine Bow Peak and rimmed with wildflowers and subalpine firs, this large lake is well worth some time to admire even though it is right beside the busy highway and quite crowded.

The paved trail leads to the East Lake Marie Trailhead at the northeast end of the lake where you go left (northwest) on a footpath to a junction with the paved loop road through the Mirror Lake Picnic Area. Turn left and walk about 150 yards up this road to a sign identifying the resumption of trail. The trail now sets off through an alpine wonderland of meadows, rocks, and a few struggling conifers. Marmots, a nearly constant companion along this section, provide musical entertainment with a chorus of cheeps and whistles from the nearby rocks. You soon reach the southern extension of large Lookout Lake, another gorgeous gem that sits beneath the majestic ramparts of Medicine Bow Peak.

The trail slowly climbs away from Lookout Lake into an above-treeline landscape of rocks, snow, and alpine wildflowers. The impressive variety of blossoms here in late July and early August includes alpine buttercup, lousewort, elephant head, paintbrush, pink

TAKE THIS TRIP

The appropriately named Snowy Range, a cluster of sky-scraping peaks that overlook dozens of stunning mountain lakes and grassy meadows, represents the crowning glory of the Medicine Bow Mountains. Located not far to the west of growing Laramie, this compact group of peaks is popular with weekend hikers and is small enough so that every highlight can be reached by dayhikers. But backpackers should not overlook this range, because spending a night (or two or three) amid the glories of these mountains is an experience not to be missed. The figure-eight described here visits most of the range's best scenery and even takes you to the top of Medicine Bow Peak, the highest point in southern Wyoming, and with a view to match.

Snowy Range High Lakes Loop

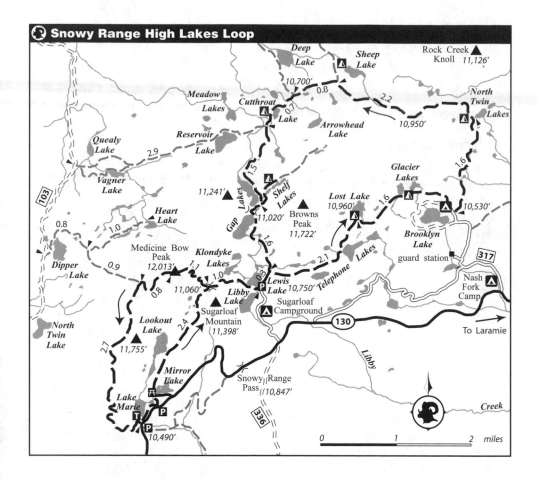

heather, blue columbine, marsh marigold, moss campion, glacier lily, bistort, aster, and many others. Top out at 2.4 miles at a junction in a rocky pass between Medicine Bow Peak on your left and much lower Sugarloaf Mountain to the right. Straight ahead, to the north, you can see flat-topped Browns Peak, which your route encircles.

If you are doing the recommended figure-eight, you will return to this junction before heading up Medicine Bow Peak. For now go straight (downhill) on a rocky trail past several fine viewpoints of the Klondyke Lakes to lovely Lewis Lake and its popular trailhead.

Take the trail north from the parking lot here, and hike 0.3 mile to a junction that forms another key point in the figure-eight. Bear right on Lost Lake Trail and pass a stunning array of scenic but unnamed little lakes, all reflecting the rounded mass of nearby Browns Peak and most also featuring good views back to the west of Medicine Bow Peak. At 5.8 miles you reach Lost Lake, which is no prettier than the others you have passed, but has a name because it's larger. There are good campsites at the lake's southwest end.

The trail almost immediately turns right (away from Lost Lake), crosses the lake's intermittent outlet creek, then descends to the two Glacier Lakes, where there are more good campsites. From here more downhill, mostly in forest, leads to a junction with the gravel road beside Brooklyn Lake. Walk 0.1 mile down this road going south-southeast past the Brooklyn Lake Campground, then turn left on the Sheep Lake Trail.

This gentle trail stays in forest for 0.8 mile and then rather abruptly leaves the trees and enters rolling alpine terrain as it passes a small lake and takes you to some good campsites above the two North Twin Lakes at 9 miles. There is superior fishing for cutthroat trout at these lakes, although brook trout are found in most of the other lakes in this range.

The trail now gradually ascends through very beautiful open country with views to the north of rounded Rock Creek Knoll. Although this north side of the Snowy Range is much less rugged and dramatic than the cliff-edged east face, it is still quite beautiful with larger meadows and abundant displays of wildflowers. After topping a rise at nearly 11,000 feet descend through alpine meadows above large Sheep Lake, which you can see to the north, and come to a junction at 11.2 miles.

The trail that goes straight ahead (north) passes campsites near Sheep Lake before continuing to Sand Lake and several other destinations. For this loop, however, turn left and walk through meadows and past small lakes toward the craggy northeast ridge of Medicine Bow Peak, which rises impressively to the southwest. After 0.8 mile the trail forks, where you veer left and wander past a nice campsite at Cutthroat Lake before climbing to yet another junction.

Lake Marie

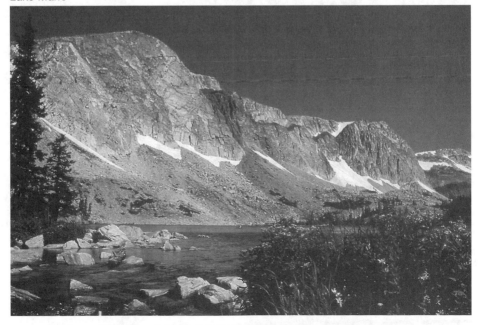

To do the recommended loop, and to visit the spectacular Gap Lakes, go left at this junction and continue uphill through a couple of gorgeous mountain meadows to rock-lined North Gap Lake. To describe it as "outstanding" simply does not do this lake justice. The towering cliffs of the 11,241-foot northeast ridge of Medicine Bow Peak rise directly above the west shore of the irregularly-shaped lake, making this a dramatically scenic spot. Unfortunately, good campsites far enough from the water to avoid environmental damage are hard to find. For better camping options, follow the main trail to the south end of North Gap Lake where there is a signed junction. Turn left (uphill) and hike 0.2 mile to the two narrow Shelf Lakes. Campsites are a little easier to find here although these smaller lakes are not up to the high scenic standards of North Gap Lake.

To continue the loop, return to North Gap Lake, turn left (south), and soon climb over a low rocky pass where you can look down on South Gap Lake. To say that this lake is not quite as spectacular as its northern twin is certainly not intended as a criticism—you won't be disappointed. The trail takes you the short distance down to this lake and then follows its eastern shoreline, whose rockiness severely limits camping possibilities. After pulling away from South Gap Lake, the circuitous trail winds downhill for 1 mile back to the junction with Lost Lake Trail you passed earlier in the trip. Go straight, return to the Lewis Lake trailhead, and then turn right and climb back up to the pass and junction below Medicine Bow Peak.

Pack goats below North Gap Lake

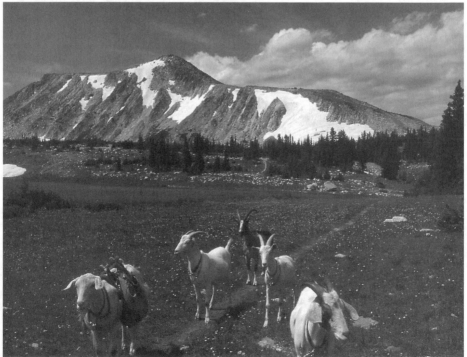

Weather permitting, it is time to do the south half of the figure-eight. So turn right and climb steeply on a rocky trail with fantastic views to the south along the rugged Snowy Range to the distant peaks of Colorado. The trail eventually tops out at the 12,013-foot summit of Medicine Bow Peak. From here you can see not only almost the entire route of this trip, but for nearly 100 miles in every direction.

WARNING: The area around Medicine Bow Peak is well above treeline and very exposed. Do not attempt this climb if the weather is iffy and especially if any thunderclouds are starting to build, something that occurs almost every afternoon in the summer.

After soaking in the view, take the trail down Medicine Bow Peak's south ridge and follow it for 0.8 mile to a junction with Dipper Trail. Veer left (south) and go gradually up and down across open slopes of tundra and rocks. After a little more than 1.5 miles of this view-packed rambling, the trail descends in a series of switchbacks over rocky slopes. Pass a tremendous viewpoint almost directly above Lake Marie and then finish the trip with another 0.8 mile of downhill to your starting point at the West Lake Marie Trailhead.

POSSIBLE ITINERARY

	CAMPS & SIDE TRIPS	MILES	ELEVATION GAIN
DAY 1	Lost Lake	5.8	800'
DAY 2	Shelf Lakes	8.7	900'
DAY 3	Out	7.8	1700

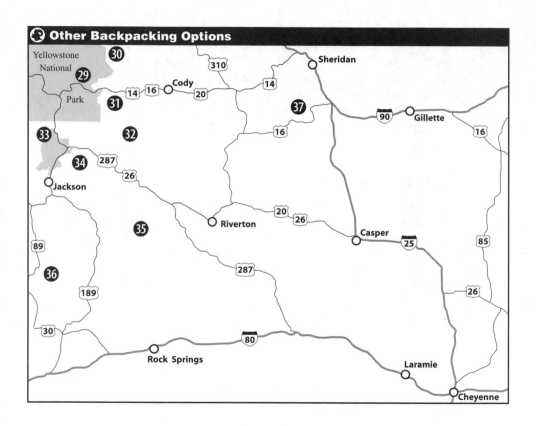

OTHER BACKPACKING OPTIONS

Although this book highlights my choices for the best long backpacking trips in Wyoming, there are countless other options for the adventurous backpacker. With some creativity and a good set of topographic maps, a backpacker could spend several lifetimes exploring the mountains, canyons, and deserts of the Cowboy State. What follows is an overview of some additional recommended trips, with just enough description to whet the appetite.

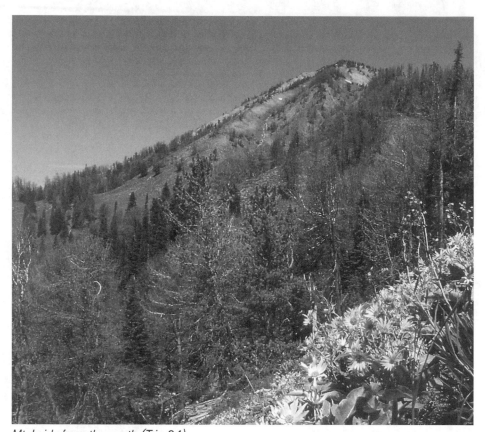

Mt. Leidy from the south (Trip 34)

29

PELICAN VALLEY & WAPITI LAKE LOOP

RATINGS: Scenery 6   Solitude 6   Difficulty 5

MILES: 31 (plus several challenging side trips)

ELEVATION GAIN: 900´

DAYS: 3–6

MAPS: Trails Illustrated *Yellowstone Lake & SE Yellowstone National Park* and *Tower/Canyon & NE Yellowstone National Park*

USUALLY OPEN: July 5 to October

BEST: Mid-July to early August

PERMIT: Required. Advanced reservations may be helpful.

CONTACT: Yellowstone National Park

SPECIAL ATTRACTIONS: Lots of wildlife; cross-country access to some unique and rarely visited backcountry thermal features

CHALLENGES: Grizzly bears are very common—camp and act accordingly. There are plenty of mosquitoes in July.

From a trailhead on the northeast shore of Yellowstone Lake, you hike up the Pelican Creek Trail through the wildlife-rich Pelican Valley. After a long but enjoyable side trip to the lookout building atop view-packed Pelican Cone, hike north past the Mushpots Thermal Area to campsites at Wapiti Lake. From here adventurous hikers can continue cross-country north about 2.5 miles on dusty, confusing bison trails to the Hot Spring Basin Group Thermal Area. *Extremely* dedicated hikers can bushwhack downstream along Broad Creek for 4.5 tough miles to the colorful and wildly scenic hot springs, geysers, and weird pinnacles around Josephs Coat Spring and Fairyland Basin. To return from Wapiti Lake, walk south past Fern Lake on the Astringent Creek Trail to Pelican Valley, then turn right (southwest) on the Pelican Creek Trail and back to the trailhead.

WARNING: Hydrothermal features are beautiful but uniquely dangerous with scalding water, deceptively thin soils, and unpredictable eruptions. Stay on the trail in these areas and remain well back from all hot water pools, springs, geysers, and other features.

Much of this hike travels through bear management zones where the access trails are closed before July 4. Once the trails open, overnight camping is not allowed on the lower portions of the Pelican Creek Trail, so you face a *very* long day to the first allowable campsites near Wapiti Lake. Bear-related restrictions mean that some off-trail areas beyond Wapiti Lake are only open to day users. Check the latest park regulations for details.

30

CRANDALL CREEK
& PAPOOSE RIDGE LOOP

RATINGS: Scenery 8   Solitude 8   Difficulty 8

MILES: 43

ELEVATION GAIN: 8900´

DAYS: 4–6

MAPS: USGS *Hunter Peak, Hurricane Mesa;* Trails Illustrated *Tower/Canyon & NE Yellowstone National Park*

USUALLY OPEN: Mid-July to October

BEST: August and September (for lower water in the streams)

PERMIT: Required to enter and to camp along that portion of the loop in Yellowstone National Park

CONTACT: Clarks Fork Ranger District, Shoshone National Forest; Yellowstone National Park

SPECIAL ATTRACTIONS: Lots of wildlife; plenty of solitude amid huge mountains and grand scenery

CHALLENGES: Grizzly bears are very common and unusually aggressive in this area—travel in a noisy group and camp and act accordingly. Some of the stream crossings are very difficult.

NOTE: This trip is recommended only for strong and experienced backpackers who travel in groups and don't mind being around an abundance of bears.

Loop lovers sometimes look at a map of the northern Shoshone National Forest and salivate over what appears to be a nearly perfect loop that goes up and down above the steep canyons of Crandall and Timber Creeks, visits scenic Canoe Lake (see Trip 3, p. 31) and Bootjack Gap in Yellowstone National Park, and returns via the view-packed Papoose Ridge Trail. And while the scenery is indeed impressive and the wildlife abundant, for years "problem" grizzly bears were transported here from Yellowstone National Park. The bears here are both extremely common and unusually aggressive, which will make many hikers queasy about traveling here and lead to some sleepless nights.

The trail also requires a couple of potentially dangerous stream crossings, which are not typically feasible until late July or early August. Even in late summer a heavy thunderstorm may pick up dirt from the easily eroded soils of this range and turn the creeks into muddy maelstroms. Side trails abound, but the enticing one up Closed Creek, although very scenic, is particularly famous for its bruin population. The trail starts near the Crandall Ranger Station on State Highway 296.

31

EAGLE CREEK TO EAGLE PASS

RATINGS: Scenery 7   Solitude 7   Difficulty 6

MILES: 33

ELEVATION GAIN: 2700´

DAYS: 3–6

MAPS: USGS *Eagle Creek, Eagle Peak,* and *Pinnacle Mountain*

USUALLY OPEN: Mid-July to October

BEST: Late-July to September

PERMIT: None required, unless you continue into Yellowstone National Park

CONTACT: Wapiti Ranger District, Shoshone National Forest

SPECIAL ATTRACTIONS: Lots of solitude; the chance to visit the highest peak in Yellowstone National Park; large meadows; plenty of wildlife

CHALLENGES: Grizzly bears are common—camp and act accordingly. At least one stream crossing is potentially difficult.

Eagle Creek, a major tributary of the North Fork Shoshone River, drains a large area across from the southeast border of Yellowstone National Park. The trail along this stream passes beneath tall peaks and ridges, goes through huge and glorious Eagle Creek Meadows, and eventually climbs all the way to Eagle Pass. At the pass you are right on the border of Yellowstone Park and a stone's throw from Eagle Peak, which at 11,358 feet is the highest point in the park.

In addition to its scenic treasures, the trail boasts the same assortment of abundant wildlife as the park, including grizzly bears, so act accordingly. Most of the 16.5 miles to the pass are quite gentle and relatively easy, with the majority of the elevation gain coming in the last couple of miles. The biggest potential obstacles are a couple of difficult stream crossings, so save this trip for later in the summer.

The trail starts from either Eagle Creek Campground right along U.S. Highway 14/16/20 west of Cody, or, to avoid a very difficult ford of North Fork Shoshone River, from Buffalo Bill Camp a couple of additional hiking miles to the east.

32

ISHAWOOA CREEK & DEER CREEK PASS LOOP

RATINGS: Scenery 8   Solitude 6   Difficulty 7
MILES: 46, plus an 8.4-mile roadwalk or car shuttle
ELEVATION GAIN: 7200´
DAYS: 4–7
MAPS: USGS *Clouds Home Peak, Ptarmigan Mountain, Thorofare Buttes, Valley,* and *Yellow Mountain*
USUALLY OPEN: July to October
BEST: Mid-July and August
PERMIT: None required
CONTACT: Wapiti Ranger District, Shoshone National Forest
SPECIAL ATTRACTIONS: Huge mountains, high passes, waterfalls, grand views, abundant wildlife, rolling meadows . . . well, you get the idea.
CHALLENGES: This huge, rugged, and extremely wild country is unsuitable for novice hikers. Grizzly bears are common—camp and act accordingly. This route is used fairly heavily by horses. Some stream crossings are potentially difficult in early summer.

Starting off the South Fork Shoshone River Road (Wyoming Highway 291) southwest of Cody, the trail goes west up the deep, rugged mountain valley of boisterous Ishawooa Creek, past two fine waterfalls, to Ishawooa Pass at 17 miles. Descend southwest along Pass Creek to a junction at Thorofare Creek, then turn east and ascend along Butte Creek to Deer Creek Pass next to the impressive ramparts of Kingfisher Mountain. Continue east another 10 miles beside Deer Creek back to the road. The loop is long and rugged, but well worth it for hardy backpackers. Be prepared to encounter grizzly bears almost anywhere along this trail.

33

MOOSE CREEK & OWL CREEK LOOP

RATINGS: Scenery 8   Solitude 8   Difficulty 8
MILES: 26, from the Glade Creek Trail entry
ELEVATION GAIN: 4100´
DAYS: 3–5
MAP: Trails Illustrated *Grand Teton National Park*
USUALLY OPEN: Late July to early October
BEST: August and September (for lower water at stream crossings)
PERMIT: Required
CONTACT: Grand Teton National Park
SPECIAL ATTRACTIONS: Lots of wildlife; plenty of solitude; outstanding wildflowers; fine mountain scenery
CHALLENGES: Grizzly bears are common—camp and act accordingly. Some stream crossings are very difficult. Trails receive little maintenance.

The trails in the central and southern Teton Range are wildly popular and are justifiably packed with hikers and backpackers, who typically have to reserve a permit well in advance. At the same time, the paths in the northern part of the same range remain virtually unknown. The mountains here are slightly less spectacular than the more famous southern peaks, but the meadows and wildflowers are better and the wildlife is more abundant, including a healthy population of grizzly bears, a species that is rare elsewhere in Grand Teton National Park. This area receives relatively little trail maintenance, and several of the creek crossings are very challenging early in the summer.

Start the recommended loop trip by either canoeing across the north end of Jackson Lake or hiking 6.9 miles south from the Glade Creek Trailhead on the Reclamation Ranch Road west of Flagg Ranch. From a junction near the patrol cabin at Berry Creek, hike southwest up scenic Webb Canyon along Moose Creek to impressive Moose Basin Divide, and then return along the Owl Creek Trail. Off-trail side trips abound, but they are quite rugged and should be left to only the most experienced and athletic among us.

34

MOUNT LEIDY HIGHLANDS

RATINGS: Scenery 6   Solitude 8   Difficulty 4

MILES: Variable

ELEVATION GAIN: Variable, but most trails are fairly gentle

DAYS: 3–9

MAPS: USGS *Green Mountain, Grizzly Lake, Mount Leidy,* and *Shadow Mountain*

USUALLY OPEN: Late June to October

BEST: Late June, July, and late September

PERMIT: None required

CONTACT: Jackson Ranger District, Bridger-Teton National Forest

SPECIAL ATTRACTIONS: Lots of wildlife; plenty of solitude; outstanding meadows and wildflower displays; mostly gentle and inviting hiking

CHALLENGES: Grizzly bears are present—camp and act accordingly. Poorly marked trails and routes can be confusing. This area receives significant ATV (all-terrain vehicle) use with the usual resulting trail damage and confusion.

There are a number of possible hiking options in this large, undesignated wild area east of Jackson Hole. Most of the trails are gentle routes through sagebrush flats, high meadows, and rolling, partly forested hills. Aspen groves add to the appeal, especially in late September when the leaves change color. Wildlife is abundant, as this area serves as a critical migration corridor between Yellowstone National Park and the Gros Ventre and Wind River ranges to the south. Sadly, lack of wilderness protection has allowed this otherwise pristine land to be overrun by the ATV crowd, so be prepared for machine-related aggravation. A typical itinerary is to start from the Gros Ventre Road near Red Hills Campground and hike north up Slate Creek toward ruggedly scenic Mt. Leidy. Numerous other options exist, however, so use your imagination and enjoy.

35

WIND RIVER HIGHLINE TRAIL

RATINGS: Scenery 10   Solitude 5   Difficulty 8
MILES: 72.5, plus all kinds of enticing side trips
ELEVATION GAIN: Variable but significant
DAYS: 8–20
MAP: Earthwalk Press *Northern Wind River Range* and *Southern Wind River Range*
USUALLY OPEN: Mid-July to early October
BEST: Late July and August
PERMIT: None required—sign in at the trailhead.
CONTACT: Pinedale Ranger District, Bridger-Teton National Forest
SPECIAL ATTRACTIONS: Glorious mountain scenery; hundreds of beautiful mountain lakes; plenty of good fishing; enough side trips to fill a month of spectacular hiking
CHALLENGES: The route requires a long car shuttle, has mosquitoes in July, and frequently experiences thunderstorms.

Comparable to the famous John Muir Trail through California's Sierra Nevada, the Highline Trail is the classic long-distance ramble in the Wind River Range. Usually begun at the Big Sandy Trailhead in the south (Trip 17, see p. 153) and completed at the Green River Lakes in the north (Trip 15, see p. 131), this magnificent adventure traces a wildly scenic course through the heart of these mountains. Along the way it accesses so many outstanding side trips that you could easily spend a month seeing only a portion of the many wonders. If scenery is your goal, then whenever possible, it is better to follow the *old* Highline Trail (now called the Fremont Trail) rather than the newer, rerouted Highline Trail. The old trail stays closer to the high peaks, although it passes somewhat fewer lakes and the campsites are generally more exposed. Regardless of which route you select, bring a fishing pole, a camera, and a good map to scout out the countless great side trips along the way.

36

LAKE ALICE
& FONTENELLE MOUNTAIN LOOP

RATINGS: Scenery 6   Solitude 6   Difficulty 7

MILES: 27

ELEVATION GAIN: 4900´

DAYS: 3–5

MAPS: USGS *Graham Peak* and *Porcupine Creek*

USUALLY OPEN: Mid-June to October

BEST: Late June to mid-July

PERMIT: None required

CONTACT: Kemmerer Ranger District, Bridger-Teton National Forest

SPECIAL ATTRACTIONS: Open ridges with excellent views; a scenic, geologically interesting lake with excellent fishing

CHALLENGES: The area around Lake Alice is fairly popular, even though it has only limited camping areas. Some trails elsewhere are faint and/or disappearing. Some trails are muddy and often very badly chewed up by horses.

At the south end of the Salt River Range in the Bridger-Teton National Forest, this loop explores a land of rolling open forests, numerous small creeks, view-packed ridges, interesting beaver dams, and extremely colorful Commissary Ridge. A highlight is Lake Alice, which was formed by an ancient landslide. Although a shorter, more popular trail reaches Lake Alice from the southwest, for this trip it is better to begin at the less crowded Poker Creek Trailhead off Forest Service Road 10138 west of Big Piney.

Begin by hiking 2.2 miles south up Little Corral Creek to a junction at a pass on Commissary Ridge and the start of the loop. Turn southeast and walk a view-packed ridgeline past the radio towers on Graham Peak to Fontenelle Mountain. Then go west on a sketchy path to Coantag Creek, White Saddle, and Lake Alice, and turn north along Poker Creek back to the pass and junction on Commissary Ridge.

37

CIRCLE PARK LOOP

RATINGS: Scenery 7   Solitude 3   Difficulty 5
MILES: 9, plus many miles of off-trail exploring
ELEVATION GAIN: 1600´
DAYS: 2–4
MAP: Trails Illustrated *Cloud Peak Wilderness*
USUALLY OPEN: July to October
BEST: Mid-July and August
PERMIT: Required—free at the trailhead
CONTACT: Powder River Ranger District, Bighorn National Forest
SPECIAL ATTRACTIONS: Lots of lakes with good fishing; a relatively easy loop suitable for families; possible side trips to some great off-trail lakes and climbing areas
CHALLENGES: Rather crowded at lakes with trails; mosquitoes in July.

Located in the southeastern Bighorn Mountains not far off U.S. Highway 16, this short, relatively easy loop is a nice sampler of what this impressive range offers. The trail ascends 1.8 miles to a junction at Sherd Lake and then loops counterclockwise past Otter and Trigger Lakes before returning to Sherd Lake via the South Fork Ponds. Most of the main loop route is in forest with limited views, but excellent short side trails offer access to Willow and Old Crow lakes where you can catch nice views of the high peaks to the west.

If you have the time and energy, visit some of those enticing peaks on a rugged but wildly scenic off-trail side trip. To do so, go west from the pleasant campsite at Old Crow Lake, climb gently to large Lame Deer Lake, then keep going up past a string of progressively more spectacular mountain pools, appropriately called the Chill Lakes, into a tremendous canyon with towering cliffs and grand scenery. The route offers climbers access to both Bighorn and Darton peaks, each higher than 12,000 feet and with views to match. Reaching any of these off-trail destinations requires plenty of boulder hopping and calorie burning, but it's worth it.

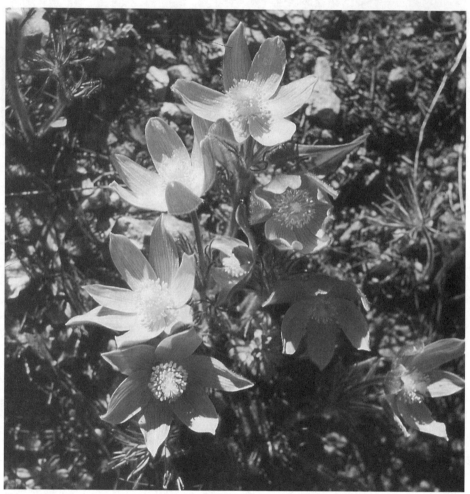

Pasqueflower

APPENDIX:
ORGANIZATIONS & AGENCIES

HIKING AND CONSERVATION ORGANIZATIONS

Biodiversity Conservation Alliance
www.voiceforthewild.org
P.O. Box 1512
Laramie, WY 82073
(307) 742-7978

Buffalo Pathfinders
(no website)
1197 North Burritt Avenue
Buffalo, WY 82834
(307) 684-9160

Cheyenne High Plains Wanderers
(no website)
P.O. Box 2025
Cheyenne, WY 82003
(307) 638-9979

Greater Yellowstone Coalition
www.greateryellowstone.org
P.O. Box 1874
13 S. Wilson, Suite 2
Bozeman, MT 59771
(406) 586-1593

Jackson Hole Conservation Alliance
www.jhalliance.org
685 South Cache Street
Jackson, WY 83001
(307) 733-9417

Wyoming Chapter of the Sierra Club
http://wyoming.sierraclub.org
P.O. Box 12047
Jackson, WY 83002
(307) 733-4557

Wyoming Outdoor Council
www.wyomingoutdoorcouncil.org
262 Lincoln Street
Lander, WY 82520
(307) 332-7031

Wyoming Wilderness Association
www.wildwyo.org
Box 6588
Sheridan, WY 82801
(307) 672-2751

LAND AGENCIES

Bighorn National Forest
www.fs.fed.us/r2/bighorn/

Powder River Ranger District
1415 Fort Street
Buffalo, WY 82834
(307) 684-7806

Black Hills National Forest
www.fs.fed.us/r2/bhnf/

Bearlodge Ranger District
121 South 21st Street
P.O. Box 680
Sundance, WY 82729
(307) 283-1361

Bridger-Teton National Forest
www.fs.fed.us/r4/btnf (although the website is practically useless for hikers)

Big Piney Ranger District
315 South Front Street
P.O. Box 218
Big Piney, WY 83113
(307) 276-5800

Buffalo Ranger District
Highway 26/287
P.O. Box 278
Moran, WY 83013
(307) 543-2386

Greys River Ranger District
671 North Washington Street
P.O. Box 339
Ashton, WY 83110
(307) 886-5300

Jackson Ranger District
25 Rosencrans Lane
P.O. Box 1689
Jackson, WY 83001
(307) 739-5400

Kemmerer Ranger District
308 Highway 189
Kemmerer, WY 83101
(307) 877-4415

Pinedale Ranger District
29 East Fremont Lake Road
P.O. Box 220
Pinedale, WY 82941
(307) 367-4326

Bureau of Land Management: Rawlins District
Note: The website is useless for hikers—don't bother.
1300 North Third
Box 2407
Rawlins, WY 82301
(307) 328-4200

Grand Teton National Park
www.nps.gov/grte/
P.O. Drawer 170
Moose, WY 83012
(307) 739-3300

Medicine Bow National Forest
www.fs.fed.us/r2/mbr/

Brush Creek/Hayden Ranger District
Saratoga Office
South Highway 130/230
P.O. Box 249
Saratoga, WY 82331
(307) 326-5250

Shoshone National Forest
www.fs.fed.us/r2/shoshone/

Clarks Fork Ranger District
203A Yellowstone Avenue
Cody, WY 82414
(307) 527-6921

Greybull Ranger District
Note: Greybull is in the same office as Clarks Fork.
203A Yellowstone Avenue
Cody, WY 82414
(307) 527-6921

Wapiti Ranger District
Note: Wapiti is in the same office as Clarks Fork.
203A Yellowstone Avenue
Cody, WY 82414
(307) 527-6921

Washakie Ranger District
333 East Main Street
Lander, WY 82520
(307) 332-5460

Wind River Ranger District
P.O. Box 186
1403 West Ramshorn
Dubois, WY 82513
(307) 455-2466

Targhee National Forest
www.fs.fed.us/r4/caribou-targhee/

Ashton/Island Park Ranger District
Ashton Office
460 South Highway 20
P.O. Box 858
Ashton, ID 83420
(208) 652-7442

Yellowstone National Park
www.nps.gov/yell/
Mammoth Hot Springs
Yellowstone National Park
P.O. Box 168
Yellowstone National Park, WY 82190
(307) 344-7381

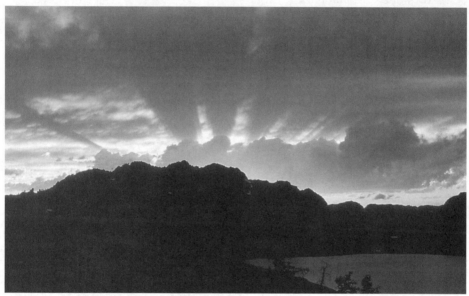

Sunset at Upper No Name Lake (Trip 15), Wind River Range

INDEX

A

Absaroka Range, trips within 73–85, 248, 249, 250
Absaroka Trail 84
Adams Pass 170
Alaska Basin 109, 110
Albino Lake 62
altitude sickness 7, 207
Antoinette Peak 126
Appaloosa Meadows 33
Arrowhead Lake (Beartooth Mountains) 61
Arrowhead Lake (Wind River Range) 161
Atlantic Creek 100, 101
August Lake 146
Avalanche Divide 108–109

B

Bannock Peak 19
Baptiste Creek 158, 159
Baptiste Lake 153, 159
"Barbara" Lake 147
Barren Lake 160
Basco Creek 178
Basin Creek 52, 53
Battleship Mountain 109
bear canisters 9, 77, 104
Bear Creek 28
Bear Creek Pass 85
Bear Lakes 171
Bear Lodge Mountains 223–229
Bears Ears Mountain 171
Bears Ears Trail 159, 162, 169
Beartooth Butte 60
Beartooth Creek 60, 65

Beartooth High Lakes Trail 60, 62
Beartooth Highway 58
Beartooth Lake 60, 62
Beartooth Mountain 62
Beartooth Mountains 55, 58
Beauty Lake 62
Beaver Creek 47
Beaver Park 136
Bechler River country 16
Becker Lake 62
Berry Creek 251
Beth Lake 147
"Big Balls of Cowtown" Trail 124
Big Chief Mountain 159
Big Game Ridge 51, 53
Big Meadows 167
Big Sandy Lake 156, 161, 162
Big Sandy Pass 161
Big Sandy River 156, 162
Big Sandy Trailhead 153, 155, 253
Big Springs 102
Bighorn Mountains 207–221, 255
Bighorn Pass 19
Bighorn Peak 255
bighorn sheep 19, 27
Billie Creek 236
Bills Park 178
Billys Lake 160
bison 16, 32
Bitch Creek 90, 92
Bitch Creek Narrows 92
black bear 8, 10, 160, 161, 173
Black Canyon of the Yellowstone River 24–28
Black Hills 207, 223, 226
Black Joe Lake 161

Black Peak 121, 126
Blackman Creek 117
Blacktail Bridge 28, 29
Blacktail Deer Creek 29
Bobs Lake 143
Bomber Basin 164
Bomber Falls 164
Bonneville Lake 150
Bonneville, Mount 150, 157
Boot Lake 180
Bootjack Gap 37, 248
Bootjack Gap Trail 37
Boulder Creek 118
Boulder Lake Trailhead 151
Boundary Lake 142
Box Canyon 196
Box Canyon Creek 236
Box Canyon Pass 196
Box Lake 115
Bradley Lake 112
Brewster Lake 120, 124, 127
Bridger Wilderness, trips within 131–162, 253
Broad Creek 247
Brooklyn Lake 241
Brown Basin 82, 83
Brown Rock Canyon 84
Browns Peak 240
Buck Mountain Pass 109–110
Buffalo Bill Camp 249
Burro Flat 166
Burwell Creek 76
Burwell Pass 83–84
Butte Creek 250

C

Cache Creek 33
Cache Lake 23
Cache Peak 117
Caldwell Creek 84
Calfee Creek 33
Calfee Creek Patrol Cabin 33
Camp Lake 92, 93
Canoe Lake 36, 248
Canyon Creek 66
Cascade Creek (Encampment River) 236
Cascade Creek (Teton Range) 108
Castle Creek 101
Castle Rock Glacier 60
Cathedral Lake 173
Cathedral Peak 171
cattle 5, 118
Chateau Lake 124
Chauvenet, Mount 171
Chicken Ridge 47
Chief Joseph Scenic Highway 58, 64
Chill Lakes 255
Chipmunk Creek 50
Circle Park Loop 255

Cirque of the Towers 153, 156, 160, 161, 162, 169, 172
Clarks Fork Canyon 66–67, 68
Clarks Fork Yellowstone River 55, 64
Clay Butte 60
Clear Creek (Teton Wilderness) 97
Clear Creek (Wind River Range) 133
Clear Creek Falls 133
Clear Creek Natural Bridge 133
Clear Lake 161
Cliff Creek 189
Cliff Creek Falls 189
Cliff Creek Pass 189
Cliff Lake 213, 214
Cloud Peak 218
Cloud Peak Wilderness, trips within 209–221, 255
Closed Creek 248
Cloverleaf Lakes (Beartooth Mountains) 61
Cloverleaf Lake (Wind River Range) 173
Coantag Creek 254
Coffin, Mount 195
Commissary Park 234, 237
Commissary Ridge 254
Conant Basin 94
Conant Creek 94
Cook Lake 173
Coon Lake 179
Corner Peak 126
Corral Creek 202
Corral Creek Lake 201, 202
Cottonwood Creek 28
Cow Creek 83
Coyote Creek 92
Coyote Meadows 91
Crandall Creek 248
Crane Lake 62
Crater Creek 92
Crater Lake (Teton Wilderness) 102
Crater Lakes (Bighorn Mountains) 213–214
Crescent Lake 143
Crescent Top Mountain 76
Crevice Creek 28
Crevice Lake 28
Crow Creek 197
Crow Creek Lakes 203
Crowfoot Ridge 19
Crystal Lake (Beartooth Mountains) 60
Crystal Lake (Bighorn Mountains) 213
Crystal Spring 94
Cube Rock Pass 137
Cutthroat Lake (Snowy Range) 241
Cutthroat Lake (Wind River Range) 139

D

Dads Lake 157
Dale Lake 137
Darton Peak 255

Darwin Peak 121, 124
Dead Indian Trail 68, 69
Deadman Mountain 190
Death Canyon 110–111
Death Canyon Shelf 110
Deep Creek 180
Deep Creek Lakes 180
Deep Draw 235
Deep Lake 161
Deer Creek 250
Deer Creek Pass 250
Deer Ridge 121
Delacy Creek 44
Dennis Lake 147
Devils Lake 212
Devils Tower 223
Dickinson Park 173
Dickinson Park Work Center 169
Dillworth Bench 67
Dinwoody Creek 166, 167
Dinwoody Glacier 167
Dishpan Butte 173
Divide Lake 143
Dodge Creek 139
Dogtooth Mountain 172
Double Cabin 74
Double Lake 166
Doubletop Mountain Trail 138–139
Downs Fork 167
Downs Fork Meadows 167
Dragon Head Peak 149
Dream Creek 150, 151
Dream Lake 150, 151
Dudley Creek 237
Duncan Lake 212
Dunkard Creek 236
Dunrud Pass 85
Dunrud Peak 85

E
Eagle Creek 249
Eagle Creek Meadows 249
Eagle Pass 249
Eagle Peak 249
East Fork Big Goose Creek 212
East Fork River 157
East Torrey Creek 164
Edelman Creek 212
Edelman Pass 211
Edge Trail 228
Elbow Creek 138
Elbow Lake 138
Electric Divide 23
Electric Peak 23
elk 19, 33, 43, 77, 139, 190
Elk Creek 204
Emerald Creek 76
Emerald Lake (Absaroka Range) 74, 77

Emerald Lake (Bighorn Mountains) 211
Encampment River 233–237
Europe Canyon 147–148

F
Factory Hill 46
Fairyland Basin 247
Fall Creek 146
Fan Creek 22
Fawn Pass Trail 19, 23
Fayette Fire 151
Fern Lake 247
Ferry Lake 102
Firehole River 40–41, 42
First Creek 190
Fish Creek Park 157
Fitzpatrick, Mount 201, 202, 203
Fitzpatrick Wilderness 164–167
Flat Creek 117
Flat Rock Lake 60
Florence Canyon 216, 218
Florence Lake 218
Florence Pass 218
Floyd Wilson Meadows 167
Fontenelle Mountain 254
Fortress Lake 218
Fourth Creek 190
Fox Creek Pass 110, 112
Fox Creek Patrol Cabin 51
Fremont Creek 138
Fremont Crossing 138
Fremont Trail 143, 146, 150, 156, 253
Frontier Creek 74, 77
Frozen Lakes 219, 220

G
Gallatin Bear Management Area 17
Gallatin Range 18
Gallatin River 19
Gannett Creek 167
Gannett Peak 164, 167
Gardiner 25, 30
Gardner River 23, 26
Gardners Hole 23
Garnet Canyon 112
Geneva Pass 213
geysers 39, 40, 41, 42, 47, 247
Ghost Creek 65
Glacier Lakes 241
Glacier Peak 93
Glacier Trail 163–167
Glade Creek Trailhead 251
Glen Creek 23
Goat Flat 166
Golden Gate Trailhead 23
Golden Lake 61
Graham Peak 254

Grand Teton 108, 109
Grand Teton National Park 87, 89, 93,
    104–112, 251
Granite Creek 114, 115, 120
Granite Falls 114
Granite Highline Trail 114, 117–118
Granite Hot Springs 114
Granite Lake 136
Grants Pass 42, 44
Grave Creek 159
Grave Lake 159
Grayback Ridge 188
Green Lake 77
Green River 133
Green River Lakes 253
Greybull Pass 83
Greybull River 83
Grizzly Basin 124
grizzly bears 6, 8–11, 36, 37, 40, 45–46, 55–56,
    71, 103, 247, 248, 249, 250, 251
Grizzly Creek 94
Gros Ventre Range 87, 114–127
Gros Ventre River 124, 125, 127
Gros Ventre Wilderness, trips within 113–127
Grouse Creek 47
Gunboat Lake 218

H
Hailey Pass 158
Halls Butte 146
Halls Creek 143, 146, 149
Halls Lake 149
Hancock, Mount 51
Harebell Creek Patrol Cabin 53
Hat Pass 146
Hawks Rest 101
Hawks Rest Patrol Cabin 101
Hay Pass 147
Haystack Mountain 161
Heart Lake 46, 47, 52, 53
Heart Lake Geyser Basin 47
Heart Lake Ranger Station 47, 52
Hellroaring Creek 29
Hellroaring Trailhead 25, 29
Hidden Corral Basin 92
Hidden Lake 94
High Meadows Creek 172
Highline Trail 133, 137, 143, 151, 253
Hog Park Creek 237
Holly Lake 107
Honeymoon Lake 166
Hoodoo Basin 37–38
Hooker, Mount 157, 159
Horse Creek 85
Horse Heaven Meadows 189
Horseshoe Ridge 148, 149
Hot Springs Basin Group Thermal Area 247
hunting seasons 6

Hurricane Pass 109
hypothermia 7

I
Ice Lakes 179, 180
Icefloe Lake 109
Indian Basin 138
Indian Creek 19
Indian Creek Campground 18
Ishawooa Creek 250
Ishawooa Pass 250
Island Lake 138

J
Jackass Pass 161
Jackson Lake 251
Jasper Lake 62–63
Jedediah Smith Wilderness 89–94, 109
Jenny Lake 107
John Muir Trail 253
Jojo Creek 79
Josephs Coat Spring 247

K
Kingfisher Mountain 250
Kirwin 82, 85
Klondike Creek 167
Klondyke Lakes 240
Knowles Falls 28

L
Lake Alice 254
Lake Angeline 219, 220
Lake Barstow 203
Lake Creek (Wind River Range) 139
Lake Creek (Wyoming Range) 194, 195
Lake Elsa 214
Lake Eunice 213, 214
Lake Geneva 212–213
Lake Helen 217
Lake Marie 239, 243
Lake Marion 217
Lake Sequa 146
Lake Solitude (Bighorn Range) 218
Lake Solitude (Teton Range) 108
Lake Victor 147
Lakeside Trail 133, 140
Lamar River 33
Lamar Valley 32
Lame Deer Lake 255
Lee Lake 149
Leidy, Mount 252
Lewis Lake 240
Lewis River Channel 43
Lightning Lakes 143

Little Bear Creek 60, 62
Little Bonneville Lake 150
Little Corral Creek 254
Little Cottonwood Creek 28
Little Divide Lake 143
Little Granite Creek 117
Little Greys River 186, 190, 191
Little Wind River 159
Lizard Head Meadows 161, 162, 172
Lizard Head Peak 171
Lone Star Geyser 41, 44
Lonesome Lake 153, 160, 161, 172
Lonesome Mountain 62
Lookout Lake 239
loon, common 47
Lost Lake 240
Lost Temple Spire 161
Lost Twin Lakes 220
Lower Green River Lake 133, 140
Lower Jean Lake 137
Lower Paint Rock Trailhead 210, 214
Lunch Creek 194
Lupine Meadows Trailhead 105, 112

M
MacLeod Lake 126
Macon Lake 159
Mae's Lake 157
Marion Lake 110, 112
Mariposa Lake 51
marmots 110, 239
Marms Lake 157
Marston Pass 102, 103
Martin Lake 60, 61
Mason Gulch 236
Medicine Bow Mountains 231, 239
Medicine Bow Peak 239, 241, 243
Medicine Lodge Creek 210, 211
Medicine Park 218
Medina Mountain 148
Middle Fork Boulder Creek 143
Middle Fork Lake 143, 149
Middle Lake 173
Middle Popo Agie River 178, 179, 180, 181
Middle Tensleep Creek 221
Middle Teton 108, 109
Miller Creek 33, 36, 37
Mirror Lake (Bighorn Mountains) 221
Mirror Lake (Wind River Range) 157
Mistymoon Lake 217, 218, 221
moose 22, 106, 115, 139, 172, 212, 216
Moose Basin Divide 251
Moose Creek (Teton Range) 251
Moose Creek (Yellowstone Park) 43
Moose Mountain 93
Moose Ponds 106
mosquitoes 96, 101, 132, 153, 166, 195
Mount Hunt Divide 112

Mount Meek Pass 110
mountain pine beetle 7–8, 237
Mud "Lake" 97
Mushpots Thermal Area 247

N
Native Lake 60
Navajo Tarn 60
New Fork Park 139
New Fork River 139
1988 Yellowstone fires 18, 33, 40, 43, 46, 100
No Name Lakes 139
Nord, Mount 93
Nord Pass 93
North Absaroka Range 55–56, 248
North Bitch Creek 92, 93
North Buffalo Fork 97, 103
North Clear Creek 218, 219
North Cow Creek 83
North Fork Boulder Creek 146, 147
North Fork Cascade Creek 108
North Fork Crow Creek 202
North Fork Lake 146
North Fork Meadows 97
North Fork Shoshone River 249
North Fork Yellowstone River 103
North Gap Lake 242
North Hidden Lake 60
North Lake 161
North Paint Rock Creek 213, 214
North Piney Creek 193, 197
North Piney Lake 195
North Piney Meadows 197
North Popo Agie River 169, 172
North Three Forks Creek 203
North Twin Lakes 241

O
Ogden Creek 228, 229
Old Crow Lake 255
Old Faithful backcountry office 39
Open Canyon 112
osprey 27
Otter Lake 255
Outlet Creek 47
Outlet Lake 47
Owl Creek Trail 251

P
Pacific Creek 100
Paintbrush Canyon 107
Paintbrush Divide 108
Palmer Canyon 139
Palmer Lake 139
Palmer Peak 124
Panther Creek 19

Papoose Ridge Trail 248
Parker Peak 37
Pass Creek 250
Passage Creek 50, 51
Peak Lake 137
Pelican Cone 247
Pelican Valley 247
Penny Lake 139
Periodic Spring 200–201
permits 3, 15, 105
Phelps Lake 111, 112
Phelps Lake Overlook 111
Phillips Lake 166
Pickle Pass 188
Pingora Peak 160
Pinion Creek 197
Pipestone Lakes 146
Plateau Creek 51, 53
Poison Lake 179
Poker Creek 254
Popo Agie Wilderness, trips within 168–181
Porcupine Creek 139–140
Porcupine Creek Falls 140
Porcupine Pass 139
Purgatory Gulch 236
Pyramid Lake 157
Pyramid Peak (Gros Ventre Range) 115
Pyramid Peak (Wind River Range) 157, 158

Q

Quadrant Mountain 19

R

Rachel Lake 61
Raid Lake 150
Rainbow Lake (Bighorn Mountains) 213
Rainbow Lake (Wind River Range) 149
Rammel Mountain 92
Rattlesnake Butte 30
Red Creek 94
Red Mountains 46–47
Rescue Creek 29
Rescue Creek Trail 25, 29–30
Reuter, Emil gravesite 228
Richardson Creek 229
Richardson Fire Trail 229
Roaring Fork Creek (Wind River Range) 175
Roaring Fork Creek (Wyoming Range) 197
Roaring Fork Lake (Wind River Range) 175
Roaring Fork Lakes (Wyoming Range) 197
Roaring Fork Mountain 178
Robin Lake 213
Rock Creek 203
Rock Creek Knoll 241
Rock Lake 205
Rock Lake Peak 201, 204
Roosevelt Meadows 190

Round Top Mountain 146
Rumbaud Lake 146
Rustic Geyser 47

S

Salt River Range 183, 198–205, 254
Sand Creek 171
Sand Pit Trail 228
sandhill cranes 30, 50
Sandpoint Lake 143
Sanford Park 172
Scab Creek Trailhead 142, 151
Schideler, Mount 193
Schoolroom Glacier 109
Second Creek 190
Seven Brothers Lakes 219
Shadow Lake 153, 157, 160, 162
Shannon Pass 137
Sheep Bridge 181
Sheep Lake 241
Sheep Steps 110
Sheep Nose Trail 229
Sheila Lake 150
Shelf Lakes 242
Sherd Lake 255
Sheridan Lake 52
Sheridan, Mount 47, 52
Shoal Creek 121
Shoal Falls 121
Shoal Lake 121, 127
Shoestring Lake 149
Shoshone Creek 42
Shoshone Geyser Basin 42, 44
Shoshone Lake 40, 42–44
Shoshone Lake Ranger Station 43
Sickle Creek 51
Sierra Madre 231, 234
Silver Tarn 62
Skull Lake 157, 159, 162
Slate Creek 252
Smith Lake 169, 173
Smith Lake Creek 173
Snake River 51, 52, 53
Sniffel, Mount 82
Snowdrift Lake 109
snowpack information 5
Snowy Range 231, 238–243
Soda Butte Creek 32
Soda Fork 102, 103
Soda Fork Meadows 97
Soda Mountain 102
Soda Springs 103
Solitude Trail 212, 218, 221
South Absaroka Range 71
South Bitch Creek 92
South Boundary Trail 51, 53
South Fork Boulder Creek 143, 150, 151
South Fork Cascade Creek 108

South Fork Crow Creek 202
South Fork Ogden Creek 229
South Fork Ponds 255
South Fork Teton Creek 110
South Fork Yellowstone River 103
South Gap Lake 242
South Teton 108, 109
South Three Forks Creek 203
Sportsman Lake 22
Squaretop Mountain 133, 136
Star Lake 166
Static Peak Divide 110
Steamboat Peak 124
Steeple Peak 161
Steer Creek 83
Stough Creek 178
Stough Lakes 178
String Lake 107
Stroud Peak 137
Sugarloaf Mountain 240
Summit Lake 137, 138
Sundance Campground 226
Sunrise Lake 150
Sunset Lake 109
Surprise Creek 47
Sweetwater Gap 178
Swift Creek (Gros Ventre Range) 120, 126
Swift Creek (Salt River Range) 199, 201

T
Table Creek 66
Table Mountain 108
Taggart Lake 112
Tayo Creek 179
Tayo Lake 179
Tayo Park 179
Teepee Pole Flats 214
Teewinot Mountain 107
Temple Lake 161
Temple Pass 161
Tent Canyon 229
Teton Range 87, 88, 89–94, 104–112, 251
Teton Wilderness 46, 53, 87, 95–103
Texas Lake 160
Texas Pass 160
Thayer Lake 212
The Meadows 79
Third Creek (Teton Wilderness) 100
Third Creek (Wyoming Range) 190
Thorofare Creek 250
Three Forks Park (Green River) 136–137
Three Forks Park (Popo Agie River) 180
thunderstorms 7, 132
ticks 235
Timber Creek 248
Timico Lake 146
Titcomb Basin 137, 138
Toboggan Lakes 142

Torrey Creek 164
Trail Creek (Teton Wilderness) 97
Trail Creek (Wind River Range) 137
Trail Creek Park 137
Trail Creek Trail 97
Triangle Peak 124
Trigger Lake 255
turkey 228
Turkey Pen Peak 30
Turquoise Lake 114, 116
Twin Lakes (Green River) 140
Twin Lakes (Hailey Pass) 158
Two Bits Lake 62
Two Ocean Bear Management Area 45–46
Two Ocean Pass 100
Two Ocean Plateau Trail 50, 53

U
Upper Crow Creek Lake 203
Upper Falls 125
Upper Green River Lake 133
Upper Jean Lake 137, 138
Upper Miller Creek Patrol Cabin 37
Upper Titcomb Lake 138

V
Valentine Lake 159, 162, 171
Valley Lake 147
Valley Trail 111
Varve Lake 60
Vista Pass 137

W
Wapiti Lake 247
Warren Peak 228
Washakie Creek 157, 159, 160
Washakie Lake 159, 162
Washakie Pass 159, 162
Washakie Wilderness, trips within 73–85
Webb Canyon 251
West Lake Marie Trailhead 239
West Shoal Creek 121
West Tensleep Creek 216, 217
West Tensleep Lake 216
White Saddle 254
Wiggins Fork 74–75, 84
Willow Creek 188
Willow Lake 255
Wind River Indian Reservation 148, 159, 169
Wind River Peak 179
Wind River Range 129, 253
Wind River Range, trips within 131–181, 253
Witch Creek 47
wolves 19, 33, 50
Wood River 79, 82, 85
Woodard Canyon 102

Worthen Meadow Reservoir 175, 181
Wright Lake 60
Wyoming Peak 195
Wyoming Range 183, 185–197
Wyoming Range National Recreation Trail
  188, 190, 195

Y
Yellow Creek 83
Yellow Ridge 83
Yellowstone Lake 50, 53, 247
Yellowstone National Park 15
Yellowstone National Park, trips within 17–53,
  247, 248
Yellowstone River 26–28, 46, 101
Youngs Point 94

ABOUT THE AUTHOR

DOUGLAS LORAIN's family moved to the Northwest in 1969, and he has been obsessively hitting the trails of his home region ever since. With the good fortune to grow up in an outdoor-oriented family, he has vivid memories of countless camping, biking, birdwatching, and other trips in every corner of this spectacular area. Over the years he calculates that he has logged well over 30,000 trail miles in this corner of the continent, and despite a history that includes being bitten by a rattlesnake, shot at by a hunter, charged by grizzly bears (twice!), and donating countless gallons of blood to "invertebrate vampires," he happily sees no end in sight.

Lorain is a photographer and recipient of the National Outdoor Book Award. His books cover only the best trips from the thousands of hikes he has taken throughout Oregon, Washington, Idaho, and Wyoming. His photographs have been featured in numerous magazines, calendars, and books, and his other guidebooks include *100 Classic Hikes in Oregon, Backpacking Oregon, Backpacking Idaho, Backpacking Washington, Afoot & Afield Portland/Vancouver,* and *One Night Wilderness: Portland.*

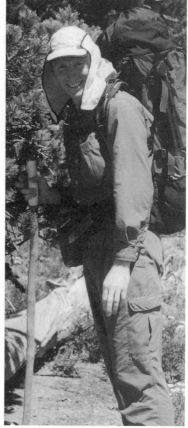

Photo by Becky Lovejoy